Metastasis Research Protocols

METHODS IN MOLECULAR MEDICINE™

John M. Walker, SERIES EDITOR

Methods in Molecular Medicine™

Metastasis Research Protocols

Volume II: Analysis of Cell Behavior In Vitro and In Vivo

Edited by

Susan A. Brooks

*Research School of Biological and Molecular Sciences,
Oxford Brookes University, Oxford, UK*

and

Udo Schumacher

*Institute for Anatomy, Department of Neuroanatomy,
University Hospital Hamburg-Eppendorf, Hamburg, Germany*

Humana Press Totowa, New Jersey

Cover Illustration: Fig. 2 from Chapter 7 in Volume I: "Surrogate Markers of Angiogenesis and Metastasis" by Girolamo Ranieri and Giampetro Gasparini.

Production Editor: Jessica Jannicelli.
Cover design by Patricia F. Cleary.

For additional copies, pricing for bulk purchases, and/or information about other Humana titles, contact Humana at the above address or at any of the following numbers: Tel.: 973-256-1699; Fax: 973-256-8341; E-mail: humana@humanapr.com; or visit our Website: www.humanapress.com

Printed in the United States of America. 10 9 8 7 6 5 4 3 2 1

Library of Congress Cataloging in Publication Data

Main entry under title:

Methods in molecular medicine™.

Metastasis research protocols/edited by Susan A. Brooks and Udo Schumacher.
    p. cm. -- (Methods in molecular medicine ; 57-58)
  Includes bibliographical references and index.
  Contents: v. 1. Analysis of cells and tissues -- v. 2. Analysis of cell behavior in vitro and in vivo.
  ISBN 0-89603-610-3 (v. 1 : alk. paper) -- ISBN 0-89603-615-4 (v. 2 : alk. paper)
    1. Metastasis--Laboratory manuals. 2. Cancer cells--Laboratory manuals. 3. Cytology--Laboratory manuals. I. Brooks, Susan A. II. Schumacher, Udo. III. Series.

  RC269.5 .M478 2001
  616.99'407--dc21

                                                                            2001016931

Preface

In Volume I, *Analysis of Cells and Tissues*, we presented a range of protocols aimed at mapping and analyzing the expression of various molecules of potential interest in metastasis research and for examining their production at the genetic level. In this second volume of metastasis research protocols, we move to the level of living cells and tissues and present methodologies applicable to examining metastatic behavior in vitro and in whole animal models.

The methods described in the first section of this volume concentrate on the separation of cell lines with high and low metastatic potential, including the genetic modification of cell lines. The assay systems to test defined aspects of the metastatic cascade are then described in Part II and include cell migration assays, assays for matrix degrading enzymes, basement membrane degrading assays, adhesion assays, and assays of angiogenesis. The role of the specific elements of the metastatic cascade assayed in each of these systems in turn must of course be put into perspective relative to their roles in entire living organisms.

To this end, a range of animal models of metastasis are described in Part III of this book. This section begins with an overview of basic principles for the study of metastasis using animal models and goes on to describe in detail a number of specific animal model systems that have proven of value in metastasis research. The selection presented is by no means comprehensive, but was planned to give a broad spectrum of models, the employment of immunodeficient animals, syngeneic and transgenic models, and orthotopic models of metastasis. Chapters on dissection of tumor and host cells from metastasized organs for testing gene expression directly ex vivo and techniques for the labeling of cells with green fluorescent protein for metastasis research are also included.

Cancer mortality will only decrease if metastases can be treated successfully. To do so, it is probably necessary to understand the metastatic cascade first at the molecular level, than at the level tissue level, and finally at the level of the whole organism. Based on comprehensive knowledge, rational—and effective—strategies to combat metastatic disease might be developed. We hope that this collection of protocols will help to work toward this goal.

Susan A. Brooks
Udo Schumacher

Introduction to Volumes I and II

Why a Collection of Metastasis Research Protocols?

A metastasis is a secondary tumor derived from a primary tumor at a distant site. The process leading to the formation of metastases is complex and, owing to its complexity, many researchers have shunned away from tackling this problem. "Science is to do the doable" and many excellent minds have tried to tackle the problem of metastases unsuccessfully, leading to a general frustration in addressing this important research topic. Metastases formation is by far the overwhelming cause of death in cancer patients and should therefore be a major issue to be addressed in cancer research. In 1971, President Nixon declared war on cancer with the aim of eradicating it as a major cause of death in the United States. Yet, at the beginning of the new millennium, cancer is still undefeated and accounts for approximately 25% of the deaths in the developed world. In contrast, mortality because of cardiovascular diseases in the age groups below 60 years has declined impressively *(1,2)*. While surgical techniques and anesthesia have made progress during the last decades, cancer mortality remains high. The primary tumor can often be removed surgically, but no surgical cure for generalized metastases can be offered to the patient. Metastatic disease is frequently resistant to other forms of treatment and may not be eradicated by even the most aggressive chemotherapy or radiotherapy. Metastatic disease is the most common cause of death in cancer patients. And even here there remain unanswered questions. If metastases erode a large blood vessel resulting in a massive bleeding or if they destroy a vital brain center, then the cause of death is clear. However, at post-mortem examinations, no such clear signs for the cause of death are detected for the vast majority of cancer victims and so the ultimate reason why cancer patients die from metastatic disease remains an unsolved problem.

Metastasis formation is a multistep process (for review, *see* **refs.** *3,4)*. The following simple description will focus on the formation of systemic metastases and will not deal with local lymph node metastasis. The process of metastasis formation starts when the transformed malignant cell starts to grow. Once the primary tumor reaches a certain size, it needs blood vessel penetration in order to grow further. Once tumor neoangiogenesis has started, tumor cells have to loosen themselves from the primary tumor, penetrate the surrounding connective tissue and basal lamina of the blood vessel. In order to proceed further, tumor cells have to invade through the endothelium into the bloodstream. Once tumor cells have entered the systemic circulation, they have to survive in this environment and have to be transported to the site of the future metastasis. Here, they have to attach to the endothelium, penetrate it, and complete the reverse of the process observed at the original site of invasion: cross the endothelium and its basal lamina and establish themselves in the connective tissue surrounding the blood vessel. Once this has been achieved, the metastatic cancer cell has to start to grow in order to form a clinically detectable metastasis.

The process of metastasis formation is often referred to as a cascade, meaning that every single step has to be successfully completed in order to proceed to the next. The cascade nature of the process makes it so difficult to analyze, and, hence, the rate-limiting step of metastasis formation is still unknown. During the last decades, a shift has occurred of what is thought to be important in this process. In the 1970s, much attention was paid to the degradation of the basal lamina as the initial step of metastasis formation *(5)*. The focus of the attention shifted then toward cell adhesion molecules. Cell adhesion molecules have a dual role to perform: First of all, their expression at the site of the primary tumor make them act as an anti-metastatic factor because they ensure that a cell with a metastatic potential remains at the site of the primary tumor. On the other hand, expression of cell adhesion molecules at the site of the future metastasis are thought to be essential for the interaction between the tumor cell in the bloodstream with the endothelial cell of the target organ. At this site, the cell adhesion molecule would act as a pro-metastatic molecule. The apparent paradox can be solved in two ways: Either two different cell adhesion molecules act at the two different sites or the behavior of one cell adhesion molecule is subject to down- and upregulation at the invasion and at the evasion sites, respectively (for dual role of a cell adhesion molecule, *see* **ref. *6***).

While the importance of the processes occurring at the evasion site has been the focus of attention in the 1970s and 1980s, processes in the bloodstream and at the invasion site are of particular interest at present. That viable tumor cells are frequently detectable within the blood of cancer patients has been known for many years. Although many tumor cells are shed into the blood, only very few tumor cells form distant metastases. Only recently, however, the molecular basis of this phenomenon has been elucidated. If tumor cells lose the contact to their basement membrane at the site of the primary tumor, they switch toward apoptosis, and only if the signaling pathway leading to apoptosis, such as the p53-mediated one, is abrogated, can tumor cells survive within the circulation in order to form metastases *(7)*. The clinical relevance of circulating tumor cells has been reinvestigated using PCR analysis for the presence of genetic material derived from tumor cells. In addition to the problem of the viability of the circulating tumor cells mentioned above, further problems such as the presence of pseudogenes *(8)* and methodological problems that occur when working at the maximum sensitivity needed for single cell detection and preanalytical and statistical influences have to be considered *(9)*. Hence, the clinical significance of detecting pieces of circulating tumor derived DNA by PCR amplification remains unclear and has to be assessed more vigorously.

Another issue of fundamental importance is the question how the metastatic process is initiated and regulated. At the molecular level, the best understood model of carcinogens is the colorectal one. This famous model of colorectal carcinogenesis worked out by Vogelstein and his coworkers implies that a specific mutation occurs prior to the formation of metastasis *(10)*. This theory would imply that metastasis is primarily a somatic mutation which is not or to a lesser extent subject to regulatory processes. Using the serial analysis of gene expression (SAGE) technique, Vogelstein's group has screened the expression of at least 45,000 different genes in colorectal cancer, colon cancer cell lines, and colonic mucosa *(11)*. The result of this extensive survey was surprising: Few genes were differently expressed and no specific metastasis-associated gene was described. Hence, the opposite proposition that the formation of metastases is subject to cell regulatory mechanisms may at least in some cancers be true.

That regulatory mechanisms are indeed governing metastasis is best illustrated in solid neoplasms. Cancers are malignant tumors of epithelial origin. In simple epithelia such as the ones lining the gut lumen, lining cells are characterized by their attachment to the basement membrane. This attachment to the basement membrane mediated by hemidesmosomes and cell adhesion molecules such as integrins renders the cells immotile. This cellular behavior is in contrast to the mesenchymal cells: These are the cells of the embryonic connective tissue that are characterized by their ability to migrate. Tumor cells that are to become metastatic are undergoing the epithelial–mesenchymal transition: This implies that regulatory mechanisms are present which enable tumor cells to change their phenotype from an epithelial to a mesenchymal one, which represents the migrating tumor cell in the bloodstream *(12)*. At the evasion site, the tumor cells have to reverse their behavior and form epithelial formations. Evidence for the shift of antigen expression during the sequence epithelial phenotype-mesenchymal phenotype-epithelial phenotype in the mature large metastasis has been shown for the cell adhesion molecule epithelial glycoprotein-2 *(13)*.

In vitro systems by their very nature can only mimic limited steps of the metastatic cascade, which can, however, be studied in depth. Since the rate-limiting step of the metastatic cascade is not known, it is often difficult to meaningfully interpret the results of an in vitro assay for the metastatic cascade as a whole. Hence, old fashioned animal models of metastasis, for which there is an increased demand *(14,15)*, are included in these volumes. While the in depth analysis is better done in an in vitro system, animal models of metastases offer not only the great advantage of analyzing the process as a whole but also reflect the biological diversity of tumors much better than in vitro systems. Owing to cell culture conditions in general and the two-dimensional growth pattern in particular, the heterogeneity of antigen expression as seen in vivo is most often not fully reflected in cell culture systems, but is much better observed in vivo in experimental animals *(16)*. However, the clinical significance of animal models has to be assessed critically as well. In murine breast cancer, the mammary tumor virus induces hormone-independent breast cancer. This does not reflect the clinical situation, where many breast cancers are hormone sensitive and where no evidence for a viral cause exists *(17)*.

Despite this complexity, the problem of metastasis formation can be resolved. It may well be that relatively few mechanisms are rate-limiting in this complex process and, hence, simple ways of predicting metastasis formation can be found which ultimately lead to novel therapies once a through road has been established. We hope that these two volumes provide some tools wih which to do this.

References

1. Bailar, J. C. and Gornik, H. L. (1997) Cancer undefeated. *N. Engl. J. Med.* **336,** 1969–1574.
2. Sporn, M. B. (1996) The war against cancer. *Lancet* **347,** 1377–1381.
3. Hart, I. R., Goode, N. R., and WIlson, R. E. (1989) Molecular aspects of the metastatic cascade. *Biochim. Biophys. Acta* **989,** 65–84.
4. Hart, I. R. and Saini, A. (1992) Biology of tumour metastasis. *Lancet* **339,** 1453–1457.
5. Liotta, L. A., Rao, N. C., Barsky, S., and G. Bryant (1984) The laminin receptor and basement membrane dissolution: role in tumour metastasis. *Ciba Foundation Symposium* **108,** 146–154.
6. Takeishi, M. (1993) Cadherins in cancer: implications for invasion and metastasis. *Current Opin. Cell Biol.* **5,** 806–811.

7. Nikiforov, M. A., Hagen, K., Ossovaskaya, V. S., Connor, T. M. F., et al. (1996) p53 modulation of anchorage independent growth and experimental metastasis. *Oncogene* **13,** 1709–1719.

8. Nollau, P., Jung, R., Neumaier, M., and Wagener, C. (1995) Tumour diagnosis by PCR-based detection of tumour cells. Scand. *J. Clin. Lab. Invest. Suppl.* **221,** 116–121.

9. Jung, R., Ahmad-Nejad, P., Wimmer, M., Gerhard, M., Wagener, C., and Neumaier, M. (1997) Quality management and influential factors for the detection of single metastatic cancer cells by reverse transcriptase polymerase chain reaction. *Eur. J. Clin. Chem. Clin. Biochem.* **35,** 3–10.

10. Fearon, E. R. and Vogelstein, B. (1990) A genetic model for colorectal tumorigenesis. *Cell* **61,** 759–767.

11. Zhang, L. Zhou, W., Velculescu, V. E., Kern, S. E., Hruban, R. H., Hamilton, S. R., Vogelstein, B., and Kinzler, K. W. (1997) Gene expression profiles in normal and cancer cells. *Science* **276,** 1268–1272.

12. Birchmeier, C., Birchmeier, W., and Brand-Saberi, B. (1997) Epithelial-mesenchymal transitions in cancer progression. *Acta Anat.* **156,** 217–226.

13. Jojovic, M., Adam E., Zangemeister-Wittke, U., and Schumacher, U. (1998) Epithelial glycoprotein-2 (EGP-2) expression is subject to regulatory processes in epithelial-mesenchymal transitions during metastases: an investigation of human cancers transplanted into severe combined immunodeficient mice. *Histochem. J.* **30,** 723–729.

14. Tannock, I. F. (1998) Conventional cancer therapy: promise broken or promise delayed? *Lancet* **351** (Suppl. II), 9–16.

15. Lane, D. (1998) The promise of molecular oncology. *Lancet* **351** (Suppl II), 17–20.

16. Schumacher, U., Mohamed, M., and Mitchell, B. S. (1996) Differential expression of carbohydrate residues in human breast and colon cancer cell lines grown in vitro and in vivo in SCID mice. *Cancer J.* **9,** 247–254.

17. Van de Vijver, M. J. and Nusse, R. (1991) The molecular biology of breast cancer. *Biochem. Biophys. Acta* **1072,** 33–50.

Contents

CONTENTS OF THE COMPANION VOLUME

Metastasis Research Protocols

Volume 1: Analysis of Cells and Tissues

Contributors

ROY BICKNELL • *Molecular Angiogenesis Laboratory, Imperial Cancer Research Fund, Weatherall Institute of Molecular Medicine, University of Oxford, John Radcliffe Hospital, Oxford, UK*

TOM BOTERBERG • *Laboratory of Experimental Cancerology, Department of Radiotherapy, Nuclear Medicine and Experimental Cancerology, University Hospital Gent, Gent, Belgium*

MARC E. BRACKE • *Laboratory of Experimental Cancerology, Department of Radiotherapy, Nuclear Medicine and Experimental Cancerology, University Hospital Gent, Gent, Belgium*

ERIK A. BRUYNEEL • *Laboratory of Experimental Cancerology, Department of Radiotherapy, Nuclear Medicine and Experimental Cancerology, University Hospital Gent, Gent, Belgium*

PETER C. BROOKS • *Department of Biochemistry and Molecular Biology, Norris Cancer Center, The University of Southern California School of Medicine, Los Angeles, CA*

SUSAN A. BROOKS • *Research School of Biological and Molecular Sciences, Oxford Brookes University, Oxford, UK*

NICHOLAS S. BROWN • *Molecular Angiogenesis Laboratory, Imperial Cancer Research Fund, Weatherall Institute of Molecular Medicine, University of Oxford, John Radcliffe Hospital, Oxford, UK*

GIZELA CARDOSO • *Ardais Corporation, Lexington, MA*

CATHERINE CLARKE • *LICR/UCL Breast Cancer Laboratory, Department of Surgery, Royal Free and University College Medical School, London, UK*

HILARY COLLINS • *Academic Unit of Cancer Studies, University of Nottingham, Nottingham, UK*

DEREK DAVIES • *FACS Laboratory, Imperial Cancer Research Fund, London, UK*

SUSAN DAVIES • *LICR/UCL Breast Cancer Laboratory, Department of Surgery, Royal Free and University College Medical School, London, UK*

SUZANNE A. ECCLES • *CRC Centre for Cancer Therapeutics, McElwain Laboratories, Institute of Cancer Research, Surrey, UK*

SÜLEYMAN ERGÜN • *Institute for Anatomy, University Hospital Hamburg-Eppendorf, Hamburg, Germany*

CHISATO FUJIYAMA • *Molecular Angiogenesis Laboratory, Imperial Cancer Research Fund, Institute of Molecular Medicine, University of Oxford, John Radcliffe Hospital, Oxford, UK*

ANGELA GAROFALO • *LBTM, Department of Oncology, Mario Negri Institute for Pharmacological Research, Bergamo, Italy*

RAFFAELLA GIAVAZZI • *LBTM, Department of Oncology, Mario Negri Institute for Pharmacological Research, Bergamo, Italy*

CHANTALE T. GUY • *Ardais Corporation, Lexington, MA*

ARAYO HAGA • *Tumor Progression and Metastasis Program, Karmanos Cancer Institute, Wayne State University School of Medicine, Detroit, MI and Department of Public Health, Gifu Pharmaceutical University, Gifu, Japan*

STEPHEN HAGUE • *Molecular Angiogenesis Laboratory, Imperial Cancer Research Fund, Institute of Molecular Medicine, University of Oxford, John Radcliffe Hospital, Oxford, UK*

DEBBIE M.S. HALL • *Research School of Biological and Molecular Sciences, Oxford Brookes University, Oxford, UK*

MARY J. C. HENDRIX • *Department of Anatomy and Cell Biology and The Holden Comprehensive Cancer Center, College of Medicine, University of Iowa, Iowa City, IA*

ROBERT M. HOFFMAN • *AntiCancer, Inc. and Department of Surgery, University of California, San Diego, CA*

YUICHIRO HONJO • *Departments of Pathology, Wayne State University, Detroit, MI*

JIN HUA • *Department of Pathology and Laboratory Medicine, University of Pennsylvania School of Medicine, Philadelphia, PA*

ADAM JONES • *Molecular Angiogenesis Laboratory, Imperial Cancer Research Fund, Institute of Molecular Medicine, University of Oxford, John Radcliffe Hospital, Oxford, UK*

NERBIL KILIC • *Department of Clinical Chemistry, University Hospital Hamburg-Eppendorf, Hamburg, Germany*

MARC M. MAREEL • *Laboratory of Experimental Cancerology, Department of Radiotherapy, Nuclear Medicine and Experimental Cancerology, University Hospital Gent, Gent, Belgium*

DANIEL MCWILLIAMS • *Academic Unit of Cancer Studies, University of Nottingham, Nottingham, UK*

TERESA M. MORRIS • *Academic Unit of Cancer Studies, University of Nottingham, Nottingham, UK*

RUTH J. MUSCHEL • *Department of Pathology and Laboratory Medicine, University of Pennsylvania School of Medicine, Philadelphia, PA*

PRATIMA NANGIA-MAKKER • *Tumor Progression and Metastasis Program, Karmanos Cancer Institute, Wayne State University School of Medicine, Detroit, MI*

YASUFUMI NIINAKA • *Tumor Progression and Metastasis Program, Karmanos Cancer Institute, Wayne State University School of Medicine, Detroit, MI and Department of Oral and Maxillofacial Surgery (I), Faculty of Dentistry, Tokyo Medical and Dental University, Tokyo, Japan*

ERIC PETITCLERC • *Department of Biochemistry and Molecular Biology, Norris Cancer Center, The University of Southern California School of Medicine, Los Angeles, CA*

JANET E. PRICE • *Department of Cancer Biology, University of Texas M. D. Anderson Cancer Center, Houston, TX*

G. ED RAINGER • *Cardiovascular Rheology Group, Department of Physiology, University of Birmingham Medical School, Birmingham, UK*

AVRAHAM RAZ • *Tumor Progression and Metastasis Program, Karmanos Cancer Institute, Wayne State University School of Medicine, Detroit, MI*

MARIAN ROCHA • *Deutsches Krebsforschungszentrum, Abteilung Zelluläre Immunologie, FSP Tummorimmunologie, Heidelberg, Germany*

VOLKER SCHIRRMACHER • *Deutsches Krebsforschungszentrum, Abteilung Zelluläre Immunologie, FSP Tummorimmunologie, Heidelberg, Germany*

UDO SCHUMACHER • *Institute for Anatomy, Department of Neuroanatomy, University Hospital Hamburg-Eppendorf, Hamburg, Germany*

ELISABETH A. SEFTOR • *Department of Anatomy and Cell Biology and The Holden Comprehensive Cancer Center, College of Medicine, The University of Iowa, Iowa City, IA*

RICHARD E.B. SEFTOR • *Department of Anatomy and Cell Biology and The Holden Comprehensive Cancer Center, College of Medicine, University of Iowa, Iowa City, IA*

VICTOR UMANSKY • *Deutsches Krebsforschungszentrum, Abteilung Zelluläre Immunologie, FSP Tummorimmunologie, Heidelberg, Germany*

SUE A. WATSON • *Academic Unit of Cancer Studies, University of Nottingham, Nottingham, UK*

I

SELECTION/SEGREGATION OF CELL POPULATIONS FOR IN VITRO AND IN VIVO ASSAYS OF METASTATIC BEHAVIOR

1

Cell Separations by Flow Cytometry

Derek Davies

1. Introduction
1.1. Cell Analysis by Flow Cytometry

Flow cytometry is a means of measuring the physical and chemical characteristics of particles in a fluid stream as they pass one by one past a sensing point. The modern flow cytometer consists of a light source, collection optics and detectors, and a computer to translate signals into data. In effect, a flow cytometer can be described as a large and powerful fluorescence microscope in which the light source is of a highly specific wavelength, generally produced by a laser, and the human observer is replaced by a series of optical filters and detectors that aim to make the instrument more objective and more quantitative. As a cell passes through the laser beam, light is scattered in all directions, and also at this point any fluorochromes present on the cell are excited and emit light of a higher wavelength. Scattered and emitted light is collected by two lenses—one set in front of the light source and one set at right angles to it. By a series of beam splitters, optical filters, and detectors the wavelengths of light specific for particular fluorochromes can be isolated and quantitated—up to six fluorochromes can be measured in some flow cytometers. A simplified diagram of the optical setup for two-color analysis is shown in **Fig. 1.** The theory of operation of flow cytometers is well documented, and there are several good general books on the subject *(1–3)*.

1.2. Cell Sorting by Flow Cytometry

Flow sorting may be defined as the process of physically separating particles of interest from other particles in the sample. Sorting can be accomplished by two flow cytometrically based methods: the electrostatic deflection of charged droplets (so-called "stream-in-air" sorters) *(2,4)* or mechanical sorting *(5)*. Most

From: *Methods in Molecular Medicine, vol. 58:*
Metastasis Research Protocols, Vol. 2: Cell Behavior In Vitro and In Vivo
Edited by: S. A. Brooks and U. Schumacher © Humana Press Inc., Totowa, NJ

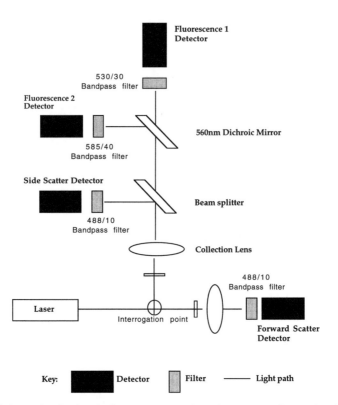

Fig. 1. Schematic of a simple four-parameter detection system: forward and right angle light scatter and two fluorescence parameters set to detect FITC (Fluorescence 1) and PE (Fluorescence 2) emission spectra.

commercially available cell sorters use the electrostatic method, which is based on the principles of droplet formation, charge, and deflection analogous to those used in ink-jet printers. Any fluid stream in the atmosphere will break up into droplets but this is not a stable process. However, by applying vibration at certain frequencies it is possible to stabilize the point at which droplets break off from the stream, the droplet size, and the distance between the drops. Therefore the time between the point at which the cell passes through the laser beam and is analyzed until its inclusion in a droplet as it breaks from the stream—the drop delay—is known and constant (**Fig. 2**). By calculating this time period, the droplet containing the cell of interest can be specifically charged through the fluid stream the moment that the drop is forming. To avoid cell loss, the duration of the charging pulse can be altered to include either or both the preceding and the following drop. Charged droplets will then pass through an electrical field created by two plates—one charged positively, the other charged negatively. Droplets containing a charge will be attracted toward the plate of opposite charge and in this way will be separated from the stream.

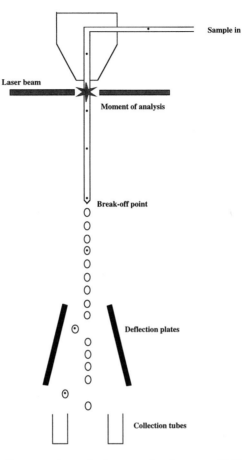

Fig. 2. Schematic diagram of a typical stream-in-air sorter. Cells are analyzed at the laser intersection ("moment of analysis"), enclosed in droplets at the breakoff point, and are charged at this point if they are to be sorted. High-voltage deflection plates attract cells of the opposite polarity.

Mechanical sorters do not use the droplet method but rather employ a motor-driven syringe to aspirate the fluid containing the cell of interest *(6)*. From a practical point of view mechanical sorters are relatively slow (maximum sorting speed of 500 cells/s) but they do have advantages: The system is enclosed, preventing both contamination and evaporation, and it is easier to set up and perform a sort and therefore a skilled operator is not a prerequisite.

The sorting speed of stream-in-air flow cytometers varies depending on the manufacturer and the design of the machine from 5000 cells/s up to 20,000 cells/s. However, this is still relatively slow compared with bulk isolation methods such as cell filtration techniques or cell affinity techniques, as even at top speeds no more than 10^8 cells may be sorted in an hour. However in comparison with other techniques flow sorting achieves the highest cell purity and recovery. In addition, such stream-in-air sorters are capable of sorting one, two, three, or four subsets which may be defined by quantitative and qualitative measurements of multiparametric cell characteristics, the number of which is limited only by the configuration of the flow sorter. It is also possible to adjust the mode of sorting depending on whether high purity (the default mode), high recovery (if a small, precious population is needed) or high count accuracy (for single cell sorting for cloning or polymerase chain reaction [PCR]) is required.

1.3. Applications of Flow Cytometry

Anything that can be tagged with a fluorescent marker can be examined on a flow cytometer. This can be a structural part of the cell such as protein, DNA, RNA, an antigen (surface, cytoplasmic, or nuclear), or a specific cell function (apoptosis, ion levels, pH, membrane potential). As long as a specific cell population can be identified by its fluorescence characteristics it can be sorted. Examples of the applications of flow analysis and sorting are given in **Table 1**.

The fluorochrome of choice will to a large extent depend on both the intended application and the illumination wavelengths available in the cytometer. The most common laser wavelengths and the fluorochromes that can be used with these are given in **Table 2**. The choice will depend on the number of cell characteristics being examined, as well as the spectral overlap between the fluorochromes and their commercial availability.

The most common application of cell sorting is to separate a subpopulation of cells based on their specific phenotype, whether this be, for example, tumor cells from normal cells or cells expressing a particular antigen after transfection.

To be able to successfully sort a subpopulation of cells, a sample must be in a single-cell suspension. This is generally achieved by enzymatic or mechanical dissociation. Once in a single-cell suspension, the cells of interest should be prepared by labeling with fluorochromes, to detect either antigenic determinants, structural components, or functional status that will allow them to be specifically identified.

2. Materials

1. Trypsin–versene: 0.02% EDTA (known as versene by many cell culturists; store at room temperature), 0.25% trypsin (store at –20°C). Add 4 mL of trypsin to 16 mL of versene. This mixture can be used for up to 1 wk if stored at 4°C. Warm the solution to 37°C before use.
2. Phosphate-buffered saline (PBS): 8 g of NaCl, 0.5 g of KCl, 1.43 g of Na_2HPO_4, 0.25g of KH_2PO_4. Dissolve in 1 L of distilled water. Check that the pH is 7.2. Autoclave for 20 min.

Table 1
Examples of Flow Analysis of Mammalian Cells

Phenotyping (surface, cytoplasmic or nuclear antigen) *(7,8)*
Cell cycle analysis (DNA or kinetics via bromodeoxyuridine) *(9,10)*
Functionality, e.g., calcium flux, pH, membrane potential *(11–13)*
Apoptosis and cell death *(14,15)*
Enzyme activity *(16,17)*
Monitoring drug uptake *(18)*
Measurement of RNA or protein content *(19)*
Fluorescence *in situ* hybridization (FISH) *(20,21)*

Sterile sorting for reculture *(2,6)*
Sorting of rare populations *(22)*
Single cell sorting for cloning or PCR *(23,24)*
Sorting for protein, RNA or DNA extraction *(25)*
Chromosome sorting for production of chromosome-specific paints *(26,27)*
Isolation of defined populations, e.g., tumor cells from normal cells *(28)*

Table 2
Common Fluorochromes

Laser wavelength	Examples
488 nm	Fluorescein isothiocyanate (FITC)
	R-Phycoerythrin (PE)
	PerCP (peridinin chlorophyll protein)
	PE-Cy5 tandem conjugates, e.g., TriColor, Cychrome
	Propidium iodide
	Ethidium bromide
	Acridine orange
	Fluo-3
UV (ca. 350 nm)	Aminomethyl coumarin
	DAPI (4,6-diamidino-2-phenylindole)
	Hoechst (33258 or 33342)
	Indo-1
	Monochlorobimane
635 nm	Allophycocyanin
	TO-PRO-3
	Cy5

3. Propidium iodide (PI; 50 µg/mL in PBS). This is light sensitive so should be stored in an opaque container at 4°C (*see* **Note 1**).
4. Trypan blue (0.4% w/v).

5. Cell culture medium appropriate to the cell used, both with and without phenol red.
6. Fetal calf serum.
7. 70% Ethanol. Take 700 mL of absolute ethanol and add 300 mL of distilled water.
8. Nylon mesh: 35 μm and 70 μm (Lockertex, Warrington, Cheshire, UK; Small Parts Inc., Miami, FL).

3. Methods

3.1. Preparation of Cells for Flow Cytometry

3.1.1. Suspension Cells, for Example, Cultured or Primary Blood Cells

1. Perform a viable cell count using PI or trypan blue. Live cells will exclude the dye, whereas it will be taken up by cells whose membranes have been compromised.
2. Select the desired number of cells and decant into a sterile container.
3. Centrifuge at 800*g*. The length of centrifugation will depend on the volume of fluid. For small volumes (up to 100 mL), 10 min is sufficient; increase this for larger volumes (*see* **Note 2**).
4. Carefully pour off the supernatant, taking care not to disturb the pellet.
5. Resuspend the pellet in medium at a cells density of approx 10^6 cells/mL.
6. Perform antigen staining (*see* **Subheading 3.2.**).

3.1.2. Adherent Cell Lines or Primary Cultures

1. Remove culture medium by suction using a sterile pipet.
2. Add an appropriate amount of trypsin–versene (e.g., 10 mL per 10-cm dish, 20 mL per 250-mL flask). Wash the fluid around and discard all but a small volume (5 mL per flask, 2 mL per dish) (*see* **Note 3**).
3. Examine the cell monolayer microscopically at regular and frequent intervals and tap the vessel gently to aid the dispersion of cells. Incubate at 37°C if the progress is slow.
4. When the cell sheet is sufficiently dispersed, add an appropriate amount of growth medium with serum (e.g., 10 mL per dish, 20 mL per flask) and carefully resuspend the cells in the medium. The addition of medium serves to neutralize the effect of the enzyme (*see* **Note 4**).
5. Perform a viable cell count using PI or trypan blue. Resuspend the pellet in medium at a cell density of approx 10^6 cells/mL (*see* **Note 5**).
6. Centrifuge at 800*g* for 10 min and again resuspend the pellet in medium at a cell density of approx 10^6 cells/mL.
7. Once cells are in suspension, antigen staining can be performed (*see* **Subheading 3.2.**).

3.1.3. Solid Tissue

1. Place tissue in a 10-cm sterile tissue culture plate and add 20 mL of enzyme (trypsin–versene) solution.
2. Leave for 15 min at 37°C, checking constantly for cell release.
3. If cell release is slow, tease gently using sterile forceps or a scalpel. Repeat this as necessary.

4. Add medium containing 10% fetal calf serum to neutralize the enzymatic action.
5. Decant cells solution into a sterile 50-mL tube and centrifuge at 800g for 10 min.
6. Discard supernatant, perform a viable cell count, and resuspend cells at a density of approx 10^6 cells/mL. Repeat the centrifugation step.
7. Finally resuspend cells at a density of approx 10^6 cells/mL before antigen staining (*see* **Subheading 3.2.**).

3.2. Antigen Staining
3.2.1. Directly Conjugated Antibody

1. Take cells at 10^6/mL and centrifuge at 800g for 10 min. Carefully pour off the supernatant.
2. Add appropriate amount of fluorochrome-labeled antibody (*see* **Note 6**); incubate for 15 min at 37°C (*see* **Notes 7** and **8**).
3. Add medium to a cell density of 10^6/mL. Centrifuge, discard supernatant and repeat.
4. Resuspend at 10^6/mL in phenol red free medium containing a low level of serum or protein (no higher than 2%; *see* **Note 9**) in a sterile container before flow cytometry.

3.2.2. Indirect Staining of Antigen

1. Take cells at 10^6/mL and centrifuge at 800g for 10 min.
2. Add appropriate amount of primary antibody (*see* **Note 6**); incubate for 15 min at 37°C (*see* **Note 8**).
3. Add medium to a cell density of 10^6/mL. Centrifuge at 800g for 10 min, discard supernatant, and repeat.
4. Add fluorochrome-labeled secondary antibody at a dilution of between 1:10 and 1:20 (If the primary antibody is a monoclonal, this will generally be a rabbit antimouse antibody). Incubate for 15 min at 37°C.
5. Add medium to cell density of 10^6/mL. Centrifuge, discard supernatant, and repeat.
6. Resuspend at 10^6/mL in phenol red free medium containing a low level of serum or protein (no higher than 2%; *see* **Note 9**) in a sterile container before flow cytometry.

3.3. Preparation of the Flow Cytometer for Sterile Sorting

1. Sterilize the cytometer by passing 70% ethanol through all sheath and sample lines for 60 min. Wash out by replacing ethanol in the sheath container with sterile deionized water for 30 min, then replace this with sterile sheath fluid (PBS; *see* **Notes 10** and **11**).
2. Wash down all exposed surfaces—sample lines, nozzle holder, nozzle, deflection plates, tube holders—with 70% ethanol.
3. Define cell population within the sample using the scatter characteristics of the particles in suspension (**Fig. 3A**) (*see* **Notes 12** and **13**).
4. Define the population to be sorted on the basis of fluorescence characteristics (*see* **Fig. 3B,C**).
5. Decide whether purity, recovery, or count accuracy is the most important factor and adjust the mode of sorting accordingly. Cells may be sorted into tubes; 96-, 24-, or 6-well plates- or directly onto slides (*see* **Notes 14–18**).

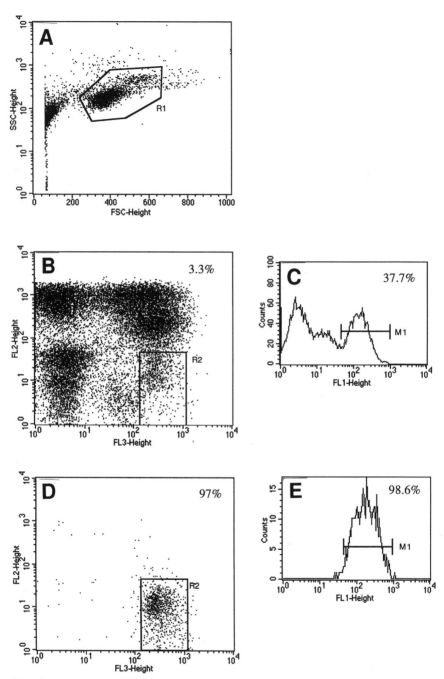

Fig. 3. A typical three-color sort setup: cells have been stained with three fluoro-chrome labeled antibodies—FITC, PE, and TriColor. (A) Scatter characteristics of cells. A region (R1) is selected to exclude debris and include the single cell-population. (B) PE (*y*-axis) and TriColor (*x*-axis) fluorescence from this cell population. On the basis of these characteristics, a subpopulation is selected (R2) and the FITC fluorescence of these cells is shown in C. (D,E) These populations after sorting with the percentage purity.

4. Notes

4.1. Preparation of Cells

1. Always wear gloves when handing potentially mutagenic chemicals such as propidium iodide.
2. When centrifuging it is advisable to avoid braking, as this can lead to cell loss. This also applies during subsequent antigen staining.
3. For some experiments, the use of trypsin may be contraindicated, for example, if the antigen under consideration is known to be cleaved by enzymatic action. In this case the cell sheet may be scraped from the vessel using a sterile cell scraper. This should be aseptic and only one cell scraper should be used for each vessel.
4. Phenol red in media may interfere with subsequent procedures, so it is generally advisable to use media without this when harvesting cells and subsequent antibody staining.
5. If the cells still look clumped when examined microscopically, it is advisable to pass the cell suspension through a 21-gauge needle, which will help to disperse these but should have only a minimal effect on cell viability.

4.2. Antibody Staining

6. The amount of antibody added will depend on the number of cells to be stained and the concentration of antibody in the staining solution. This is best determined empirically in positive control cells by a pilot experiment of test dilutions to determine the optimal concentration. Always do these experiments on equivalent numbers of cells and remember to scale up the amount of antibody used when doing bulk staining. The dilutions required for optimal staining using commercial antibodies will vary widely. Also, in general, the dilution for flow cytometry is lower than for slide-based immunofluorescence, that is, a higher protein concentration is needed. Also it is important after washing steps to remove as much fluid as possible to avoid subsequent dilution of antibodies.
7. All pipets, tips, and containers should either be purchased sterile or should be autoclaved.
8. The length of time taken for antigen staining can vary—most antibody binding is very rapid (seconds), but some low-density, low-affinity antigens may take longer. The optimal temperature for staining is either 37°C unless using lymphocytes or other cells where antigen capping may occur in which case 4°C is preferable—in these cases the incubation time should be increased (doubled).
9. Immediately before flow sorting, cells should be suspended in low-serum or low-protein medium. Protein has a tendency to coat the sides of the sample lines in the cytometer and this can lead to blockages, which are best avoided. Collection medium, however, should contain serum and antibiotics.

4.3. Sorting

10. PBS is generally used as a sheath fluid, although any ionized fluid will be suitable. Obviously this needs to be sterile for sterile sorting; sterility is achieved by

alcohol washing of all fluid containers and fluid lines in the cytometer and may be improved by having an in-line 0.22-μm filter in the sheath line.

11. Sterilization will add to the preparation time of the cytometer, and it is important to ask whether the sort will be sterile (if cells are to be recultured) or nonsterile (if cells are required for RNA extraction for example).

12. Cells, especially adherent cells or cells recovered from solid tumors, have a tendency to clump which will lead to machine blockages. These can be reduced by prefiltering cells to be sorted through sterile gauze of a pore size appropriate to the cells being used—35 μm for small cells (e.g., blood or bone marrow), 70 μm for epithelial or tumor cells. Gauze may be sterilized by autoclaving or by brief washing in 70% ethanol.

13. Clumping may also be due to high levels of cell death leading to nuclear breakup. The addition of a small amount of DNase (5 Kunitz units/mL) to the cell suspension can be beneficial.

14. Owing to the possibility of coincidence of a wanted and an unwanted cell in either the same droplet or consecutive droplets, a decision as to whether these droplets should be sorted can be made by the operator, depending on the desired purity and recovery for the cell fraction. Sorting a one-drop envelope will give high purity but will lead to reduced recovery; increasing the size of the deflection envelope will increase recovery at the expense of purity.

15. It is advisable to collect cells into medium, especially if they are to be recultured after sorting. This medium should also contain double-strength antibiotics—cells may be centrifuged out of this medium after sorting and recultured in normal medium.

16. Viability of sorted cells is usually good—there should be no significant reduction in viability of pre- and post-sorted cells. There may be loss of viability if the cells are not kept in optimal conditions, and this may mean keeping them at 37°C during the duration of the sort.

17. There are a number of practical considerations to be addressed before embarking on a sort. How numerous is the population of interest? How many cells are required at the end of the sort? How long will the sort take? The first two questions will enable the third to be determined. It may be that if a large number of cells of a minor population is required, flow sorting may actually be impractical. In these circumstances, it is possible to pre-enrich for the population of interest by a prior step such as Magnetic Activated Cell Sorter (MACS)®-bead separation *(29,30)* (*see* Chapter 2 by Clarke and Davies).

18. At the end of the sort, a small aliquot of sorted cells should be reanalyzed to determine the sort purity. **Figures 3** and **4** show examples of sorts based on triple- and single-color staining. If sorting using a purity mode, purity should always be >96%. Cell sorting is a highly skilled procedure that can be learned only through experience. Therefore it is important to emphasize the necessity for a trained and experienced flow cytometer operator who can advise on the practical considerations of cell preparation and be aware of the subtleties of flow sorting.

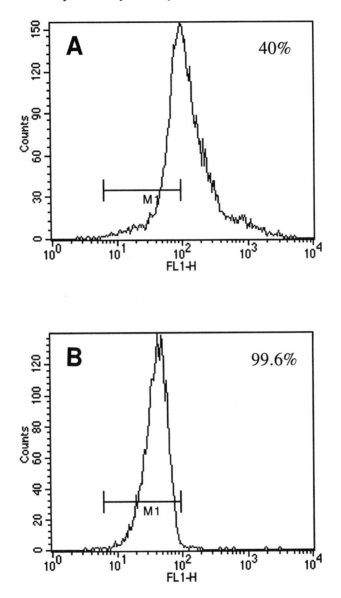

Fig. 4. A single-color sort. Here cells have been treated with an FITC-labeled antibody. The lower 40% of the histogram has been selected (**A**, M1) and sorted. Post-sort purity is >99% (**B**).

References

1. Ormerod, M. G., ed. (2000) *Flow Cytometry: A Practical Approach*, Third Edition. IRL Press, Oxford.
2. Shapiro, H. M. (1994) *Practical Flow Cytometry*. John Wiley & Sons, New York.
3. Longobardi-Givan, A. (1992) *Flow Cytometry. First Principles*. Wiley-Liss, New York.
4. Herzenberg, L. A., Sweet, R. G., and Herzenberg, L. A. (1976) Fluorescence activated cell sorting. *Science* **234,** 108–117.
5. Duhnen, J., Stegemann, J., Wiecorek, C., and Mertens, H. (1983) A new fluid switching cell sorter. *Histochemistry* **77,** 117–121.
6. Orfao, A. and Ruiz-Arguilees, A. (1996) General concepts about cell sorting. *Clin. Biochem.* **29,** 5–9.
7. Carter, N. P. (1990) Measurement of cellular subsets using antibodies, in *Flow Cytometry: A Practical Approach,* Ormerod, M. G. (ed.), IRL Press, Oxford, pp. 45–67.
8. Tough, G. F. and Sprent, J. (1994) Turnover of naive- and memory-phenotype T cells. *J. Exp. Med.* **179,** 1127–1135.
9. Krishan, A. (1975) Rapid flow cytofluorometric analysis of mammalian cell cycle by propidium iodide. *J. Cell Biol.* **66,** 188–193.
10. Crissman, H. A. and Steinkamp, J. A. (1987) A new method for rapid and sensitive detection of bromodeoxyuridine in DNA-replicating cells. *Exp. Cell Res.* **173,** 256–261.
11. Shapiro, H. M., Natale, P. J., and Kamentsky, L. A. (1979) Estimation of membrane potentials of individual lymphocytes by flow cytometry. *Proc. Natl. Acad. Sci. USA* **76,** 5728–5730.
12. Rijkers, J. T., Justement, L. B., Griffioen, A. W., and Camber, J. C. (1990) Improved method for measuring intracellular Ca^{++} with Fluo-3. *Cytometry* **11,** 923–927.
13. Wieder, E. D., Hang, H., and Fox, M. H. (1993) Measurement of intracellular pH using flow cytometry with carboxy-SNARF 1. *Cytometry* **14,** 916–921.
14. Darzynkiewicz, Z., Bruno, S., Del Bino, G., Gorzyca, W., Hotz, M. A., Lassota, P., and Traganos, F. (1992) Features of apoptotic cells measured by flow cytometry. *Cytometry* **13,** 795–808.
15. Ormerod, M. G., Sun, X. M., Brown, D., Snowden, R. T., and Cohen, G. M. (1993) Quantification of apoptosis and necrosis by flow cytometry. *Acta Oncolog.* **32,** 417–424.
16. Nolan, G. P., Fiering, S., Nicolas, J. F., and Herzenberg, L. A. (1985) Fluorescence activated cell analysis and sorting of viable mammalian cells based on β-D-galactosidase activity after transduction of *Escherichia coli lacZ. Proc. Natl. Acad. Sci. USA* **85,** 2603–2607.
17. Maftah, A., Huet, O., Gallet, P. F., and Ratinaud, M. H. (1993) Flow cytometry's contribution to the measurement of cell functions. *Biol. Cell* **78,** 85–93.
18. Leonce, S. and Burbridge, M. (1993) Flow cytometry: a useful technique in the study of multidrug resistance. *Biol. Cell* **78,** 63–68.
19. Darzynkiewicz, Z., Evenson, D., Staiano-Coico, L., Sharpless, T., and Melamed, M. R. (1979) Relationship between RNA content and progression of lymphocytes through S phase of the cell cycle. *Proc. Natl. Acad. Sci. USA* **76,** 358–362.

20. Bauman, J. G. J., Bayer, J. A., and van Dekken, H. (1990) Fluorescent in situ hybridization to detect cellular RNA by flow cytometry and confocal microscopy. *J. Microsc.* **157,** 73–81.
21. Wieckiewicz, J., Krzeszowiak, A., Ruggiero, I., Pituch-Nowarolska, A., and Zembala, M. (1998) Detection of cytokine gene expression in human monocytes and lymphocytes by fluorescent in situ hybridization in cell suspension and flow cytometry. *Int. J. Mol. Med.* **1,** 995–999.
22. Leary, J. F. (1994) Strategies for rare cell detection and isolation. *Methods Cell Biol.* **42,** 331–357.
23. Horan, P. K. and Wheeless, L. L. (1977) Quantitative single cell analysis and sorting. *Science* **198,** 149–157.
24. Williams, C., Davies, D., and Williamson, R. (1993) Segregation of ΔF508 and normal CFTR alleles in human sperm. *Hum. Mol. Genet.* **2,** 445–448.
25. Dunne, J. F., Thomas, J., and Lee, S. (1989) Detection of mRNA in flow-sorted cells. *Cytometry* **10,** 199–204.
26. Green, D. K. (1990) Analysis and sorting of human chromosomes. *J. Microscop.* **159,** 237–245.
27. Davies, D. C., Monard, S. P., and Young, B. D. (2000) Chromosome analysis and sorting by flow cytometry, in *Flow Cytometry: A Practical Approach*, 3rd ed. Ormerod, M. G. (ed.), IRL Press, Oxford, pp. 189–201.
28. Berglund, D. L. and Starkey, J. R. (1989) Isolation of viable tumor cells following introduction of labeled antibody to an intracellular oncogene product using electroporation. *J. Immunol. Methods* **125,** 79–87.
29. Miltenyi, S., Müller, W., Weichel, W., and Radbruch, A. (1990) High gradient magnetic cell separation with MACS. *Cytometry* **11,** 231–238.
30. Pickl, W. F., Majdic, O., Kohl, P., Stöckl, J., Riedl, E., Scheinecker, C., et al. (1996) Molecular and functional characteristics of dendritic cells generated from highly purified CD14+ peripheral blood monocytes. *J. Immunol.* **157,** 3850–3859.

2

Immunomagnetic Cell Separation

Catherine Clarke and Susan Davies

1. Introduction

In metastasis research, it may sometimes be necessary to separate populations of tumor cells from a mixed cell population such as a tumor, peripheral blood, or bone marrow. In addition, the normal counterparts of populations of tumor cells can be separated to allow direct comparisons to be made (1). In recent years magnetic bead separation techniques have become increasingly popular for these purposes.

Immunomagnetic separation methods are based on the attachment of small magnetizable particles to cells via antibodies or lectins. When the mixed population of cells is placed in a magnetic field, those cells that have beads attached will be attracted to the magnet and may thus be separated from the unlabeled cells.

Several makes of bead are available, some of which are designed specifically for cell sorting, and others that are designed for purifying molecules (particularly nucleic acids) but that may be adapted for cell sorting if necessary. The different types of beads work on the same principle, but the strength of the magnetic field required to separate the cells differs depending on the size of the beads. Of the larger beads (>2 µm), the most commonly used type is the range produced by Dynal (Dynal [UK] Ltd., Wirral, Mersyside, UK; Dynal, Inc., Lake Success, NY). The smaller beads (<100 nm) represented by the MACS system produced by Miltenyi Biotech (Miltenyi Biotech Ltd., Bisley, Surrey, UK; Miltenyi Biotech Inc., Auburn, CA) require a more complicated separation apparatus. Details of each type of bead together with advantages and disadvantages of each system are described below.

Dynabeads are 4.5-µm superparamagnetic beads; that is, they have no residual magnetism outside a magnetic field. An iron-containing core is surrounded by a thin polymer shell to which biomolecules may be adsorbed.

From: *Methods in Molecular Medicine, vol. 58:*
Metastasis Research Protocols, Vol. 2: Cell Behavior In Vitro and In Vivo
Edited by: S. A. Brooks and U. Schumacher © Humana Press Inc., Totowa, NJ

The beads can be coated in primary antibodies, species-specific antibodies, lectins, enzymes, or streptavidin. The beads may be attached to cells via a coating of primary antibodies specific for the cell type using beads bought ready coated, or using beads coated by the user with their own antibody. Alternatively the cells, rather than the beads, may be labeled with a primary antibody, and then species-specific secondary antibody-coated beads added. Similarly, streptavidin-coated beads can be used in conjunction with biotinylated primary or secondary antibodies. The cells, surrounded by a "rosette" of beads, may then be separated from the unlabeled population in a magnetic field using a relatively small (but powerful) magnet produced by Dynal.

If no antibody is available that specifically identifies a cell type in a heterogeneous population, the cells may still be separated using the "negative sorting" method. In this case, all the unwanted cell types are immunomagnetically labeled, a process that may require a cocktail of antibodies. The labeling procedure is the same as for positive sorting except that the unlabeled fraction of the cell population is retained and the labeled cells are discarded.

The range of precoated beads available includes those coated in antibodies specific for human B (CD19) and T cells (CD2 and CD3) and T-cell subsets (CD4 and CD8), hematopoietic progenitor cells (CD34), and monocytes (CD14). For metastasis research two types of beads are available to separate tumor cells from blood or bone marrow. For epithelial tumors, beads coated with antibodies against the human epithelial antigen are available. Nonepithelial tumors, however, require negative selection using anti-CD45-coated beads to remove all the leukocytes. It is possible to separate cells not only from blood, but also from a primary tumor and/or arising metastases by first disaggregating the tumor to form a single-cell suspension and then labeling the cells with a suitable antibody. Frequently in tumor samples only a small number of cells are present, and the process of cell sorting, requiring several washing steps, may result in unacceptable cell losses. In this case, it is worth precoating the beads with the antibody rather than labeling the cells and then using species-specific secondary antibody-coated beads, to limit the number of washing steps required, and thus reduce possible cell loss.

The beads may be left attached to the cells even if the cells are to be subsequently cultured. If the density of the beads is too great, however, they may interfere with cell attachment and growth, and should be removed. It is also desirable to remove the beads from the cell surface if the cells are subsequently to be used in experiments to investigate cell–cell interactions. Several options are available for removing the beads. First, some precoated beads (anti-human CD4, CD8, CD19, CD34, and antimouse CD4) may be removed using a polyclonal anti-Fab antibody, DETACHaBEAD, which competes with antibody–antigen binding to release the antibody and bead from the cell. Second, a new type of bead has been produced that may be used for any cell separation, and that is specifically designed to be released from the cells. CELLection beads are available both primary antibody coated and for use with any mouse primary antibody or biotinylated antibody. Antibodies are attached to the surface of these beads via a DNA linker, which may be cleaved after the cells have been isolated by the addition of a DNase releasing buffer. Thus, although the beads are removed, the cells retain attached antibodies.

The MACS separation system (2) uses particles consisting of iron oxide and polysaccharide. These beads are approx 50 nm in diameter, and they require a far stronger magnetic field than that provided by the Dynal magnet to separate cells. As with Dynabeads, cells may be negatively or positively sorted from a population using the MACS separation system. A large range of primary antibody-coated beads is available to sort leukocyte subsets, fibroblasts, endothelial cells, epithelial cells, and apoptotic cells. Alternatively, the cells may be labeled with primary antibodies followed by species-specific antibody-coated MACS beads. The labeled cell suspension is then placed in a separation column in a strong magnetic field. The column contains a plastic-covered ferromagnetic core through which the cell suspension can flow. The flow rate is governed by the size of the hole at the base of the column or by an attached needle (depending on the column type). The labeled cells are retained within the column as long as it remains in the magnetic field, and unlabeled cells flow through and can be collected. The column may then be removed from the magnetic field, allowing the positive cells to be eluted. Following cell separation, MACS beads are internalized by the cells, and so they do not need to be removed because they do not interfere with cell attachment to the culture surface or with cell–cell interactions. It may be necessary to remove the beads, however, if a subset of cells are to be resorted from a population already sorted using MACS beads. A bead removal reagent is available for this purpose that enzymatically removes the MACS beads and allows the cells to be relabeled with another marker and sorted again.

The two bead separation systems have advantages and disadvantages. Until recently, it was preferable to separate cells using the MACS system if they were to be subsequently used in studies of cell–cell interactions. The development of removable types of Dynabeads means that this is no longer the case. Dynabeads are not suitable for every type of cell separation, however, because, in rare cases, they have been shown to strip the antigen off the surface of cells, making cell separation impossible (3). The main disadvantage of the MACS system is that initial costs are higher to purchase the separation magnet, and running costs include not only the price of the beads, but also replacement columns. In comparison to the running costs of a fluorescence-activated cell sorter (FACS) (methodology described in Chapter 1 by Davies), however, both systems are relatively cheap because no servicing is required. Furthermore, the bead separation systems do not require an operator as skilled as the one required for the FACS system. It should be noted, however, that magnetic separation is far more limited than FACS because immunomagnetic techniques can only separate cells into positive and negative populations and not, for example, into high and low expressors of a molecule, as is possible with FACS sorting *(4)*. Furthermore, only cell surface molecules can be used as markers for magnetic separation of live cells, and not markers that distinguish cells by other means such as the expression of green fluorescent protein in transfected cells *(5)*.

The purity of cell populations obtained by immunomagnetic sorting is dependent on producing a single-cell suspension, as any unwanted cell attached to a labeled cell will also be retained in the positively labeled fraction. Large clumps of cells may be removed from a suspension by passing the cell suspension through a 35–40-μm mesh; however, some cell doublets may still remain. In FACS sorting, the gating parameters may be set to sort only single cells, and thus a high level of purity is achieved, but at the expense of a reduction in cell numbers. In immunomagnetic sorting, cell doublets that contain only the desired phenotype can be retained while those that contain unwanted cells can be removed by using a double sorting method. Several approaches may be used to remove the unwanted cell types:

1. Label the "contaminating" cell type and remove these cells (including doublets containing only one of this phenotype). Retain the unlabeled cells and then positively sort the desired phenotype.
2. Positively sort the desired cell phenotype using removable beads. Remove these beads, resort using a marker of the unwanted cells, and then keep the final negative fraction and discard the positive cells.
3. Positively sort the desired cell type using MACS beads and then remove contaminating cells using Dynabeads (the small MACS beads are not sufficient to cause cells to be attracted to the Dynal magnet). In this case it is essential that the antibody on the Dynabeads does not recognize the antibody used for MACS sorting; otherwise, all the cells will become coated in Dynabeads.

Although the type of separations that can be carried out by immunomagnetic sorting are not as extensive as those by FACS sorting, it can prove a useful and relatively simple technique that can yield large numbers of highly purified cells.

2. Materials

1. Primary antibody: The correct dilution of the primary antibody should be determined by the user.
2. Biotinylated secondary antibody: A biotinylated secondary antibody directed against the primary antibody should be used if the only beads available for sorting are streptavidin coated, and the primary antibody is not already biotinylated.
3. Buffer: Phosphate-buffered saline (PBS), 0.5% w/v bovine serum albumin (BSA).

4. Magnetic beads: Dynabeads or MACS beads coated in appropriate primary or secondary antibodies or streptavidin.
5. Separation columns: Positive or negative selection columns are required for MACS separation, and the type of column should be chosen accordingly. The size of column to be used is determined by the number of cells to be separated.
6. Bead detachment: If Dynabeads are to be removed, DETACHaBEAD may be required, or if CELLection beads are used, DNase solution (supplied as part of a kit) will be required.

3. Methods

If the cells are going to be cultured, carry out all procedures in a laminar flow cabinet.

3.1. Cell Preparation

1. Prepare a single-cell suspension by standard methods depending on whether the cells are from tissues, blood, or cell cultures (*6*) (*see* **Note 1**).
2. If cell clumps are present, pass the cell suspension through a 35–40-μm mesh.
3. Count the cells using a hemacytometer (*see* **Note 2**).

3.2. MACS Separation

1. If using directly conjugated beads, then proceed to **step 5**. Suspend the cell pellet in a small volume (approx 200 μL/10⁷ cells) of primary antibody diluted in buffer. The correct dilution should be determined by titration, with a likely concentration of antibody being 5–10 μg/mL.
2. Incubate the cell suspension at 4°C (on ice) for 40 min to 1 h with rocking or regular inversion to mix the cell suspension (*see* **Note 3**).
3. Wash cells with 5 mL of buffer and centrifuge at 300*g* for 5 min.
4. Repeat **step 3** twice (*see* **Note 4**).
5. Suspend cell pellet in appropriate amount of buffer according to bead manufacturer's instructions and add appropriate amount of beads (*see* **Note 5**). For most types of MACS microbead, resuspend cells in 80 μL of buffer plus 20 μL of beads per 10⁷ cells (for fewer than 10⁷ cells, still use 100 μL of total volume).
6. Mix and incubate for 15 min at 6–12°C (refrigerator) or 40 min at 4°C (on ice).
7. Wash cells with 5 mL of buffer and centrifuge at 300*g* for 5 min.
8. Resuspend cells in 500 μL of buffer.
9. Prepare a MACS column of appropriate size (*see* manufacturer's instructions). Columns are available that are designed specifically for positive or negative selection and should be chosen accordingly. Columns for positive selection are ready to use; those for negative selection should be attached via a three-way tap to a "flow regulator" (syringe needle) and a syringe filled with buffer.
10. Rinse the column with cold buffer (*see* **Note 6**).
11. Apply cells to the MACS column in a magnetic field.
12. Allow unlabeled cells to flow through the column and collect the effluent as the "negative fraction" (*see* **Note 7**).

13. If using a positive selection column, rinse the cells 3× by applying buffer to the column (within the magnetic field) using a volume appropriate to the column size (*see* manufacturer's instructions). For a negative selection column, turn the three-way tap to the "fill" position (i.e., open to the syringe and column but not the needle), remove the whole column assembly from the magnet, and back-flush the cells into the column with buffer from the syringe. Replace the column in the magnetic field and change the flow resistor to a higher gauge. Allow the cells to flow through once more and collect the effluent as the wash fraction. This fraction may contain both negative and weakly positive cells and is usually discarded.

14. Fill the column once more with buffer and elute the positive cells outside the magnetic field using the supplied plunger for positive selection columns or by attaching the syringe to the top of a negative selection column and removing the flow resistor.

3.3. Dynabead Separation

1. If using directly conjugated Dynabeads, proceed to **step 2** below. If using a primary antibody followed by secondary antibody-coated beads, follow **steps 1–4** of **Subheading 3.2.,** then proceed to **step 2** below.

2. Suspend a cell pellet in an appropriate amount of PBS–BSA according to bead manufacturer's instructions and add an appropriate amount of beads (*see* **Note 8**).

3. Mix and incubate for 15–30 min at 2–8°C with rocking or occasional inversion.

4. Add 5 mL of buffer to the cell suspension, mix gently, and then place the tube into the Dynal magnet and leave for 1 min, during which time the beads and any attached cells are drawn to one side of the tube.

5. Carefully aspirate off the buffer containing unlabeled cells, making sure that the beads and labeled cells are not disturbed, and retain this as the negative fraction.

6. Remove the tube from the magnetic field and repeat **steps 4** and **5** (*see* **Note 9**).

7. Suspend the beads and labeled cells in buffer and retain this as the positive fraction.

8. If the beads are to be detached from the positively selected cells, follow **steps 9–13** for removal with DETACHaBEAD (certain types of beads only) or **steps 14–16** where CELLection beads have been used.

9. Suspend the positively labeled cells in 100 μL of buffer (this will suffice for 10^6–10^7 cells).

10. Add 1 U (10 μL) of DETACHaBEAD and incubate at room temperature with tilting and rotation for 45–60 min (*see* **Note 10**).

11. Place the tube in the Dynal magnet and leave for at least 1 min.

12. Carefully aspirate off the buffer containing the cells and retain.

13. Resuspend the beads and repeat **steps 11–12** to release any trapped cells.

14. Where CELLection beads are to be removed, resuspend the rosetted cells in 200 μL of buffer prewarmed to 37°C. This is sufficient for up to 5×10^7 beads, that is, approx 10^7 cells.

15. Add 4 μL of DNase solution (provided by Dynal as part of the CELLection bead kit). This is sufficient for up to 10^8 Dynabeads.

16. Incubate at room temperature, with tilting, for 15 min.

17. Flush rosettes through a pipet several times.

18. Follow **steps 11–13** above.

4. Notes

1. Exposure of the cells to trypsin should be minimized to reduce cell damage. Overtrypsinized cells are particularly fragile and may be more easily damaged by the labeling procedure.
2. It can be helpful to assess the number of dead cells in the suspension by carrying out a trypan blue dye exclusion test. Both Dynabeads and MACS beads can stick to dead cells nonspecifically, and it may be worth removing the dead cells at this stage by density gradient centrifugation.
3. All solutions should be kept cold to avoid antibody internalization by the cells.
4. Any remaining free primary antibody must be completely removed or it may bind to the beads and hinder their attachment to the cells.
5. If the primary antibody is biotinylated and streptavidin-coated beads are to be used for separation, ensure that the buffer used is biotin free.
6. Passing the buffer through the column both precools it and may reduce nonspecific interactions of the cells with the column material.
7. A negative selection column may become blocked because of trapped air bubbles. These may be released by gently applying pressure to the side syringe.
8. Dynabeads are provided in a buffer containing azide which should be removed before use. The azide may be removed by placing the bead solution in the separation magnet, removing the bead-free buffer and resuspending the beads.
9. The purity of positively sorted cells can be improved by repeating this step up to 3× to release trapped cells.
10. Check an aliquot of cells microscopically to ensure that the beads have been removed. If beads remain, the cells can be incubated for longer, or more DETACHaBEAD added.

References

1. Clarke, C., Titley, J., Davies S. C., and O'Hare, M. J. (1994) An immunomagnetic separation method using superparamagnetic (MACS) beads for large-scale purification of human mammary luminal and myoepithelial cells. *Epithel. Cell Biol.* **3**, 38–46.
2. Miltenyi S., Müller W., Weichel W., and Radbruch A. (1990) High gradient magnetic cell separation with MACS. *Cytometry* **11**, 231–238.
3. Manyonda, I. T., Soltys, A. J., and Hay, F. C. (1992) A critical evaluation of the magnetic cell sorter and its use in the positive and negative selection of CD45RO⁺ cells. *J. Immunol. Methods* **149**, 1–10.
4. Harris, R. A., Eichholtz, T. J., Hiles, I. D., Page, M. J., and O'Hare, M. J. (1999) New model of ErbB-2 over-expression in human mammary luminal epithelial cells. *Int. J. Cancer* **80**, 477–484.
5. Wiechen, K., Zimmer, C., and Dietel, M. (1998) Selection of a high activity c-erbB-2 ribozyme using a fusion gene of c-erbB-2 and the enhanced green fluorescent protein. *Cancer Gene Ther.* **5**, 45–51.
6. Freshney, R. I. (1994) *Culture of Animal Cells: A Manual of Basic Technique,* 3rd ed., Alan R. Liss, New York.

3

Genetic Modification of Cell Lines to Enhance Their Metastatic Capability

Daniel McWilliams and Hilary Collins

1. Introduction

1.1. Matrix Metalloproteinases and Transfection

Metastasis is the final step in tumor progression from a benign cell to a fully malignant cell. The metastatic phenotype results from a wide range of phenotypic changes in the cell from the expression of proteinases, to adhesion molecules, the loss of proteinase inhibitors and tumor suppressor gene function, to name a few. However, the molecular basis for this progression has long been investigated and there does not appear to be a specific genetic alteration responsible for influencing all the changes which occur in a metastatic cell. As mentioned, the proteolytic ability of the cell is a key factor in the malignant phenotype and the expression of matrix metalloproteinases (MMPs) is known to contribute to metastases *(1)*. The gelatinase group (MMP-2 and MMP-9) within this enzyme family has been associated with tumor progression and the active form of MMP-2 has the strongest correlation with the metastatic phenotype in colorectal cancer *(2)*.

Genetic manipulation of MMP-2 and MMP-9 in vitro has correlated with an increase in metastatic ability in vivo. Bernhard et al. (1990) demonstrated that overexpression of gelatinase B (MMP-9) in rat fibroblasts was strongly associated with the increased metastatic ability of these cells when injected into nude mice *(3)*, while inhibition of this enzyme using ribozymes decreased lung colonization. Transfection of gelatinase A (MMP-2) into a bladder cell line has increased the area of lung metastases *(4)* while transfection of its activator MT-MMP-1 has enhanced the survival of lung carcinoma cells in the lungs of intravenously injected mice *(5)*. The ability of MMPs to degrade the basement

From: *Methods in Molecular Medicine, vol. 58:*
Metastasis Research Protocols, Vol. 2: Cell Behavior In Vitro and In Vivo
Edited by: S. A. Brooks and U. Schumacher © Humana Press Inc., Totowa, NJ

membrane and extracellular components has contributed to the effects seen in the experimental and spontaneous models of metastasis described. This view has been confirmed by in vitro studies demonstrating the increased invasive abilities of cells through Matrigel when transfected with these MMPs. The participation of MMPs in the invasive process has also been confirmed by targeted disruption of genes controlling their inhibitors. Disruption of tissue inhibitor of metalloproteinasen-1 (TIMP-1) in mesenchymal cells increased their invasive ability in vitro (*6*), while transfection of TIMP-1 or TIMP-2 decreased invasive potential (*7*).

Owing to the extensive evidence in the literature that MMPs alter the invasive ability of carcinoma cells, we will concentrate on the introduction of MT-MMP-1 into an adenoma cell line. This may be considered as a model system, which is applicable to the introduction of other genes of interest in metastasis research. The cell line used has been profiled for MMPs and possesses a wide range of the enzymes, but no invasive activity has been detected related to active MMP-2 (determined by substrate gel electrophoresis, zymography). By altering the levels of MT-MMP-1, we hoped to achieve an increase in active MMP-2 which has been linked to metastasis and therefore alter the invasive potential of this cell line.

In this chapter, a method is described to confirm stable transfection by culture in selective media. Stable transfection can also be confirmed by reverse transcriptase-polymerase chain reaction (RT-PCR), described in Chapter 19 by Haack et al. in the companion volume. The application of gene transfection experiments to produce clones of increased metastatic potential and their subsequent use in tumorogenesis and metastasis assays in nude mice are covered in Chapter 17 by Muschel and Hua, and the reader is directed to consult this chapter also.

1.2. Definition of Transfection

Transfected cell lines, known as transfectants, can be either stable or transient. In transient transfection, no selection pressure is applied to the cells to encourage them to incorporate the vector into their own genome. Most transient transfections are lost within 1 wk, and so all assays must be performed before then, usually within 48–72 h of transfection. To assess the metastatic potential of transfectants, it is normally necessary to perform assays lasting much longer than this, especially in vivo studies. Therefore, it is essential to establish stable transfectants. Once the plasmid has been incorporated into the genotype, then the cell line will, theoretically, express the sequence in question in the conditions required (constitutively or upon stimulation).

1.3. Methods of Transfection

Several different transfection methods have been developed, such as calcium phosphate-mediated, DEAE-dextran, electroporation, and adenovirus infection. This chapter focuses on liposome mediated transfection, describing the use of the Tfx reagents from Promega. This method is efficient and of minimal toxicity, and useful for establishing pools of stable transfectants within about 3–4 wk. In brief, cells are incubated with media, liposomes, and plasmid DNA for 1–2 h and then cultured for 2 d. After that, selection begins to establish stable transfectants.

1.4. Establishment of Stable Transfectants

Most commercially available vectors have antibiotic resistance genes incorporated into the plasmid to allow for selection of bacterial clones. In the cases of the neomycin resistance genes, these may be used to select for plasmid expression in mammalian cells as well. An analog of neomycin called geneticin (G418) is available from GIBCO and is toxic to mammalian cells as well as bacteria. By culturing the transfectants in media containing the chosen antibiotic at a predetermined concentration, it is possible to kill any cells lacking the plasmid and induce a selection pressure upon the cells to incorporate the vector into their genomes. This process will normally last about 2–3 wk, but can take longer as is the case for slow growing adenoma cells.

1.5. Dosage Determination of Antibiotic

It is necessary to discover the doses at which the antibiotic will kill mammalian cells. This is accomplished by seeded 5×10^4 cells per well into a 96-well plate and culturing with complete media plus various concentrations of antibiotic. For geneticin (G418) or mycophenolic acid (MPA), the cells should be tested with concentrations from 100 µg/mL to 1 mg/mL. Normally increments of 100 µg/mL are sufficient. After 4–7 d, the cells can be counted using a tetrazolium-based assay or else manually, and a dosage curve can be plotted. Generally, the concentration required to kill >90% of cells is that which is used for selection of stable transfectants. However, we have found that no more than approx 65–75% of NIH3T3 cells, for example, were killed by 1 mg/mL of geneticin. Increased concentrations did not result in increased mortality of NIH3T3s. However, when selecting transfectants, these concentrations have been shown to be perfectly adequate, killing all control wild-type NIH3T3.

1.6. Confirmation of Stable Transfection

After 2–3 wk of selection and expansion, the cells growing in the wells can be tested for stable incorporation of the plasmid. Once cells have begun to grow well in the selective media, after 2 wk they may be harvested and split. Cells are then seeded into nonselective, complete media and cultured as normal. After 1–2 wk, they are seeded back into selective media and then checked after two passages to see whether all, or some, of the cells are still viable. If the cells have not lost the resistance to the antibiotic, then it follows that they must be stably transfected. The cell lines should not lose their antibiotic resistance after that, although samples should be tested throughout the study to confirm this.

A DNA extraction from a sample of the cells can also be tested by RT-PCR (described in Chapter 19 by Haack et al. in the companion volume). Using one primer from the insert and one from the plasmid will confirm that the cells have the correct genotype.

2. Materials

1. Transfection Kit- Tfx™-50 (Promega). Solution to be made up 24 h prior to use by adding 400 μL of nuclease free water. Stable at –20°C for up to 8 wk.
2. Plasmid DNA. Stored at –20°C. The gene for MT-1-MMP was cloned into the mammalian expression vector pGW1HG (method not described). Use GPT selective media for selection procedure.
3. Antibiotic GPT selection media. To one 500-mL bottle of growth media, add 12.5 mL of 50X HT supplement, 12.5 mL of 50X xanthine, 12.5 mL of 50X MPA. Adjust to normal pH level of media with 1 M HCl. Adjust antibiotic MPA levels according to results of tetrazolium-based assay on each cell line. Stock stored at –20°C, media stored at 4°C.
4. Standard tissue culture conditions employed for growth of cells, 37°C, 5% CO_2 in humidified conditions. RPMI growth media +10% fetal calf serum (FCS) + L-glutamine. Harvest cells using 0.025% EDTA.

3. Methods

3.1. Transfection

The method for transfection using the liposome-mediated method of Tfx-50 (Promega) is as follows:

1. The cells for transfection are seeded onto a 24-well plate between 24 and 48 h before transfection. The cells need to be approx 70–80% confluent to minimize the toxicity of the liposome reagent. Excessively confluent cells appear to reduce the transfection efficiency (*see* **Note 1**).
2. Plasmid DNA should be accurately quantified and as pure as possible. Endotoxin free purification methods (such as QIAGEN's Endo-free Maxiprep kit) should be used to obtain plasmids from bacterial clones. Ideally, when measured on a spectrophotometer, the A_{260}/A_{280} ratio of the purified plasmid should be 1.6–1.8. The gene for MT-1-MMP was cloned into the mammalian expression vector pGW1HG (method not described). As well as the vectors containing inserts, a control consisting of a self-ligated plasmid can be included in the procedure. This will control for any phenotypic effects of transfection that are not due to the expression of the desired insert. This may also present a use for the products of any unsuccessful cloning experiments! Prepare the plasmids using sterile tubes and tips, or contamination will be present in the cell cultures during transfection.

3. The medium is eluted from the cells and the transfection mix is added (*see* **Notes 2** and **3**). After ensuring that the mix covers all the cells, the cells incubate at 37°C for 1 h.
4. A volume of 1 mL of complete media is added to the cells and they are incubated in normal cell culture conditions for approx 2 d. Selection procedures may begin.

3.2. Selection Procedure

1. The medium is eluted and the cells are harvested and split into different dilutions. The cells should be harvested using EDTA, if possible, as trypsin is more harmful. Most cell lines require a few minutes at 37°C in 0.025% EDTA to remove them from the flask.
2. Prepare several dilutions of the transfectants in complete, selective media. A range from 1:5, 1:10, 1:50, and 1:100 can be used to establish cell colonies and, in the case of the lower dilutions, fairly rapid confluency (2 wk is optimal for the fast-growing NIH3T3 cells, allow longer time frame for slow growing cells). Complete media containing the required concentration of antibiotic is added and the cells are cultured changing the media every 3–4 d (i.e., twice a week) (*see* **Note 4**).

3.3. Confirmation of Stable Transfectants

1. Once the transfectants are growing well, they may be split and plated into both selective and nonselective media at equal concentrations.
2. After 1–2 wk of growth in both media the cells from the nonselective media are harvested. Half are cultured in selective media while the other half continue to be grown in nonselective conditions. If both halves survive, then the cells are stably transfected. If the selective media kills the cells, then stable incorporation has not occurred and further selection is required.
3. The cells grown in nonselective media during this experiment act as a backup in case the incorporation of the plasmid has not occurred.
4. Subject all cell cultures to this test, as it will eliminate any possibly unstable transfectants.

4. Notes

1. For slower growing cells, for example, adenoma cell lines, it may be necessary to seed cells in T75 flasks and allow to reach 50–70% confluence before transfection.
2. The charge ratio of liposome/DNA needs to be carefully controlled. There must be sufficient liposomes present to result in a 2:1 to 4:1 charge ratio once the reagents are mixed. A charge ratio of 3:1 has been used for transfection of NIH3T3 fibroblasts, but optimization of the ratio from 2:1 to 4:1 may be necessary in some cell lines.
3. Normally 1 µg of DNA is used per well for transfection. Again, this may need to be optimized as quantities of 0.5 µg are optimal in some cell lines. The plasmid is diluted in 200 µL of media, which may contain serum. Liposomes are added to give the required charge ratio (4.5 µL/µg of DNA to give 3:1) and the mix is immediately vortexed to remove any clumping before a 15-min room temperature incubation.

4. If the cells reach confluency, they may be harvested similarly to their parent cells and this can begin the expansion necessary for other procedures, such as the confirmation of stability experiments and the freezing down of stock.

References

1. Stetler-Stevenson, W. G., Aznavoorian, S., and Liotta, L. A. (1993) Tumor cell interactions with the extracellular matrix during imvasion and metastasis. *Annu. Rev. Cell Biol.* **9,** 541–573.
2. Parsons, S. L., Watson, S. A., Collins, H. M., et al. (1998) Gelatinase (MMP-2 and -9) expression in gastrointestinal malignancy. *Br. J. Cancer* **78,** 1495–1502.
3. Bernhard, E. J., Muschel, R. J., and Hughes, E. N. (1990) Mr 92,000 gelatinase release correlates with the metastatic phenotype in transformed rat embryo cells. *Cancer Res.* **50,** 3872–3877.
4. Kawamata, H., Kameyama, S., Kawai, K., et al. (1995) Marked acceleration of the metastatic phenotype of a rat bladder carcinoma cell line by the expression of human gelatinase A. *Int. J. Cancer* **63,** 568–575.
5. Tsunezuka, Y., Kinoh, H., Takino, T., et al. (1996) Expression of membrane-type matrix metalloproteinase (MT-1-MMP) in tumor cells enhances pulmonary metastasis in an experimental metastasis assay. *Cancer Res.* **56,** 5678–5683.
6. Alexander, C. M. and Werb, Z. (1992) Targeted disruption of the tissue inhibitor of metalloproteinases gene increases the invasive behaviour of primitive mesenchymal cells derived from embryonic cells in vitro. *J. Cell Biol.* **118,** 727–739.
7. Khokha, R., Zimmer, M. J., Graham, C. H., et al. (1992) Suppression of invasion by inducible expression of tissue inhibitor of metalloproteinase-1 (TIMP-1) in B16-F10 melanoma cells. *J. Natl. Cancer Inst.* **84,** 1017–1022.

II

In Vitro Assays of Metastatic Behavior

4

Cell Aggregation Assays

Tom Boterberg, Marc E. Bracke, Erik A. Bruyneel, and Marc M. Mareel

1. Introduction

Invasion of carcinoma cells is the result of a disequilibrium between invasion promoter and invasion suppressor gene products (*1*). The E-cadherin/catenin complex is the most potent invasion suppressor at the cell membrane of epithelioid cells (*2*). This complex consists of E-cadherin, a transmembrane glycoprotein of 120 kDa, which is linked to the actin cytoskeleton via the catenins (*3*). Downregulation of the complex is a common feature in invasive carcinoma cells, and has been recognized at several levels, ranging from genomic mutations to functional deficiencies of an apparently intact complex (*4*). Cell aggregation assays have been set up to test the functionality of the complex in epithelioid tumor cells. Functional integrity of the complex is a prerequisite for cell–cell adhesion between epithelial cells, and measuring cell aggregation in vitro has thus become another elegant tool to study differences between invasive and noninvasive cell types.

One type of assay for cell aggregation is done in microtiter plates (*5*). The bottom of the wells is covered with an agar layer to prevent cell–substratum adhesion. On top of this agar layer a cell suspension is incubated under static culture conditions, and aggregate formation can be evaluated microscopically after several hours or days of incubation. This "slow" aggregation assay is easy to perform, does not require sophisticated equipment, and allows the screening at minute quantities of agents that may affect cell–cell adhesion (*6*). The E-cadherin specificity of the aggregation can be evidenced by antibodies that block the function of this molecule. A disadvantage of the assay is its lack of quantitative information: the result is scored microscopically in a semiquantitative way.

Another assay for cell aggregation is coined "fast" (30 min) and allows numerical analysis (*5*). This assay is a modification of the technique described

From: *Methods in Molecular Medicine, vol. 58:*
Metastasis Research Protocols, Vol. 2: Cell Behavior In Vitro and In Vivo
Edited by: S. A. Brooks and U. Schumacher © Humana Press Inc., Totowa, NJ

by Kadmon et al. *(7)*. For the preparation of a single-cell suspension, this assay requires a cell detachment procedure that preserves E-cadherin on the cell membrane and its linkage to the catenins. Simple trypsinization without Ca^{2+} would remove the extracellular 80-kDa part and make E-cadherin-mediated aggregation impossible. Cell aggregation is measured with a particle size counter, which yields a particle volume distribution curve as a function of the particle diameter. At time 0 min, the particle volume distribution of a well-dispersed cell suspension is measured, and after 30 min incubation in a calcium-containing aggregation buffer solution, this measurement is carried out on the aggregate suspension. The calculations are based on the diffraction model of Fraunhofer *(8)*. This model can be applied when the diameter of the particles lies between 0.4 and 2000 μm and the wavelength of the laser light is around 750 nm. In those conditions, the diffraction angle (which is measured by the detectors in the machine) is related to the diameter of the particle, which can thus be calculated. This numerical evaluation allows statistical evaluation of the results in a Kolmogorov–Smirnov test *(9)*. Because of the short incubation period, this assay can also be used to test effects of tool molecules (e.g., kinase and phosphatase inhibitors), that interfere more or less specifically with signaling pathways, but are no longer specific or cytotoxic on the long run *(10)*.

The slow and fast aggregation assays have been used to study the E-cadherin dependent cell–cell adhesion of human colonic and mammary cancer cells. In the case of the HCT-8 colon cancer cells mutations in the α-catenin gene can lead to altered expression of the protein. The functional repercussions of these mutations are loss of aggregation and acquisition of the invasive phenotype *(11)*. MCF-7/6 mammary carcinoma cells, however, possess a complete E-cadherin/ catenin complex that is yet not functional in cells in suspension: These cells poorly aggregate and are invasive *(12)*. Aggregation assays with MCF-7/6 cells have proven to be useful for the detection of aggregation-promoting agents, which are able to activate the complex. Examples of such agents, which also appear to possess an anti-invasive activity, are insulin-like growth factor-I *(5)*, retinoic acid *(12)*, tamoxifen *(13,14)*, and the citrus flavonoid tangeretin *(15)*. In general, we believe that the use of aggregation assays to detect agents that can maintain or restore the functional integrity of the E-cadherin/catenin complex in epithelioid cells offers a new strategy in the search for possible anti-invasive molecules.

2. Materials
2.1. Slow Aggregation Assay

1. Ringer's salt solution: Dissolve in 900 mL of distilled water: 8.6 g of NaCl, 330 mg of $CaCl_2 \cdot 2H_2O$, 300 mg of KCl; adjust pH to 7.4 with NaOH and add distilled water to make 1 L. Sterilize by filtration and store at 4°C. All filtrations are done with 0.22-μm filters.

2. Semi-solid agar medium: Dissolve 100 mg of Bacto-agar (Difco Laboratories, Detroit, MI, USA) in 15 mL of sterile Ringer's salt solution in a sterile 50-mL Erlenmeyer flask, and boil 3× during 10 s to sterilize the solution. Cool the solution to about 40–50°C and pour immediately into a 96-well microtiter plate as indicated in **Subheading 3.1.** Take care when boiling the first time: The solution may boil over (this usually does not happen the second and third time). Fifteen milliliters is sufficient to fill three 96-well microtiter plates. Do not fill the outer wells.

3. Culture medium appropriate for the cells used.

4. Moscona solution: Dissolve in 900 mL of distilled water: 8.0 g of NaCl, 0.3 g of KCl, 0.05 g of $Na_2HPO_4 \cdot H_2O$, 0.025 g of KH_2PO_4, 1.0 g of $NaHCO_3$, 2.0 g of D(+)-glucose (dextrose); adjust the pH to 7.0–7.4 with normal HCl and add distilled water to make 1 L. Sterilize by filtration. Store at –20°C.

5. Calcium- and magnesium-free Hank's balanced salt solution (CMF-HBSS): Dissolve in 900 mL of distilled water: 8 g of NaCl, 0.4 g of KCl, 0.06 g of KH_2PO_4, 0.35 g of $NaHCO_3$, 0.112 g of $Na_2HPO_4 \cdot 12H_2O$; adjust pH to 7.4 with 2 M NaOH and add distilled water to make 1 L. Sterilize by filtration and store at 4°C.

6. Trypsin–EDTA solution (e.g., Gibco BRL, Paisley, Scotland) consisting of 0.5 g of trypsin and 0.2 g of ethylenediaminetetraacetic acid tetrasodium salt (Na_4EDTA) per liter of CMF-HBSS. Store at –20°C.

7. Laminar air flow cabinet in which all procedures should be carried out.

8. Sterile Erlenmeyer flask (50 mL).

9. Sterile microtiter 96-well plate (Nunc, Roskilde, Denmark).

10. Bürker hemocytometer.

11. Sterile tips (10–1000 µL) and pipetors.

12. Sterile glass Pasteur pipets.

13. Air-passing tape (Micropore®, 3M Health Care, St. Paul, MN).

2.2. Fast Aggregation Assay

1. Dulbecco's phosphate buffered saline (PBS^D): Dissolve in 900 mL of distilled water: 8 g of NaCl, 0.2 g of KCl, 0.2 g of KH_2PO_4, 1.15 g of Na_2HPO_4; adjust pH to 7.4 with 2 M NaOH and add distilled water to make 1 L. Sterilize by filtration and store at 4°C.

2. Calcium- and magnesium-free Hank's balanced salt solution (CMF-HBSS): Dissolve in 900 mL of distilled water: 8 g of NaCl, 0.4 g of KCl, 0.06 g of KH_2PO_4, 0.35 g of $NaHCO_3$, 0.112 g of $Na_2HPO_4 \cdot 12H_2O$; adjust pH to 7.4 with 2 M NaOH and add distilled water to make 1 L. Sterilize by filtration and store at 4°C.

3. CMF-HBSS with glucose: Dissolve 1 g of D(+)-glucose (dextrose) per liter of CMF-HBSS. Prepare prior to use.

4. Isoton® II solution (Coulter Euro Diagnostics, Krefeld, Germany) consisting of 7.9 g of NaCl, 1.9 g of Na_2HPO_4, 0.4 g of Na_4EDTA, 0.4 g of KCl, 0.2 g of NaH_2PO_4 and 0.3 g of NaF per liter of distilled water; pH = 7.4. Store at room temperature.

5. 1 mM $CaCl_2$ stock solution: Dissolve 11 mg of $CaCl_2$ in 100 mL of CMF-HBSS. Sterilize by filtration and store at 4°C.

6. Collagenase solution: Dissolve 0.1 U/mL of *Clostridium histolyticum* Collagenase A (Boehringer Mannheim, Mannheim, Germany) in PBS^D. Sterilize by filtration, aliquot per 3 mL, and store at –20°C. Use within 6 mo after preparation.

7. Trypsin–EDTA solution (Gibco BRL, Paisley, Scotland) consisting of 0.5 g of trypsin and 0.2 g of Na_4EDTA per liter of CMF-HBSS. Store at –20°C.

8. Collagenase–Ca^{2+} (0.04 mM Ca^{2+}; *see* **Note 1**) solution (100 mL): Take 10 U of *Clostridium histolyticum* Collagenase A. Add 4 mL of a 1 mM $CaCl_2$ stock solution, and add CMF-HBSS with glucose to make 100 mL. Sterilize by filtration, aliquot per 3 mL and store at –20°C. Use within 6 mo after preparation.

9. Trypsin–Ca^{2+} (0.04 mM Ca^{2+}, *see* **Note 1**) solution (100 mL): Take 10 mg of bovine pancreas trypsin type I (Sigma, St. Louis, MN). Add 4 mL of 1 mM $CaCl_2$ stock solution, and add CMF-HBSS with glucose to make 100 mL. Sterilize by filtration, aliquot per 3 mL, and store at –20°C. Once dissolved trypsin may lose 75% of its potency within 3 h at room temperature. Use within 6 mo after preparation.

10. Trypsin inhibitor solution: Dissolve 0.1 g of soybean trypsin inhibitor type II-S (Sigma) in 100 mL of CMF-HBSS with glucose. Sterilize by filtration, aliquot per 1 mL, and store at –20°C. Use within 6 mo after preparation.

11. Aggregation–Ca^{2+} (1.25 mM Ca^{2+}, *see* **Note 1**) buffer: Dissolve in 100 mL of CMF-HBSS with glucose: 100 mg of bovine serum albumin (BSA) fraction V (Sigma), 0.26 g 4-(2-hydroxyethyl)-1-piperazineethanesulfonic acid (HEPES), 10 mg of deoxyribonuclease (DNase) I (Sigma), and 13.75 mg of $CaCl_2$. Sterilize by filtration, aliquot per 1.5 mL and store at –20°C. Prior to storage (and use) check Ca^{2+} concentration (should be approx 1.25 mM ± 0.2) and osmolality (approx 290 mOsm). Any deviation from the target Ca^{2+} concentration higher than 0.2 mM may affect the reproducibility of the assay. Use within 6 mo after preparation.

12. Glutaraldehyde 2.5% w/v fixation solution: Add 10 mL of a 25% w/v glutaraldehyde solution (e.g., Janssen Chimica, Geel, Belgium) to 90 mL of Isoton® II solution. Store at 4°C and do not use longer than 1 mo. Glutaraldehyde is irritating to respiratory system, skin and eyes. Do not breathe fumes or spray and avoid contact with eyes.

13. BSA coating solution: Dissolve 10 mg of BSA per milliliter of CMF-HBSS. Sterilize by filtration. Heat at 75°C for 30 min. Cool the suspension to room temperature.

14. Cell culture medium appropriate for the cells used.

15. Laminar air flow cabinet in which at least the detachment of cells in E-cadherin degenerating conditions should be carried out. If necessary, the other manipulations can be done at an ordinary bench. Always use sterile solutions and material to avoid bacterial or fungal interference.

16. Sterile tips (10–5000 µL) and pipetors.

17. Glass Pasteur pipets.

18. Pipets with a volume of 2–3 mL and with an inner tip diameter of at least 3 mm. Pasteur pipets from which the fine end is broken off and the opposite end is used to aspirate are appropriate for this purpose.

19. Plastic or glass tubes of 10–15 mL.

20. BSA-coated 24-well plates: Incubate the 24-well plate (Nunc) with BSA coating solution (1 mL per well) at room temperature for 1 h. Rinse the wells 3× with PBS^D. Leave 1 mL of PBS^D in every well after the last washing. Seal the plate (put it back in its package) and store at 4°C up to 2 mo. Dried plates should be discarded. The BSA coating solution may be recycled, stored at 4°C, and reused a couple of times, up to 6 mo.
21. Particle Size Counter with a sizing range between 0.4 and 1500–2000 μm, for example, Coulter LS 200 (Coulter Company, Miami, FL).
22. Gyrotory shaker (e.g., New Brunswick Scientific Co., New Brunswick, NJ).

3. Methods
3.1. Slow Aggregation Assay

1. Transfer 50 μL of the agar solution (40–50°C) into each well of a 96-well microtiter plate. Seal the plate (e.g., with its package) and place at 4°C on a horizontal surface for about 1 h to have the agar solidified (*see* **Note 2**). Prepare plates fresh prior to use.
2. Detach the cells to be tested by standard trypsinization procedures. For a 25-cm^2 cell culture flask, first wash the cell culture twice with 3 mL of Moscona solution. Then add 3 mL of trypsin–EDTA solution, and incubate at 37°C for 10–15 min. Further, add 5 mL of culture medium with FBS to inhibit the enzymatic activity of trypsin, suspend well, and count the cell number with a Bürker hemocytometer. Prepare a suspension of 200,000 cells/mL (*see* **Note 3**). Take care to work with a single-cell suspension: Check under the microscope (*see* **Note 4**).
3. Add 100 μL of cell suspension (20,000 cells) to the agar-coated wells (*see* **Note 4**).
4. Add 100 μL of medium containing the products to be tested (in a twofold concentration). So the end volume is 200 μL.
5. Seal the plate with air-passing tape and incubate at 37°C in a humidified atmosphere with 5% or 10% CO_2 in air (depending on the culture medium) for 24 h (*see* **Note 5**).
6. Evaluate the aggregation under an inverted microscope. An objective ×4 will usually be sufficient (*see* **Note 6**). Several situations are possible. The most common ones are presented in **Fig. 1**: formation of large compact aggregates (*see* **Fig. 1A**), formation of small, loose aggregates (*see* **Fig. 1B**), and absence of aggregate formation (*see* **Fig. 1C**).

3.2. Fast Aggregation Assay

This assay consists of three main steps: First, cells are detached in E-cadherin degenerating conditions (*see* **Subheading 3.2.1.**) to obtain a cell culture that can, in the second step (*see* **Subheading 3.2.2.**), be detached in E-cadherin saving conditions and yield a single-cell suspension (*see* **Note 7**). Finally, the aggregation procedure itself is carried out (*see* **Subheading 3.2.3.**).

3.2.1. Detachment of Cells in E-Cadherin Degenerating Conditions

1. Prepare as many confluent 75-cm^2 flasks of cells as required: one confluent flask yields enough cells to perform two or three experiments.

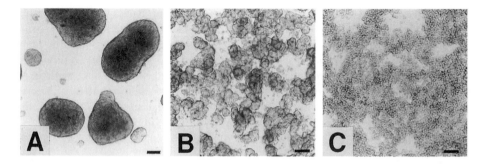

Fig. 1. (**A**) Large compact aggregates of MCF-7/AZ cells. (**B**) Small, loose aggregates of MCF-7/6 cells. (**C**) Solitary MCF-7/AZ cells, as a result of treatment with anti-E-cadherin antibody MB2. Photomicrographs were taken on an inverted microscope without phase contrast ring, after 24 h of incubation. All scale bars = 100 μm.

2. Wash the cells 3× with CMF-HBSS at 4°C.
3. Incubate the cells at 37°C in 3 mL of collagenase solution for 30 min.
4. Aspirate and remove the collagenase solution. If too many cells already detached after this procedure, keep the collagenase solution after aspiration, centrifuge at 200–250g, remove the collagenase solution, add some culture medium, and keep those cells.
5. Add 3 mL of trypsin–EDTA solution to the monolayer for a few seconds.
6. Aspirate and remove the trypsin–EDTA solution. Take care if too many cells detach. If this happens, proceed as in **step 4**, but add some calcium and serum-containing medium to block the trypsin before centrifugation.
7. Incubate the cells at 37°C for 15 min.
8. Suspend the cells in 15 mL of medium with serum.
9. Transfer the cells into a new 75-cm^2 cell culture flask. If necessary, add the recuperated cells from the collagenase or trypsin–EDTA treatment. Incubate the cells at 37°C in a humidified atmosphere with 5% or 10% CO_2 in air (depending on the culture medium) for 24 h to allow regeneration of E-cadherin at the cell surface. Afterwards, continue with the E-cadherin saving detachment procedure (*see* **Subheading 3.2.2.**).

3.2.2. Detachment of Cells in E-Cadherin Saving Conditions

1. Wash the cells 3× with CMF-HBSS at 4°C.
2. Incubate the cells at 37°C in 3 mL of collagenase–Ca^{2+} solution for 30 min.
3. Aspirate and remove the collagenase solution. If too many cells already detached after this procedure, keep the collagenase solution after aspiration, centrifuge at 200–250g, remove the collagenase solution, and add the cells to the flask again.
4. Incubate the cells at 37°C in 3 mL of trypsin–Ca^{2+} solution for 15 min.
5. Suspend the cells and add 1 mL of trypsin inhibitor solution (*see* **Note 8**).

6. Suspend the cells thoroughly (e.g., with a Pasteur pipet or with a 5-mL tip) to obtain a single-cell suspension. Divide this suspension equally in as many tubes as conditions to be tested. Do not try to test more than three conditions per 75-cm^2 cell culture flask.
7. Centrifuge the cells at 200–250g for 5 min. After this step, the cells may be kept as a pellet at 4°C for 4–6 h.

3.2.3. Aggregation Procedure

1. Add the products (e.g., anti-E-cadherin antibody to check the E-cadherin specificity of the aggregation; *see* **Note 9**) to the bottles with 1.5 mL of aggregation–Ca^{2+} buffer. Cool these bottles to 4°C.
2. Take the centrifuged cells and remove the supernatant (containing trypsin and trypsin inhibitor solution) from the cell pellet. Immediately add the precooled aggregation–Ca^{2+} buffer (supplemented with antibodies or other products as desired; *see also* **Note 1**) to the pellet and resuspend well. Incubate the cells at 4°C for 30 min. Shake the tubes every 5–10 min.
3. In the meantime, bring 1 mL of glutaraldehyde solution 2.5% in 10-mL vials for measuring the aggregation at time 0 min. Prepare as many vials as conditions to be tested (*see* **Note 10**). Remove the PBS^D from the BSA-coated 24-well plate. Two wells are needed for every condition. Now immediately proceed with **step 4** to avoid drying up of the wells.
4. Suspend the cell suspension very well. For every condition, transfer twice 400 μL of cell suspension to a BSA-coated well and once 400 μL to a 10-mL vial containing 1 mL of the 2.5% glutaraldehyde solution. Fix for at least 10 min.
5. Incubate the well-plate at 37°C on a Gyrotory shaker at 85 rpm for 30 min.
6. Fix the aggregates by adding *very carefully* 1 mL of glutaraldehyde solution 2.5% to every well. Squirt gently along the wall of the wells. Do not mix with a fine tip or Pasteur pipet, but with a tip with a broad opening (*see* **Subheading 2.2., item 18**). Fix for at least 10 min without agitation.

3.2.4. Explant Assay

1. Take two droplets of the remaining aggregation solution with the cells and transfer to a 24-well plate.
2. Add 1 mL of culture medium.
3. Check for attachment on the substratum after 2 h and for outgrowth and doubling after 24 h (*see* **Note 11**).

3.2.5. Measuring Procedure

1. Check the off-set of the laser and align laser and detectors of the particle size counter. Most machines will do this automatically (*see* **Note 12**).
2. Fill the sample module with Isoton®. Use a background measurement time of 60 s. Try to keep the background detector flux below 1500×10^3 lm (*see* **Note 12**). Load the sample to an obscuration of about 10%. Avoid deviations in obscuration between the samples higher than 2%. Use a sample measurement time of 60 s.
3. Start by measuring all samples fixed at time 0 min.

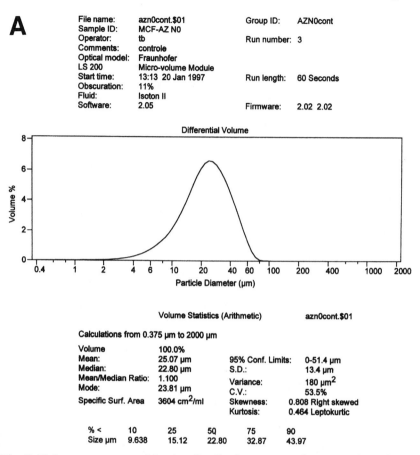

A

File name:	azn0cont.$01	Group ID:	AZN0cont
Sample ID:	MCF-AZ N0		
Operator:	tb	Run number:	3
Comments:	controle		
Optical model:	Fraunhofer		
LS 200	Micro-volume Module		
Start time:	13:13 20 Jan 1997	Run length:	60 Seconds
Obscuration:	11%		
Fluid:	Isoton II		
Software:	2.05	Firmware:	2.02 2.02

Differential Volume

Volume Statistics (Arithmetic)   azn0cont.$01

Calculations from 0.375 µm to 2000 µm

Volume	100.0%		
Mean:	25.07 µm	95% Conf. Limits:	0-51.4 µm
Median:	22.80 µm	S.D.:	13.4 µm
Mean/Median Ratio:	1.100	Variance:	180 µm²
Mode:	23.81 µm	C.V.:	53.5%
Specific Surf. Area	3604 cm²/ml	Skewness:	0.808 Right skewed
		Kurtosis:	0.464 Leptokurtic

% <	10	25	50	75	90
Size µm	9.638	15.12	22.80	32.87	43.97

Fig. 2. Volume percent particle size distribution curves of a suspension of MCF-7/AZ cells. (**A**) At time 0 min, together with its descriptive statistics.

4. For measuring the samples after 30-min aggregation, combine the contents of both wells and measure (*see* **Note 13**). Use tips or pipets as described in **Subheading 2.2., item 18**.

5. The calculations yield the volume distribution curve as a function of the particle diameter, together with its descriptive statistics (mean, median, standard deviation, skewness and curtosis) (*see* **Fig. 2A**).

6. Use the overlay function to compare different curves graphically (*see* **Fig. 2B**).

7. Use Kolmogorov–Smirnov statistics to analyze differences between cumulative distribution curves statistically (*see* **Fig. 2B**).

4. Notes

1. The Ca^{2+}concentrations in collagenase, trypsin, and aggregation buffer have been experimentally determined on two types of cell lines (MCF-7 and MDCK). The

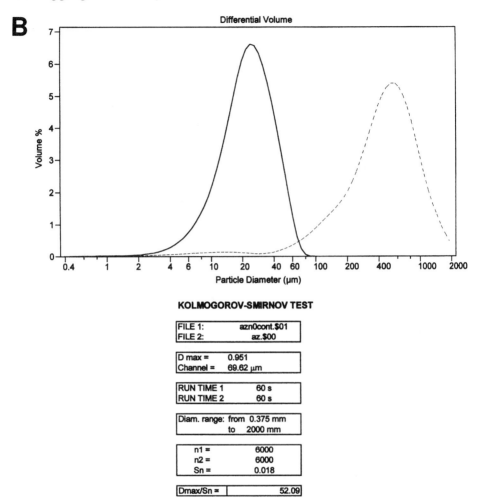

Fig. 2. *(continued)* **(B)** At time 0 min (solid line) compared with the curve at 30 min (dashed line), together with Kolmogorov–Smirnov statistics.

concentrations proposed in this chapter are the result of seeking a compromise between being able to detach the cells and allow aggregation. Although those concentrations could be used for all cell lines tested until now in the laboratory, it may be necessary to adapt them for other cell lines.

2. When covering the bottom of the wells with the agar solution, take care to cover the surface completely and equally. Avoid formation of air bubbles as they will make evaluation of the result under the microscope impossible. When transferring the agar solution into the first well, aspirate 60 µL and fill the wells with 50 µL; otherwise use a dispenser throughout. Respect the indicated temperature of 40–50°C of the agar solution when filling the wells. At higher temperatures, the well plate may

be damaged, which will lead to decreased optical clarity. At lower temperatures, the agar will solidify too early. The solidification process should take place on a perfectly horizontal surface. Otherwise, the cells may clump together in the thinnest region of the well during incubation.

3. The serum concentration is not important for the test itself, but may be important for the experimental conditions. Experiments with, for example, IGF-I should be carried out in 1% serum to reduce binding of the IGF-I by IGF-binding proteins from the serum.

4. Obtaining a single-cell suspension is essential, because the presence of preexisting cell clusters may interfere with the evaluation of aggregation. Because the result is usually evaluated after 24 h, no special detachment procedures to protect E-cadherin are necessary, in contrast to the fast aggregation assay (the turnover of E-cadherin is about 4–6 h). When transferring the cell suspension into the wells, cover the whole surface and avoid any air bubbles (*see also* **Note 2**).

5. Make sure the plate is placed in an incubator with perfectly horizontal shelves. The cells should be allowed to aggregate under static conditions and without any vibrations (e.g., caused by a centrifuge in the same room). Incubation for more than 24 h can be carried out and may give additional information about long-term effects. Always take care of drying up of the wells, even when working in a humidified atmosphere. If one knows on beforehand that a long-term incubation will be used, it may help to increase the volume of supernatant fluid.

6. An objective ×4 on an inverted phase-contrast equipped microscope is usually sufficient to score the results. Removing the phase-contrast ring may improve the quality of photographs made of the cultures.

7. The detachment procedure is the keystone of the assay. It is essential to obtain a single-cell suspension without altering cell–cell adhesion characteristics in general and E-cadherin in particular. However, not all cell lines can be treated in the same way. It will often be required to seek a compromise between an aggressive detachment procedure (which will yield a perfect single-cell suspension but may damage the cells and their E-cadherin) and a more smooth one (which will do less harm to the cells but will result in a suboptimal single-cell suspension). So the procedure may need to be adapted to every cell line. In cells that can be easily brought into a single-cell suspension by means of collagenase–Ca^{2+} and trypsin–Ca^{2+} alone (e.g., MCF-7 cells), the E-cadherin degenerating procedure (*see* **Subheading 3.2.1.**) may be omitted. With cell lines that strongly adhere to their substratum, the entire procedure should be followed carefully. However, one should not exceed the indicated incubation periods. If the cells are still adhering after the whole procedure, mechanical scraping and suspending 10–15× in a Pasteur pipet or a 5-mL tip with a pipetor should be carried out. This technique can also be used for cells that for some reason must not be treated by any enzymatic procedure. Overtreatment may occur when treating the cells longer than 30 min or keeping detached cells in the collagenase solution. The incubation periods indicated are maximum ones: Once the cells appear to be well detached the incubation can be stopped. Avoid suspending the cells too vigorously: This

will result in many dead cells. They will not only be unable to adhere, but will release their DNA which will, because of its high viscosity, result in nonspecific clumping of the cells. If vigorous suspending cannot be avoided, increase the DNase concentration in the aggregation buffer.

8. After addition of trypsin inhibitor and centrifugation, the cells should form a pellet in the tube. When cells are still floating above the pellet, not all trypsin has been blocked and this will result in loss of cells during aspiration. For the ongoing experiment, add 1 mL more of trypsin inhibitor, resuspend, and centrifuge the cells again. If the problem persists, it is advisable not to use those cells and restart the experiment with fresh trypsin inhibitor.

9. If anti-E-cadherin antibodies have to bind to the cells during the preincubation period, the suspension should by no means be allowed to reach temperatures above 4°C, to prevent internalization. When preparing the tubes, it may be advisable to put them at 4°C, especially when many samples are to be analyzed. When working with kinase or phosphatase inhibitors it may be necessary to preincubate at 37°C prior to aggregation. To avoid clumping and to allow the antibody to reach all cells, regularly (every 5–10 min) shake the tubes or hit them gently against a table.

10. Especially when starting to perform this assay, do not try to test too many conditions. Even in experienced hands, it may be rather difficult to handle more than 12 experimental conditions at a time and to respect the 30-min aggregation time.

11. The explant assay will sometimes explain "strange" results. As mentioned earlier, the presence of DNA may result in clumping of the cells, which will be measured as aggregates by the particle size counter. Inspection of the aggregates prior to measurement will readily reveal this: One just sees a clump of material in which the individual cells cannot be delineated. Moreover, antibodies against E-cadherin are unable to prevent the clump formation. After 2 h, this material will keep floating around and after 24 h no attached cells and much debris will be found. When this happens, the results of the particle size counting are irrelevant, and the experiment has to be repeated.

12. Correct settings of the particle size counter are essential to obtain reliable results and to allow comparison between different experimental conditions. The manufacturer should provide standardized control material (e.g., latex particles of a certain diameter) to allow periodic control of the instrument. Correct alignment of the laser and the detectors (usually automatically integrated in the instrument) and careful cleaning of the measuring module are prerequisites to obtain reasonably low background measurements. When background measurements are too high (i.e., flux $>1500 \times 10^3$ lm), the results are unreliable. To solve this problem, start by cleaning the module, for example, with an eyeglass detergent. Also clean the outside of the module since salt depositions or fingerprints will obscure the laser beam. A scratched module should be replaced, although it is not cheap: Be careful when handling the module! Also check if the Isoton® II buffer is not contaminated with microorganisms or dust. Sometimes realignment will help to reduce background measurements. Make sure the measurement module cannot move in its holder. Finally, wipe dust from the lenses from time to time according to the manufacturer's instructions.

13. In case of aggregating cells, always combine the contents of both BSA-coated wells. Given the same number of cells, the obscuration caused by a small number of large aggregates is relatively lower than that caused by a large number of small aggregates. When the obscuration is too low, the Fraunhofer calculations will fail owing to shortage of information, and despite obvious aggregation, the instrument will give curves indicating a very small particle size. One or more very sharp-edged peaks are most of the time also a sign of too few particles. Extra peaks may have several reasons. First of all there may really be two populations in the suspension: aggregating and nonaggregating cells. However, a second peak in, for example, the 1 μm region does not indicate cells, but usually indicates the presence of small noncellular particles, for example, vesicles originating from too vigorous manipulations or other foreign material. Finally, even after fixation some aggregation may take place. All measurements should be carried out within 2–3 h after fixation.

References

1. Mareel, M. M., Bracke, M. E., Van Roy, F. M., and de Baetselier, P. (1997) Molecular mechanisms of cancer invasion, in *Encyclopedia of Cancer*, Vol. II (Bertino, J. R., ed.), Academic Press, San Diego, pp. 1072–1083.
2. Bracke, M. E., Van Roy, F. M., and Mareel, M. M. (1996) The E-cadherin/catenin complex in invasion and metastasis, in *Attempts to Understand Metastasis Formation I* (Günthert, U. and Birchmeier, W., eds.), Springer-Verlag, Berlin, pp. 123–161.
3. Ozawa, M., Ringwald, M., and Kemler, R. (1990) Uvomorulin-catenin complex formation is regulated by a specific domain in the cytoplasmic region of the cell adhesion molecule. *Proc. Natl. Acad. Sci. USA* **87,** 4246–4250.
4. Mareel, M., Berx, G., Van Roy, F., and Bracke, M. (1996) The cadherin/catenin complex: a target for antiinvasive therapy? *J. Cell. Biochem.* **61,** 524–530.
5. Bracke, M. E., Vyncke, B. M., Bruyneel, E. A., Vermeulen, S. J., De Bruyne, G. K., Van Larebeke, N. A., et al. (1993) Insulin-like growth factor I activates the invasion suppressor function of E-cadherin in MCF-7 human mammary carcinoma cells in vitro. *Br. J. Cancer* **68,** 282–289.
6. Noë, V., Willems, J., Vandekerckhove, J., van Roy, F., Bruyneel, E., and Mareel, M. (1999) Inhibition of adhesion and induction of epithelial cell invasion by HAV-containing E-cadherin-specific peptides. *J. Cell Sci.* **112,** 127–135.
7. Kadmon, G., Korvitz, A., Altevogt, P., and Schachner, M. (1990) The neural cell adhesion molecule N-CAM enhances L1-dependent cell-cell interactions. *J. Cell Biol.* **110,** 193–208.
8. Beuthan, J., Minet, O., Helfmann, J., Herrig, M., and Muller, G. (1996) The spatial variation of the refractive index in biological cells. *Phys. Med. Biol.* **41,** 369–382.
9. Young, I. T. (1977) Proof without prejudice: use of the Kolmogorov-Smirnov test for the analysis of histograms from flow systems and other sources. *J Histochem. Cytochem.* **25,** 935–941.
10. Vermeulen, S. J., Bruyneel, E. A., Van Roy, F. M., Mareel, M. M., and Bracke, M. E. (1995) Activation of the E-cadherin/catenin complex in human MCF-7 breast cancer cells by all-trans-retinoic acid. *Br. J. Cancer* **72,** 1447–1453.

11. Vermeulen, S. J., Nollet, F., Teugels, E., Vennekens, K. M., Malfait, F., Philippé, J., et al. (1998) The αE-catenin gene (*CTNNA1*) acts as an invasion-suppressor gene in human colon cancer cells. *Oncogene* **18,** 905–915.

12. Bracke, M. E., Van Larebeke, N. A., Vyncke, B. M., and Mareel, M. M. (1991) Retinoic acid modulates both invasion and plasma membrane ruffling of MCF-7 human mammary carcinoma cells in vitro. *Br. J. Cancer* **63,** 867–872.

13. Bracke, M. E., Charlier, C., Bruyneel, E. A., Labit, C., Mareel, M.M., and Castronovo, V. (1994) Tamoxifen restores the E-cadherin function in human breast cancer MCF-7/6 cells and suppresses their invasive phenotype. *Cancer Res.* **54,** 4607–4609.

14. Charlier, C., Bruyneel, E., Lechanteur, C., Bracke, M., Mareel, M., Gielen, J., and Castronovo, V. (1996) Calcium pump modulators alter the effects of tamoxifen on E-cadherin function in human breast cancer cells. *Eur. J. Pharmacol.* **317,** 413–416.

15. Bracke, M. E., Bruyneel, E. A., Vermeulen, S. J., Vennekens, K., Van Marck, V., and Mareel, M. M. (1994) Citrus flavonoid effect on tumor invasion and metastasis. *Food Technol.* **48,** 121–124.

5

Cell Migration and the Boyden Chamber

Nicholas S. Brown and Roy Bicknell

1. Introduction

Tumors usually reach secondary sites via blood vessels or lymphatic vessels. Two processes dependent upon cell migration speed metastasis by reducing the distance between the primary tumor and these vessels. The first process is invasion, in which cancer cells migrate toward the capillaries. The second is angiogenesis, blood vessel growth into the primary tumor, which has been proved to promote blood-borne tumor spread by reducing the invasive distance, and may also aid lymphatic metastasis. Angiogenesis is dependent on endothelial cell migration. When studying the spread of tumors to secondary sites, it is therefore important to understand: (1) the response of tumor cell lines to motility boosting factors and (2) endothelial cell chemotaxis in response to tumor-derived angiogenic factors.

In the Boyden chamber an upper and a lower set of wells are separated by a cell-permeable membrane. Solutions of potential chemoattractants are added to the base wells, and a cell suspension is placed in the top wells. The number of cells that have passed through the membrane and into the bottom wells quantifies the strengths of the chemoattractants for that particular cell line.

The Boyden chamber was originally used to study the migration of inflammatory cells, which are nonadherent in vitro. Inflammatory cell migration is quantified by aspirating the medium from the bottom wells and determining the number of migrated cells using a spectrophotometer or hemocytometer. Unfortunately, using the Boyden chamber is simpler for the immunologist than for the oncologist. Whereas inflammatory cells float in vitro, endothelial and carcinoma cells sink and adhere to the base of any container. This forces us to make two changes to the simple Boyden assay. First, adherent cell migration requires the cell-permeable membrane to be coated with basement membrane components before the chamber is assembled. Second, after they have migrated

From: *Methods in Molecular Medicine, vol. 58:*
Metastasis Research Protocols, Vol. 2: Cell Behavior In Vitro and In Vivo
Edited by: S. A. Brooks and U. Schumacher © Humana Press Inc., Totowa, NJ

from the top to the bottom wells, adherent cells remain attached to the underside of the cell permeable membrane (**Fig. 1**). Migration therefore cannot be quantified by aspirating the medium from the base wells and measuring the concentration of the cell suspension. Instead, the cells fixed to the underside of the membrane must be stained, then counted using a microscope and eyepiece graticule.

2. Materials
2.1. Cell Culture Solutions

1. Migration medium: Dulbecco's Modified Eagle Medium containing 4.36 g/L of 4-(2-hydroxyethyl)-l-piperazineethanesulfonic acid (HEPES) buffer and 0.01% bovine serum albumin (BSA) or 0.1% fetal calf serum (FCS; *see* **Note 1**).
2. Trypsin solution: Phosphate-buffered saline (PBS) solution A (calcium- and magnesium-free) containing 20 mg/mL trypsin and 1 mM EDTA.
3. Neutralizing solution: Dulbecco's Modified Eagle Medium containing 4.36 g/L of HEPES buffer and 15% newborn bovine serum.

2.2. Basement Membrane Solutions

1. Collagen solution: 0.5 M acetic acid containing 100 µg/mL of collagen type IV. Solubilize 10 mg of collagen type IV powder in 5 mL of 0.5 M acetic acid, to give 2 mg/mL. Place 1 mL of this suspension in 19 mL of 0.5 M acetic acid to give 100 µg/mL of collagen type IV.
2. Fibronectin solution: PBS solution A containing 10 µg/mL of fibronectin.

2.3. Cell Fixing and Staining Solutions

1. 100% Methanol.
2. Eosin G in phosphate buffer, pH 6.6.
3. Thiazine dye in phosphate buffer, pH 6.6.
   These may be obtained from Dade International. Web address: http://www.dadebehring.com/.
4. Resin fixative (optional).

2.4. Cells

1. A 14-cm tissue culture dish must be grown to >70% confluence to yield an adequate number of cells.

2.5. Hardware

1. Migration assay specific hardware: This may be obtained from NeuroProbe Inc., 16008 Industrial Dr., Gaithersburg, MD 20877, USA. Tel: 301-417-0014. E-mail: neuroprobe@compuserve.com. Website: http://www.neuroprobe.com.
   48-well Boyden chemotaxis chamber.
   25 mm × 80 mm polyvinylpyrrolidone-free polycarbonate membranes with 8 µM or 12-µm diameter pores (*see* **Note 1**).
   Rubber scraper for removing cells from the shiny side of the membrane.

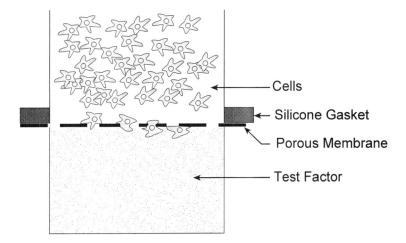

Fig. 1. Adherent cell migration in the Boyden chamber. This is one well in cross-section. The Boyden apparatus consists of 48 such wells (8 groups of 6 wells). The top and bottom halves of the chamber are separated by the silicone gasket. After migrating through the cell-permeable membrane, adherent cells do not go into suspension in the bottom wells. Instead, they remain attached to the underside of the membrane (courtesy of Rangana Choudhuri).

2. Other hardware:
   Microscope with a ×200 objective and a 10×10 grid eyepiece graticule.
   A tissue culture incubator set at 37°C and 5% or 10% carbon dioxide.
   Two pairs of forceps, timer, P200 and P1000 pipets, bulldog clip, clamp and stand, hemocytometer, and a counting device.
3. Consumables:
   30-mL plastic tubes, plastic Petri dishes, glass slides, and coverslips.

3. Methods

Time considerations: Growing an adequate number of cells will take a few days. **Steps 1–12** require between 90 min and 2 h. The cells then migrate for 4 h. **Step 17** provides a degree of flexibility—after the membrane has been removed from the chamber, it can be fixed in methanol for just 10 min, or for as long as overnight. Staining the membrane then takes 15 min. Counting the cells can be time consuming. If cells are counted in nine fields of view per treatment, it will take 20–30 min to quantify cell migration toward each treatment.

1. Identify the dull and the shiny sides of the cell-permeable membrane. They will look the same when wet, so permanently record which one is which by nicking one corner of the membrane with clean scissors. Always handle the membrane with forceps—never touch it directly.

2. The membrane must now be coated with basement membrane components to allow adherent cell migration. Place the membrane in a clean plastic Petri dish. Bathe it in 1 mL of the collagen type IV solution for 10 min. Ensure that both sides of the membrane are evenly coated. Dry thoroughly by hanging the membrane from the bulldog clip.

3. Bathe the membrane in 1 mL of the fibronectin solution for 10 min. Again ensure that both sides of the membrane are evenly coated. Using the bulldog clip, hang the membrane to air-dry.

4. Wash the membrane thoroughly in 5 mL of migration medium to remove all traces of acetic acid. Hang to air-dry.

5. Prepare the chemoattractant and control solutions that will be placed in the bottom wells. These should always be based on the same migration medium as that used for the top well cell suspension. Migration medium alone in the base wells acts as the negative control. The positive control will vary with cell type; for example, 10 ng/mL of basic fibroblast growth factor (bFGF) in migration medium stimulates migration in endothelial cell lines, while 10 ng/mL of insulin-like growth factor (IGF-1) in migration medium should be used for some carcinoma cell lines.

6. Disassemble the Boyden chamber. Unscrew the six silver thumbnuts, remove the top half of the chamber, then remove the silicone gasket that separates the top and bottom halves of the chamber. Using a P200 pipet, place 28.5 μL of chemoattractant or control solution into each base well. The solution should form a positive meniscus that protrudes from the base well. The wells are arranged in groups of six—one group may be used for each treatment. Remember to record which solution was placed in which set of wells.

7. Using two pairs of forceps, lay the membrane *rough side down* over the filled base wells. If the correct volume has been added to the base wells, the chemoattractant solutions they contain will contact the membrane without overflowing. Be careful not to drag the membrane across the base wells, as this will cause the solutions to spill. Reassemble the Boyden chamber, tighten the thumbnuts, and place it in the humidified 37°C incubator to equilibrate. Leaving the Boyden chamber in a low-humidity environment at this stage allows evaporation through the cell-permeable membrane. This may cause air bubbles to form in the base wells

8. Harvest the cells that are to be placed in the top wells. Incubate endothelial cells at 37°C for 8–10 min with 10 mL of trypsin solution (*see* **Notes 2** and **3**). Add the resulting cell suspension to 10 mL of neutralizing solution in a 30-mL plastic tube, and centrifuge for 4 min at 180*g*.

9. Dispose of the supernatant and resuspend the cell pellet in 20 mL of migration medium. Centrifuge again for 4 min at 180*g*. This washing step is essential—it ensures that the cell suspension placed in the top wells is completely serum free.

10. Dispose of the supernatant and resuspend the cell pellet in 5 mL of migration medium (*see* **Note 4**).

11. Estimate the cell concentration of this suspension using the hemocytometer. Adjust the volume of the suspension so that it contains 500,000 cells/mL. This cell concentration may be varied if previous experiments show too much, or too little, migration by a particular cell line.

12. Remove the Boyden apparatus from the 37°C incubator. Place 50 μL of the cell suspension into each of the top wells (*see* **Note 5**).

13. Return the Boyden chamber to the incubator for 4 h. Some cells will migrate to the underside of the membrane during this period.

14. Fill a small plastic Petri dish with 100% methanol and place in a refrigerator or cold room. Do this early in the 4-h period so that the methanol is cold by the end of the 4-h migration. Secure the rubber scraper in a vertical position with the stand and clamp.

15. Remove the Boyden apparatus from the incubator, unscrew the thumbnuts, and disassemble the chamber. The membrane will remain stuck to the silicone gasket. Use forceps to peel it off.

16. Using two pairs of forceps, thoroughly wipe the upper (shiny) surface of the membrane across the rubber scraper. This removes cells that have not actually migrated through the membrane. Take care not to scrape the lower (rough) side! Cells may also be removed from the upper side by stretching the membrane between the bulldog clip and a pair of forceps, then wiping it with a damp cloth.

17. Place the membrane in the Petri dish filled with ice-cold methanol. This fixes the cells adhering to the lower side. The membrane may be left in methanol for any length of time between 10 min and 24 h at 4°C.

18. During this period the Boyden apparatus should be cleaned. This must be done thoroughly to ensure that traces of chemoattractant do not remain in the base wells and affect future assays. A mild dishwashing liquid may be used to soak the chamber, but be sure to totally remove all traces of detergent afterwards. Thoroughly rinse with tap water, then the apparatus must then be rinsed twice with distilled water and dried. Never autoclave the Boyden chamber.

19. Stain the rough underside of the membrane for 3 min with eosin G (red) solution.

20. Remove the membrane from the eosin G solution. In a fresh Petri dish, stain the rough underside of the membrane for 3 min with thiazine (blue) solution.

21. Using tap water, rinse excess stain from the membrane, then hang to air-dry using a bulldog clip. Once dry, mount the membrane on a glass slide with a coverslip. Use of a resin fixative will give sharper cell definition under the microscope, but is not essential.

22. Count the number of cells in at least nine fields of view for each treatment (*see* **Note 6**). Use ×200 magnification and count only the cells within the 10 × 10 grid of the eyepiece graticule. The cells are the large pink/purple circles, while the black rings are pores in the membrane. High-quality color photomicrographs of two stained cell permeable membranes may be found at: http://bio.m.u-tokyo.ac.jp/WWW/Nature/Chemotaxis01.html. The picture on the right hand-side shows a membrane with a large number of stained cells adhering to it. The greater the number of cells fixed to the underside of the membrane, the more chemoattractive is the solution in the base well (*see* **Note 7**).

4. Notes

1. Some laboratories use migration medium containing 0.01% BSA, whereas others use migration medium containing 0.1% FCS. In most circumstances, both types of

migration medium should give good results, but in the event of repeated experiment failure, trying a change of migration medium type might be worthwhile. Similarly, variation of membrane pore size may be used to optimize an experiment. Both 8-μm and 12-μm diameter pores have been used to quantify endothelial cell migration, whereas 8 μm is more commonly used for tumor cell lines.

2. Cells do not migrate efficiently if they are incubated with trypsin–EDTA solution for an insufficient length of time. Trypsin lifts cells from their dish before separating them from each other. If the cells are still clumped together when placed in the upper wells they will be unable to migrate. One can check for cell clumping when using the hemocytometer (stage 11). If the cells are clumped together, brief agitation of the cell suspension with a vortex mixer should help to separate them.

3. Endothelial cell lines can quickly resynthesize adhesion molecules after trypsinization, whereas many carcinoma cell lines cannot. It is therefore acceptable to trypsinize endothelial cells before a migration assay, but cancer cells must not be—instead they should be removed from their culture dish with a 2 m*M* EDTA solution. This may take up to 20 min.

4. If one wishes to simply quantify cell migration toward a potential chemoattractant, all the cells should be suspended in pure migration medium, and this suspension should be added to all the top wells. If, however, one wishes to assess the effect of a second substance on the actions of a known chemoattractant, this modifier substance should be present in both the top and bottom wells (the chemoattractant should still be placed in the bottom wells only). This means that different top well sets will contain different cell suspensions. Care must be taken that the different top well cell suspensions contain the same cell concentration. One may incubate the cell suspension with the modifier substance before loading it into the chamber. If the incubation is lengthy, or the substance potentially cytotoxic, one may wish use trypan blue to test cell viability in the cell suspension left over after loading of the chamber.

5. It is, unfortunately, easy to introduce air bubbles into the top wells. To avoid this, the pipet tip must be close to the bottom of the well when the cell suspension is dispensed. Care should be taken, however, not to damage the membrane with the pipet tip. One should add cell suspension to the top wells in a random order, and frequently swirl the cell suspension during this period. This will prevent settling, helping to ensure that an equal number of cells are placed in each top well.

6. Of course, one may count more than nine fields of view for each treatment—this will give more accurate data. Counting cells manually, however, can be very time consuming. If a large number of assays are to be carried out, it may be worth automating cell counting. The majority of investigators using the Boyden assay determine the number of cells per field of view manually, although a spectrophotometer has been used to estimate the number of cells fixed to the underside of the Boyden membrane (*1*). Spectrophotometric and flourimetric determinations of cell numbers on the Boyden membrane are also discussed at: http://bio.m.u-tokyo.ac.jp/WWW/Manuals/manual56.html.

Migration assays other than the Boyden chamber allow greater automation when quantifying cell migration. The Dunn chamber allows video recording and computer analysis of cell movement *(2)*. In the phagokinetic track assay, a coverslip is coated with a monolayer of fine colloidal gold *(3)* or plastic beads *(4)*. Endothelial cells ingest these particles as they migrate and the bare tracks they leave may be computer analyzed. Cell migration under an agarose layer *(5)* is also amenable to computer analysis *(6)*. The most recently developed technique is the fluorescence-assisted transmigration, invasion and motility assay (FATIMA). The cells must be fluorescently labeled, either using lipophilic dyes or green fluorescent protein. Migration can then be quantified over as many as 24 time points. Using this system, the migration rate of a cell type labeled with a specific fluorochrome can even be measured within a mixed population of cells. More information about FATIMA can be found at http://www.tecan.com.

7. A chemotactic factor both increases cell migration and sets the direction of that migration. A substance that merely boosts cell migration in all directions is a chemokinetic factor, not a chemotactic factor. A factor chemokinetic for a carcinoma cell line will boost invasion, but efficient angiogenic factors may need to be endothelial cell chemotactic, and not just endothelial cell chemokinetic. Both chemotactic and chemokinetic factors will increase cell migration in a Boyden assay. A technique known as checkerboard analysis is required to prove that a substance is chemotactic, and not just chemokinetic. This involves placing the test chemoattractant not only in the base wells, but also in the top, cell containing, wells. A chemokinetic substance will increase cell migration when equal concentrations are present in both the top and base wells. A true chemotactic factor, however, will boost cell migration only if its concentration is higher in the base than in the top wells. A protocol for checkerboard analysis is provided in **ref. 7**.

If one merely wishes to prove that a factor is chemokinetic, one may also quantify the response using a repair assay, where a linear wound is created in a cell monolayer *(8)*. Chemokinetic factors speed cell migration and therefore speed repair of the wound.

Acknowledgments

The authors express special thanks to the laboratory of Marina Ziche, University of Florence, Italy, for valuable general advice about the Boyden chamber, and also to Hellmut Augustin, University of Gottingen Medical School, Germany, for helpful information about endothelial cell migration.

References

1. Grotendorst, G. (1987) Spectrophotometric assay for the quantitation of cell migration in the Boyden chamber chemotaxis assay. *Methods Enzymol.* **147,** 144–152.
2. Zicha, D., Dunn, G. A., and Brown, A. F. (1991) A new direct-viewing chemotaxis chamber. *J. Cell Sci.* **99,** 769–775.
3. Zetter, B. R. (1980) Migration of capillary endothelial cells is stimulated by tumor-derived factors. *Nature* **285,** 41–43.
4. Obeso, J. L. and Auerbach, R. (1984) A new microtechnique for quantitating cell movement in vitro using polystyrene bead monolayers. *J. Immunol. Methods* **70,** 141–152.

5. Orr, W. and Ward, P. A. (1978) Quantitation of leukotaxis in agarose by three different methods. *J. Immunol. Methods* **20,** 95–107.
6. Coates, T. D., Harman, J. T., and McGuire, W. A. (1985) A microcomputer-based program for video analysis of chemotaxis under agarose. *Comput. Methods Prog. Biomed.* **21,** 195–202.
7. Castellot, J. J. Jr., Karnovsky M. J., and Spiegelman, B. M. (1982) Differentiation-dependent stimulation of neovascularization and endothelial cell chemotaxis by 3T3 adipocytes. *Proc. Natl. Acad. Sci. USA* **79,** 5597–5601.
8. Lauder H., Frost, H. E., Hiley, C. R., and Fan, T.-P. D. (1998) Quantification of the repair process involved in the repair of a cell monolayer using an in vitro model of mechanical injury. *Angiogenesis* **2,** 67–80.

6

Quantification of Cell Motility

Gold Colloidal Phagokinetic Track Assay and Wound Healing Assay

Yasufumi Niinaka, Arayo Haga, and Avraham Raz

1. Introduction

Cellular migration is an integral aspect in response to extracellular stimuli, which is fundamental to numerous biological processes such as embryogenesis, inflammation, wound healing, tissue regeneration, and tumor invasion and metastasis *(1,2)*. Abundant studies centered on the identification and characterization of factors that regulate and direct cell movement have shown that host serum components and extracellular matrix breakdown products exert a chemotactic effect on various tumor cells *(3)* and that basement membrane and extracellular matrix components promote cellular haptotaxis *(4)*. Furthermore, host growth factors influence recipient cells by modulating growth and motility independently or in a coordinated manner *(2)*. Moreover, cellular migration in vitro has been reported to be correlated with tumor invasion and metastasis in vivo. A group of motility factors has been described, the primary function of which is thought to be the regulation of cellular kinesis. Motility factors have been originally distinguished by their ability to induce the random (chemokinetic) and directional (chemotactic) migration of the cells *(5)*. Therefore, quantitating the cell motility is one of the most important clues to comprehend the cellular characteristics of malignancy and/or the effect and activities of motility inducing properties. Gold colloidal method was invented to measure the random motility (chemokinesis) by Albrecht-Buehler, in which area of phagokinetic track cleared by a single cell is measured *(6)*. The Boyden chamber method, described in Chapter 5 by Brown and Bicknell, was invented to quantitate the directional motility (chemotaxis) and was modified in various ways to

From: *Methods in Molecular Medicine, vol. 58:*
Metastasis Research Protocols, Vol. 2: Cell Behavior In Vitro and In Vivo
Edited by: S. A. Brooks and U. Schumacher © Humana Press Inc., Totowa, NJ

characterize cell–extracellular matrix (ECM) interaction and invasion, in which cells migrating through a pore are counted, and this method can be applied to quantitate chemotaxis also *(7)*. Directional motility is generally classified into two categories: chemotaxis induced by soluble chemoattractant(s) and hapotaxis induced by insoluble chemoattractant(s). Wound healing assay has a unique concept, which can directly reflect the cell–cell and cell–ECM contact involving cellular migration *(8)*. In this method, the direct effect of antibody against ECM or receptors can be monitored visually *(8)*.

2. Materials
2.1. Phagokinetic Track Assay

This is the basic method to comprehend the chemokinesis of cells and/or chemoattractant. Some cells secrete the motility factor(s) that stimulate the locomotion of their own cells. In this case, no chemoattractant is necessary to induce cell motility. This method is based on the idea that the motile cell shows kinesis with phagocytosis on the uniform carpet of gold particles, in which the track of the single migrated cell is observed as an area cleared by the cell *(6)* (**Fig. 1**).

2.1.1. Apparatus
1. Sterilized flat-bottomed flask (Erlenmeyer flask).
2. Needle nose forceps.
3. 35-mm Culture dish or 6-well culture plate.
4. 22×22 mm or 18×18 mm coverglass (surface needs to be clean).
5. Whatman paper or paper towel.
6. Sterilized 10-mL glass pipet (*see* **Note 1**).
7. Hair dryer.

2.1.2. Solutions
1. 0.25% Trypsin, 0.025% EDTA (*see* **Note 2**).
2. 1% Bovine serum albumin (BSA) (solution A) that has been prepared in double-distilled water (ddH$_2$O) and filter sterilized.
3. 14.5 mM AuCl$_4$H solution (solution B): Crystallized AuCl$_4$H (hydrogen tetrachloroaurate hydrate) is available from Aldrich Chemical Co. (cat. no. 25,416-9). Carefully weigh and minimize the time because this crystal is water-absorbent. Dissolve in ddH$_2$O (*see* **Notes 3** and **4**), then store in a brown bottle at 4°C.
4. 36.5 mM Na$_2$Co$_3$ solution (solution C): Dissolve in ddH$_2$O, then store at 4°C.
5. 0.1% Formaldehyde solution (solution D) in ddH$_2$O.
6. 100% Ethanol.
7. 2.5% Glutaraldehyde in phosphate-buffered saline (PBS).

2.2. Wound Healing Assay

Cellular locomotion is a phenomenon resulting from multistep migratory mechanisms. Among them, cell–cell and cell–ECM contacts are known to

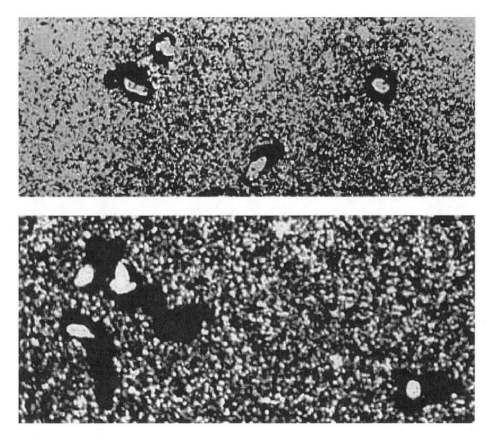

Fig. 1. Phagokinetic track assay. Cells were seeded on golden colloidal carpet and cultured with or without AMF.

affect cell motility. The phagokinetic track assay described previously, and the Boyden chamber assay described in Chapter 5 by Brown and Bicknell can rarely reflect the effect of cell–cell contact. However, wound healing assay can visualize the horizontal cellular movement caused in relation to cell–cell and cell–ECM contacts *(8)* (**Fig. 2**).

2.2.1. Apparatus

1. 24-Well plate.
2. Diamond point pen or sharply pointed pen.

2.2.2. Solutions

1. 5 μm/mL ECM component protein such as fibronectin in PBS.
2. 2.5% Glutaraldehyde in PBS.

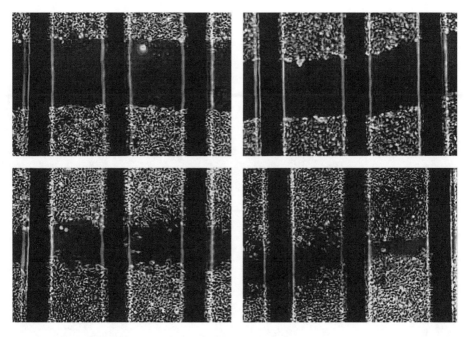

Fig. 2. Wound healing assay. Wounded cell monolayer with or without AMF were observed immediately after wounding and after 12 h.

3. Methods
3.1. Phagokinetic Track Assay
3.1.1. Preparation of Coverglass in a Hood

1. Hold coverglass with needle nose forceps and dip coverglass in solution A (*see* **Note 5**).
2. Remove excess liquid from coverglass by touching edge to Whatman paper.
3. Dip the coverglass into 100% ethanol briefly.
4. Rapidly dry the coverglass with a hot air hair dryer (*see* **Note 6**).
5. Place coverglass in 35-mm culture plate or 6-well plate.

3.1.2. Preparation of Gold Colloid

1. Mix the following solutions in the order described in a 920-mL Erlenmeyer flask (for 10 pieces of coverglass):

ddH$_2$O	11 mL
Solution C	6 mL
Solution B	1.8 mL

2. Heat the mixture on a weak flame immediately after the addition of solution B (*see* **Note 7**).
3. Immediately after the boiling point is reached, remove the flask from the flame, and add 1.8 mL of solution D, and mix well (*see* **Note 8**).

4. Layer 2 mL of the still hot (80–90°C) gold particle suspension on top of the coverglass.
5. After 45 min, wash the coverglass 3× with PBS.
6. Transfer the coverglass into another dish (well) containing 2 mL of medium.

3.1.3. Assay

1. Place 1×10^3–5×10^3 freshly trypsinized cells on the center of the coverglass and swirl gently (*see* **Notes 9** and **10**).
2. Incubate at 37°C for 24 h.
3. Fix the cells with 2.5% glutaraldehyde for 15 min and keep moist with PBS.
4. Photograph under phase-contrast microscopy.
5. Scan the photograph and measure the area of phagokinetic track cleared by a single cell using NIH-Image software (*see* **Notes 11** and **12**).

3.2. Wound Healing Assay

1. Incubate wells with 300 μL of 5 μg/mL of ECM component protein at room temperature for 1 h, or at 4°C overnight.
2. Wash with PBS 2×.
3. Make three parallel lines using diamond point pen on the back of the plate.
4. Prepare cell suspension at 2.5×10^5 cells/mL in culture medium (*see* **Notes 9** and **13**).
5. Place 400 μL of a cell suspension (1×10^5 cells/well) and swirl once (*see* **Note 14**).
6. Incubate at 37°C for 4–10 h until cell attachment.
7. Make a cell scrape in a straight line vertical to the three parallel lines using a pipet tip.
8. Remove the medium with floating cells carefully (*see* **Note 15**).
9. Add 400 μL of prewarmed culture medium with or without reagents (*see* **Note 13**).
10. Photograph under phase-contrast ×200.
11. Incubate at 37°C until closure of the line.
12. Photograph under phase-contrast ×200.
13. Fix the cells with 2.5% glutaraldehyde and keep moist in PBS.
14. Calculate the ratio of distance (*see* **Note 16**).

4. Notes

1. Sterilized plastic is acceptable, but a glass pipet is preferable.
2. Some cells are difficult to detach from the plate, in this case EDTA enables you to minimize the time.
3. Use bottles from which detergent has been completely removed.
4. Color will change to yellowish.
5. ECM can be used instead of BSA *(9)*.
6. Alternatively, burn the coverglass , and wait for 1 min for it to cool down.
7. Yellowish color will diminish as the temperature goes up to the boiling point.
8. Color will change to purplish brown. Be careful of this color in transmitted light. Purplish represents the formation of small gold particles, and dark brown the formation of large gold particles. The size of the gold formed in this method seems to be dependent on the length of boiling.

9. We routinely use cells that have reached 70–80% confluency because cell viability is a very important factor.

10. Make sure that the cells are completely dissociated from one another. Do not seed too many cells because overlap of the phagokinetic track cannot be measured. The phagokinetic track has to be cleared by a single cell.

11. NIH-Image software can be downloaded from the website (http://rsb.info.nih.gov/ij/).

12. Boyden chamber assay (*see* Chapter 5 by Brown and Bicknell) can also be used for chemotaxis, although phagokinesis track assay was invented to estimate random motility by Albrecht-Buehler. However, as shown in **Fig. 1**, motile response in phagokinetic assay has been observed to be more sensitive than the Boyden chamber.

13. Some cells need the addition of 0.1% BSA, but not all.

14. Some cells need to be recovered in normal culture medium at least 30 min prior to this application.

15. Cells are easy to detach from the well at this point.

16. At least three distances should be measured along three lines.

Acknowledgment

This work is supported by NIH Grant RO1-CA51714.

References

1. Erickson, C. A. (1990) Cell migration in the embryo and adult organism. *Curr. Opin. Cell Biol.* **2,** 67–74.

2. Stoker, M. and Gherardi, E. (1991) Regulation of cell movement: the motogernic cytokines. *Biochem. Biophys. Acta* **1072,** 81–102.

3. Erdel, M., Speiss, E., Trifz, G., Boxberger, H-J., and Ebert, W. (1992) Cell interactions and motility in human lung tumor cell lines HS-24 and SB-3 under the influence of extracellular matrix comonents and protease inhibitors. *Anticancer Res.* **12,** 349–360.

4. McCarthy, J. B. and Furcht, L. T. (1984) Laminin and fibronectin promote the haptotactic migration of B16 mouse melanoma cells in vitro. *J. Cell Biol.* **98,** 1474–1480.

5. Liotta, L. A., Mandler, R., Murano, G., Katz, D. A., Gordon, R. K., Chiang, P. K., and Schiffman, E. (1986) Tumor cell autocrine factor. *Proc. Natl. Acad. Sci. USA* **83,** 3302–3306.

6. Albrecht-Buehler, G. (1977) The phagokinetic tracks of 3T3 cells. *Cell* **11,** 359–404.

7. Albini, A., Iwamoto, Y., Kleinman, H. K., Matrin, G., Aaronson, S. A., Kozlowski, J. M., and McEwan, R. N. (1987) A rapid in vitro assay for quantitating the invasive potential of tumor cells. *Cancer Res.* **47,** 3239–3245.

8. Simon, L., Goodman, H., Vollmers, P., and Birchmeier, W. (1985) Control of cell locomotion: perturbation with an antibody directed against specific glycoproteins. *Cell* **41,** 1029–1038.

7

In Vitro Invasion Assay Using Matrigel®

Debbie M. S. Hall and Susan A. Brooks

1. Introduction

Basement membranes are specialized extracellular matrices that are comprised of several biological components including collagens, laminins, and proteoglycans. They form thin continuous sheetlike structures that separate epithelial tissues from the adjacent connective tissue stroma; thus, they form barriers, which block the passage of cells and other macromolecules. The basement membranes become permeable during tissue development, repair, and at sites of inflammation, to allow immune cells to reach the site *(1)*.

Tumor invasion of basement membranes is thought to be one of the crucial steps in the complex multistep event that leads to the successful formation of a metastasis. Tumor cells initially cross basement membranes as they begin to invade the lymphatics or vascular beds during their dissemination, and also when they penetrate into the target organ tissue, where they will eventually colonize to form secondary tumors. The penetration of the tumor cells into the basement membranes is thought to involve a series of interdependent events. These include the initial attachment (adhesion) of the cancer cells to components/receptors within the basement membrane *(2)*; degradation of the basement membranes, probably through the action of proteolytic enzymes *(2–4)*; and finally the migration of the tumor cells into the target organ tissue in response to specific chemotactic stimuli *(5,6)*.

To assess the invasive ability of tumor cells in vitro a large variety of systems have been developed that permit the assessment of their capacity to invade through basement membranes. Several of these assays utilize basement membrane extracts from tissues such as amnion *(7)*, chick chorioallantoic membranes *(8)*, lens capsule *(9)*, and bladder wall *(10)*. However, reproducibility of results using these substrata is often very difficult owing to the inherent

From: *Methods in Molecular Medicine, vol. 58:*
Metastasis Research Protocols, Vol. 2: Cell Behavior In Vitro and In Vivo
Edited by: S. A. Brooks and U. Schumacher © Humana Press Inc., Totowa, NJ

heterogeneity of the tissue preparation. Moreover, the process of extracting these substrata from the tissues is often a long and technically difficult process. To overcome these drawbacks, reconstituted, and hence more homogeneous, extracellular matrices have been developed as alternative substrata to investigate invasion in vitro.

One such example is Matrigel—a solubilized basement membrane preparation extracted from the Engelbreth–Holm–Swarm mouse sarcoma *(11)*, a tumor rich in extracellular matrix proteins. It mainly comprises laminin, collagen IV, heparan sulfate proteoglycans, entactin, and nidogen, all components of basement membranes.

Matrigel is relatively simple to handle in the laboratory in comparison to the substrata described previously. It can be dried and then reconstituted onto membranes with 8-μm pores. These Matrigel-coated membranes act as barriers to tumor cell invasion and subsequent migration through the pores in the membranes.

The invasion assay described in this chapter measures the ability of cells to attach to the matrix, invade into and through the matrix, and to migrate toward a chemoattractant. These interdependent steps are evidently crucial during the metastatic cascade.

The simple design of this assay permits easy experimental manipulation when compared to other systems such as the Boyden chamber assay described in Chapter 5 by Brown and Bicknell, and the slightly more sophisticated, and complex, version of the Matrigel assay described in Chapter 8 by Hendrix et al. Moreover, there is no need to buy any expensive (a Boyden chamber costs ~ £1000[$1600]) or specialized pieces of equipment.

The assay described in this chapter is carried out under sterile conditions, therefore allowing cells to be recovered and used for subsequent studies. This could prove difficult if tissue-extracted basement membranes were used.

Ultimately, this assay enables the researcher to screen inhibitors, which may alter the invasive phenotype of the tumor cells, thus contributing to current knowledge of the molecular events occurring during the invasive process.

Before commencing any detailed research using this assay, it is first of all important to carry out empirical studies to optimize the conditions under which the experiments will be performed. These initial studies should be carried out to determine the optimal concentration of Matrigel suitable for use in the experiments. If the concentration used is too low then it will not provide a realistic and significant enough barrier to differentiate between invasive and noninvasive cells. Conversely, if the Matrigel used is too highly concentrated, then it will be very difficult for even very invasive cells to penetrate the barrier that it provides. We suggest trying several dilutions of the Matrigel solution.

It is equally important that the experimenter determines the optimum quantity of cells for use in each of the assays. This is likely to be different for each of the cell lines assessed. Using too many cells will result in "clumping," and this will obviously give erroneous results. We suggest trying several different cell concentrations.

This part of the work takes some time, however, once completed, the assays can be done relatively quickly and can be adapted according to the researchers' needs.

2. Materials

2.1. Preparation of the Matrigel Chambers

1. Falcon multiwell companion plates (available as 6-, 12-, or 24-well).
2. Falcon cell culture inserts with 8-μm pores (also available in 6-, 12-, or 24-well format).
3. Matrigel® matrix solution (Collaborative Biomedical Products, Becton and Dickinson Labware, Bedford, UK). Stable for at least 9 mo when stored at –20°C.
4. Sterile 7-mL screw capped vials.
5. Sterile pipet tips.
6. Standard cell culture medium (e.g., Dulbecco's minimum essential medium [DMEM]) without fetal calf serum.
7. Pair of sterile forceps.

2.2. Preparation of the Cells

1. Cell lines to be analyzed (*see* **Note 1**).
2. Standard cell culture medium without fetal calf serum.
3. Phosphate-buffered saline (PBS) solution: Dissolve 8 g of sodium chloride, 0.2 g of potassium chloride, 1.44 g of sodium phosphate (bi-basic), and 0.24 g of potassium phosphate in 800 mL of distilled water. Adjust the pH to 7.2 and then adjust the volume to 1 L with distilled water. Dispense into convenient volumes and sterilize by autoclaving. Store at room temperature.
4. Ethylenediamine tetraacetic acid (EDTA) solution: Add 0.1 g of ethylenediamine tetraacetic acid disodium salt to 500 mL of PBS (*see* **step 3**). Add sodium hydroxide to adjust the pH to 8.0 and to allow the EDTA to dissolve. Dispense into convenient volumes and sterilize by autoclaving. Store at room temperature.
5. 0.05% w/v Trypsin–0.02% (w/v) EDTA solution (available from Sigma or other suitable tissue culture supplier).
6. Standard cell culture medium with 10% v/v heat-inactivated fetal calf serum.
7. Sterile 15-mL centrifuge tubes.
8. Standard cell culture medium with 0.1% w/v sterile filtered bovine serum albumin (fraction V).
9. Hemocytometer.
10. Trypan blue solution: 0.25% w/v trypan blue in PBS, filter sterilized. Stable at room temperature for several years.

2.3. Coomassie Blue Staining to Check the Matrigel Coating

1. Coomassie brilliant blue solution: Dissolve 0.25 g of Coomassie brilliant blue R-250 in a solution of 50 mL of methanol, 10 mL of acetic acid and 40 mL of distilled water. Filter sterilize.
2. Destain solution: Place 5 mL of methanol and 7.5 mL of acetic acid in 80 mL of distilled water. Filter sterilize.

2.4. Matrigel Invasion Assay

1. Standard cell culture medium with 10% v/v fetal calf serum.
2. Fixative: 4% v/v formol saline solution: Dissolve 4.25 g of sodium chloride in 500 mL of a 4% v/v formaldehyde solution in distilled water. Alternatively, use ice-cold 100% methanol.
3. 6-, 12-, or 24-well multiwell plates or companion plates (need not be sterile).
4. Sterile cotton swabs.
5. Standard cell culture medium without fetal calf serum.
6. Pair of sterile forceps.
7. Trypsin–EDTA solution (as in **Subheading 2.2., step 5**).
8. Mayer's hematoxylin solution.
9. 1% w/v Aqueous eosin solution.
10. 70% v/v Ethanol or industrial methylated spirit in distilled water.
11. 100% Ethanol or industrial methylated spirit.
12. Xylene.
13. Scalpel (no. 11 blade recommended).
14. Pair of forceps (need not be sterile).
15. Microscope slides and coverslips.
16. Depex mounting medium (xylene-based).
17. 10×10 Eyepiece graticule.

3. Methods

3.1. Preparation of the Matrigel Chambers

1. Defrost the unopened Matrigel solution for at least 6 h on ice in the refrigerator. We recommend overnight as this is more convenient (*see* **Note 2**).
2. Precool all plates, inserts, sterile pipets and 7-mL screw capped vials in the refrigerator overnight (*see* **Note 3**). **Note:** Unless otherwise indicated, all following procedures should be conducted under sterile conditions.
3. Shake the bottle to thoroughly mix the Matrigel solution. Dilute the defrosted Matrigel into a variety of concentrations for use in the empirical studies as discussed in the Introduction. Start with concentrations of 1.2 mg/mL, 0.6 mg/mL, and 0.3 mg/mL, diluted in cell culture medium without fetal calf serum. Pipet 5-mL aliquots into bijou's, refreeze, and store those not to be used immediately, at –20°C. When defrosting for later experiments this should be performed as described previously in **Subheading 3.1., step 1**.

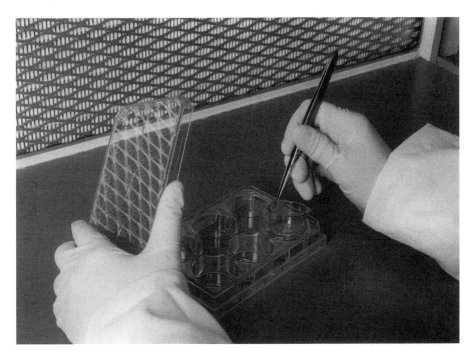

Fig. 1. An insert is placed into the housing of a companion plate using sterile forceps.

4. Using sterile forceps, remove the precooled inserts from their packaging and carefully place into the housing on the precooled companion plates (as illustrated in **Fig. 1**).
5. In a laminar flow hood (at room temperature), carefully pipet the diluted Matrigel solution on top of the insert and gently rotate the insert to ensure the entire filter is coated (for 6-well format use 300 µL; for 12-well use 100 µL, and for 24-well use 40 µL). Very carefully overlay the Matrigel with sterile double-distilled water (for 6-well format use 200 µL; for 12-well use 100 µL, and for 24-well use 50 µL) using a sterile pipet. This stage should be done in at least triplicate.
6. Control inserts should also be prepared. These are simply inserts without the Matrigel layer. To prepare these, simply place the empty inserts into the companion plate and leave in the laminar flow hood alongside the inserts that are being prepared with Matrigel. Follow all other relevant steps.
7. Leave the Matrigel layer to air-dry (in the laminar flow hood at room temperature under occasional UV light). This stage usually takes approx 1–2 d.
8. Rehydrate the dried Matrigel layer by adding warm (37°C) cell culture medium without fetal calf serum (for 6-well format, use 600 µL; for 12-well, use 200 µL, and for 24-well, use 75 µL) to the plates. Allow the Matrigel layer to rehydrate for approx 2 h in the cell culture incubator (*see* **Note 4**). Place the control inserts in the cell culture incubator with these.

3.2. Preparation of the Cells

1. Wash the cell monolayers. Pipet on cell culture medium without fetal calf serum, gently rock the flask from side to side so that the entire cell monolayer is covered. Discard the spent medium. Repeat 3×.
2. Obtain a single-cell suspension by first washing the cell monolayer with sterile PBS (4 mL for 75-cm^2 flask, 2 mL for 25-cm^2 flask). Pipet this over the monolayer and then aspirate. Next, incubate the cells with EDTA solution (volumes as PBS) for approx 10 min in the laminar flow hood. After this time, aspirate the EDTA and pipet on the trypsin–EDTA solution (2.5 mL for a 75-cm^2 flask and 1 mL for a 25-cm^2 flask). Tighten the cap on the flask and gently swirl the solution over the surface of the cells. Place the flask of cells into the cell culture incubator. After approx 30 s to 1 min, pipet off any excess solution and monitor the progress of the cells under an inverted microscope (*see* **Note 5**). Knock the flask sharply to loosen the cells from the bottom. As soon as the majority of the cells are detached from the bottom of the flask stop the action of the trypsin by the addition of cell culture medium with 10% v/v fetal calf serum (5 mL in a 75-cm^2 flask and 2 mL in a 25-cm^2 flask). Transfer the contents of the flask into a 15-mL sterile centrifuge tube and centrifuge the cells at 1100*g* for 5 min. Pipet off the medium without disturbing the cell pellet. Gently tap the centrifuge tube against the bench to loosen the cell pellet and resuspend in 5 mL of cell culture medium without fetal calf serum. Repeat twice more. The cell pellet should be resuspended in a final volume of 2.5 mL cell culture medium with 0.1% w/v bovine serum albumin.
3. Count the cell suspension using a hemocytometer (*see* **Note 6**).
4. Assess cell viability using trypan blue. Trypan blue is excluded from living cells but stains dead/damaged cells blue.

    Mix 50 µL of trypan blue solution with 50 µL of cell suspension. Transfer the mixture to a hemocytometer and observe under the microscope. The total number of viable cells can be calculated directly as follows:

$$\frac{\text{total number of viable cells}}{\text{number of squares counted}} \times 2 \times 10^4 = \text{number of viable cells/mL}$$

    Only cell suspensions that are ≥95% viable should be used in the assays.
5. Dilute the cells in culture medium with 0.1% w/v bovine serum albumin to the concentration to be used in the assays. For the empirical studies, as discussed in the Introduction, try using concentrations of between 1×10^5 and 5×10^5 cells/mL.

3.3. Coomassie Blue Stain to Check the Matrigel Coating

1. After rehydration of the Matrigel layer, carefully pipet off and discard any excess medium without disturbing the Matrigel matrix on the membrane.
2. Check the homogeneity of the Matrigel layer by using a general protein stain such as Coomassie brilliant blue. Pipet the Coomassie solution (2 mL for the 6-well; 1 mL for the 12-well, and 0.25 mL for the 24-well) onto the Matrigel layer and leave for 15 min. Analyze the stained Matrigel layer both by eye and under an inverted microscope (*see* **Note 7**). The staining should be homogeneous. Any patchy staining inserts should be discarded.

3. Before using any stained inserts in subsequent steps they must first of all be destained. Pipet the destain solution onto the stained Matrigel layer (volumes as per **step 2**), gently agitate for approx 30 s to 1 min, and discard the spent destain. Repeat until the destain solution remains clear.

3.4. The Matrigel Invasion Assay

1. In the bottom well of the chamber (below the filter), add cell culture medium with 10% fetal calf serum (*see* **Notes 8** and **9**).
2. Gently pipet the counted cell suspensions (2 mL in the 6-well format, 1 mL in the 12-well format, and 0.25 mL in the 24-well format) on top of the Matrigel matrix or onto the control insert (*see* **Notes 10** and **11**).
3. Incubate the invasion chambers in a tissue culture incubator for several timescales. For example, use timescales of 12, 24, 36, and 72 h (*see* **Note 12**).
4. Approximately 5 min before the end of the incubation period, add either ice-cold methanol or 4% v/v formol saline to the wells of a clean companion plate or multiwell plate (3 mL per well for a 6-well plate; 2 mL for a 12-well plate, and 1 mL for a 24-well plate)—need not be sterile. Place in the refrigerator until required.
5. After the required incubation time, remove any noninvading cells from the upper surface of the membrane by "scrubbing" with a sterile cotton swab (this process will not damage the invaded cells). Use gentle but firm pressure while moving the tip of the swab over the top surface of the membrane (*see* **Note 13**).
6. Discard the used swab and repeat **step 5** using a clean swab, prewetted in cell culture medium without fetal calf serum (*see* **Note 13**).
7. Wash the upper surface of the inserts by pipetting on and then aspirating two or three changes of cell culture medium without fetal calf serum.
8. If the invaded cells are to be recovered for use in subsequent experiments then, after removing the noninvaded cells, as described in **steps 5–7**, place the insert (using sterile forceps) into a clean, sterile companion plate containing trypsin–EDTA solution (500 μL for a 6-well plate, 200 μL for a 12-well plate, and 80 μL for a 24-well plate). Place the plate in the cell culture incubator for 2–3 min, by which time the majority of the cells should have detached from the surface of the membrane and will be floating in the trypsin–EDTA solution. Transfer the cells to a 25-cm^2 flask containing 5 mL of standard cell culture medium and grow the cells under standard procedures (*see* **Note 14**).
9. If the cells are to be fixed and stained for quantitative analysis, then remove the washed insert from the companion plate using forceps (need not be sterile) and fix by placing each insert into a well of the preprepared plate containing ice-cold methanol or 4% v/v formol saline. Fix the cells on the inserts for 30 min in the refrigerator.
10. Stain the cells on the membrane by immersing the insert in companion or multiwell plates which contain Mayer's hematoxylin solution (3 mL for 6-well plates, 2 mL for 12-well plates, and 1 mL for 24-well plates) for 3 min.
11. "Blue" in tap water by removing the insert from the hematoxylin and transferring to a plate containing tap water (*see* **Note 15**). Agitate the plate gently and then change the water for fresh tap water. Leave for 5 min.

12. Briefly (approx 30 s) immerse the inserts in 1% w/v aqueous eosin solution and give a quick rinse by holding the insert with forceps and dipping in and out of a dish of tap water (*see* **Note 16**).

13. Dehydrate by transferring the insert to 70%, then two changes of 100% ethanol solution, dipping in and out of the solution during each immersion to ensure equilibration.

14. Clear by transferring the insert to xylene and dipping in and out of the solvent.

15. Cut the membrane out of the insert housing using a scalpel. Insert the blade through the membrane at the edge adjacent to the housing wall. Rotate the housing against the stationary blade. Leave a very small point of attachment.

16. Using forceps, gently peel the membrane from the remaining point of attachment on the insert. Place it lower side down onto a microscope slide on which a small drop of Depex has been placed. Place a second, very small drop of Depex on top of the membrane and put a coverslip on top of it. Apply gentle pressure to expel air bubbles.

17. The simplest method of quantifying invasion is to observe and count the stained invaded cells at 100× magnification using a 10 × 10 eyepiece graticule (*see* **Note 17**). The cells are pink/purple in appearance and the pores in the membrane are small dark circles (illustrated in **Fig. 2**).

18. To calculate percent invasion the following equation should be used:

$$\frac{\text{mean number of cells invading through the membrane}}{\text{mean number of cells migrating through the control membrane}} \times 100$$

4. Notes

1. It is important that all cells are in the mid-log phase of growth when they are used in the assays. Carry out standard growth curves for all cell lines before carrying out the assays to establish at which point the cells should be harvested and used.

2. Matrigel will polymerize very quickly at temperatures between 20°C and 35°C. Be especially careful if storing it in the refrigerator as continuous opening and closing of the door can increase the temperature enough for the Matrigel to polymerize. We recommend that when it is defrosted, this should be carried out on ice, in a polystyrene ice bucket (with the lid on), in the refrigerator. This removes the likelihood of accidental polymerization.

   If the Matrigel does polymerize in the bottle, place on ice in the refrigerator for 24–48 h and it may depolymerize. If it does not, discard it, it cannot be used in the assays.

3. Take care to cool all companion plates, pipets, etc., in the refrigerator to avoid polymerization of the Matrigel on contact.

4. Some people advise constant rotation while rehydrating the Matrigel layer. We tend not to as we have found that it causes the solution to concentrate to the center of the membrane. Try with and without rotation and see which one works best for you.

5. Take care not to overdigest with trypsin as this can damage the cells and, in particular, can damage surface components on the cells, which may in turn affect the outcome of your experiments.

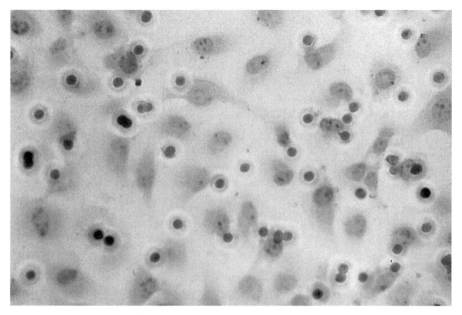

Fig. 2. Lower surface of a membrane with 8-μm pores showing cells that have invaded.

   Cells will take varying lengths of time to detach from the bottom of the flask (although it should not take longer than 3 min), keep monitoring every 30 s or so to check progress.

6. At this stage, it is easy to see whether the cells are in single-cell suspensions or not. It is very important that the cells are used in the assays are in single-cell suspensions as clumps of cells will not be able to migrate through the pores in the membrane. If this proves difficult then briefly vortex-mix the tube of cells.

7. It is not necessary to stain all the membranes. The idea of this stage is to check whether there is a homogeneous spread of the Matrigel on the membrane. If there is not, refer to **Note 4**, which may provide an answer.

8. There should be no air between the insert and the medium. If there is, then take the insert out of its housing using sterile forceps and replace it gently at an angle to expel the air.

9. The fetal calf serum acts as a source of chemoattractants.

10. To obtain reproducible results it is very important that the cell numbers in each of the wells are equal. Pipet the cells into the wells as quickly as possible, making sure that the cell suspension is well mixed between each pipetting. Do not use a multipipet as the cells will settle as they are pipetted. This will result in different numbers of cells in each of the wells.

11. If you wish to assess the involvement of specific structures on invasive ability, preincubate the cells with the relevant antibody against the structure in question for approx 15 min before adding the cell suspension to the Matrigel assay. Take care to ensure that the cells are in a single-cell suspension and that viability is still within the acceptable range for the assays.

12. You are looking for a suitable timescale where there is an obvious distinction between invasive and noninvasive cells.
13. This stage should be carried out quickly to avoid the cells drying out.
14. This process will normally give rise to a more invasive phenotype, so do not assume the cells to be of the same phenotype as they were originally.
15. Mayer's hematoxylin will change from a red to a blue/purple color on exposure to mildly alkaline conditions. In most areas, the tap water is adequately alkaline for this process to occur. If it does not, then it is likely that the tap water in your area is not sufficiently alkaline. Try using tap or distilled water with a few drops of sodium hydroxide added.
16. Since eosin is water soluble, a very brief rinse in water will suffice. If rinsed for too long the eosin stain will be washed away.
17. Count the cells in several fields, randomly chosen. It is also a good idea to ask someone else to carry out a count as well as you. This is to ensure that the results are of an objective nature.

References

1. Flug, M. and Kupf-Maier, P. (1995) The basement membrane and its involvement in carcinoma cell invasion. *Acta Anatomica* **152,** 69–84.
2. Duffy, M. J. (1996) The biochemistry of metastasis. *Adv. Clin. Chem.* **32,** 135–160.
3. Price, J. T., Bonovich, M. T., and Kohn, E. C. (1997) The biochemistry of cancer dissemination. *Crit. Rev. Biochem. Mol. Biol.* **32,** 175–253.
4. Blood, C. H. and Zetter, B. R. (1990) Tumor interactions with the vasculature: angiogenesis and tumor metastasis. *Biochim. Biophys. Acta* **1032,** 89–118.
5. Volk, T., Geiger, B., and Raz, A. (1984) Motility and adhesive properties of high and low metastatic neoplastic cells. *Cancer Res.* **44,** 811–824.
6. Hujanen, E. S. and Terranova, V. P. (1985) Migration of tumor cells to organ-derived chemoattractants. *Cancer Res.* **45,** 3517–3521.
7. Liotta, L. A., Lee, C. W., and Morakis, D. J. (1980) A new method for preparing large surfaces of intact human basement membrane for tumor invasion studies. *Cancer Lett.* **11,** 141–152.
8. Armstrong, P. B., Quigley, J. P., and Sidebottom, E. (1982) Transepithelial invasion and intramesenchymal infiltration of the chick embryo chorioallantoic by tumor cell lines. *Cancer Res.* **42,** 1826–1837.
9. Starkey, J. R., Hosick, H. L., Stanford, D. R., and Liggitt, H. D. (1984) Interaction of metastatic tumor cells with bovine lens capsule membrane. *Cancer Res.* **44,** 1585–1594.
10. Poste, G. and Fidler, I. J. (1980) The pathogenesis of cancer metastasis. *Nature (Lond.)* **283,** 139–146.
11. Kleinman, H. K., McGarvey, M. L., Liotta, L. A., Robey, P. G., Tryggvason, K., and Martin, G. R. (1982) Isolation and characterization of type IV procollagen, laminin and heparan sulfate proteoglycans from the EHS sarcoma. *Biochemistry* **21,** 6188–6193.

8

Membrane Invasion Culture System

Mary J. C. Hendrix, Elisabeth A. Seftor, and Richard E. B. Seftor

1. Introduction

Metastasis is the major cause of morbidity and death for cancer patients. A critical challenge to clinical and basic scientists is the development of improved prognostic methods to predict the metastatic aggressiveness of a patient's individual tumor and especially to control local invasion—a key step in the metastatic cascade. Before effective therapeutic regimens can be planned, we must invest more effort in understanding the pathogenesis of tumor cell dissemination in order to identify better targets for clinical intervention.

Recent advances in the field of tumor cell biology have focused on the intricate interactions between tumor cells and cellular as well as extracellular matrix barriers. A three-step hypothesis describing the sequence of biochemical events during tumor cell invasion, a critical step in metastasis, has been proposed by Liotta and co-workers (1,2) and describes: (1) tumor cell attachment to a matrix substratum; (2) local degradation of the matrix by tumor cell-associated proteases; and (3) tumor cell locomotion into the matrix modified by proteolysis. Although simple in theory, these mechanisms are quite complex to study because metastasis consists of a cascade of events, in which one event appears to trigger the onset of another.

To study aspects of invasion dynamics in vitro, a myriad of invasion assays have been developed to investigate unique metastatic properties demonstrated by specific tumor cells. Accounts of these new assays were first given in the late 1970s and have escalated exponentially since that time (3–14). A number of such assays are given in this volume, including, for example, the collagen invasion assay and chick heart invasion assay described in Chapters 9 and 10 by Bracke et al. At present, it would be difficult to imagine a novel invasion

From: *Methods in Molecular Medicine, vol. 58:*
Metastasis Research Protocols, Vol. 2: Cell Behavior In Vitro and In Vivo
Edited by: S. A. Brooks and U. Schumacher © Humana Press Inc., Totowa, NJ

assay that did not incorporate or reflect some aspect of a previously developed protocol. Probably the most controversial aspects of these assays are the qualitative and quantitative analyses associated with each. If one assumes that each assay is meritorious in its own right, then rigorous interpretation of experimental data should be applied universally. Indeed, some of these assays have been adapted for the screening of anticancer drugs, which may contribute significantly to the pool of therapeutic agents for research, development, and clinical trials *(15)*. Furthermore, these invasion assays have now been applied to genetically manipulated cells in an attempt to elucidate specific genes and gene mutations responsible for invasion and metastasis *(16–20)*. Hence, it is fair to speculate that the in vitro tumor cell invasion assays have contributed to our understanding of tumor cell dynamics and events associated with metastasis.

This section provides a complete description of a versatile and user-friendly invasion assay, named the Membrane Invasion Culture System (MICS). This assay, a slightly more sophisticated version of the assay described in Chapter 7 by Hall and Brooks, was developed for the purpose of studying tumor cell invasion in vitro through a biological barrier of consistent thickness. In this model, the application of the invasion chamber with a reconstituted matrix barrier allows one to observe the dynamics of tumor cell invasion of high and low metastatic cell populations over an extended period of time, thus simulating in vivo events of intravasation and extravasation of lymphatic and blood vessels. One of the advantages of this system is the versatility offered in terms of studying the efficacy of anticancer drugs, the influence of growth factors, and the role of immunological factors, antiadhesive agents and chemotactic attractants, to name a few, on tumor cell invasive potential. In addition, the differential analysis of specific genes important for the "invasive phenotype" can be easily assessed using this assay. Thus, the following description will provide a step-by-step protocol for the performance of the MICS assay, from the preparation stage through quantitative analysis of tumor cell invasion, including some alternative approaches and troubleshooting caveats.

2. Materials

2.1. Preparation of MICS Assay

1. Tumor cells.
2. Dulbecco's modified Eagle's medium (DMEM) (or equivalent) containing 1X MITO+ (a serum substitute from Collaborative Biomedical, Bedford, MA).
3. Matrigel (a reconstituted basement membrane matrix from Collaborative Biomedical) or purified extracellular matrix components (*see* **Note 1**).
4. Tissue culture plastic lids (that would normally cover 6-well dishes).
5. Polycarbonate filter containing 10-μm pores (one large sheet precut to fit in the MICS chamber and gas-sterilized with ethylene oxide, or autoclaved).

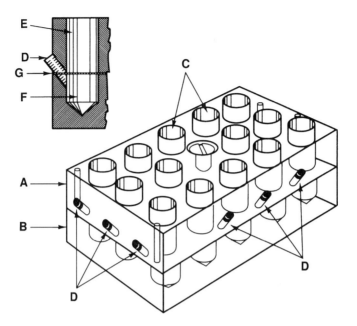

Fig. 1. Membrane invasion culture system (MICS) chamber: **A**, top plate; **B**, bottom plate; **C**, experimental wells; **D**, sampling ports; **E**, upper well; **F**, lower well; **G**, matrix-coated polycarbonate filter is interposed between top and bottom plate. Tumor cells are seeded into the upper well, allowed to attach to the coated filter, and subsequently assayed after 24–48 h in bottom wells via the side-sampling ports.

6. MICS chamber (gas- or UV-sterilized in a laminar flow hood), as shown in **Fig. 1**. MICS chambers are constructed of specially treated and stress-relieved plastics for the Hendrix laboratory and can be purchased through the Hendrix Research and Education Foundation, Iowa City, IA.
7. Glass plate (20 cm × 20 cm × 4 mm).

2.2. Sampling Post-Invasion Tumor Cells

1. Na_2-EDTA (2 mM) in phosphate-buffered saline (PBS), pH 7.4.
2. Polylysine (1 mg/mL of water).
3. Methanol (100%).
4. LeukoStat staining kit (containing malachite green methanol solution, Eosin and Wright's stain; as per the kit's instructions).
5. Large beaker containing fresh water (~150 mL).
6. Clean immersion oil.
7. Ice bucket containing crushed ice.
8. Plastic 10-mL syringe with an 18-gauge needle.
9. 12 (6-mL) Polypropylene culture tubes.
10. Minifold 1 apparatus (Schleicher and Schuell) with filter backing.

11. Polycarbonate filter containing 3-µm pores (precut to fit a glass microscopic slide).
12. Petri dish containing a filter paper blotter.
13. Vacuum and filtration tubing.

3. Methods

3.1. MICS Assay

1. In a tissue culture cabinet, place one precut, gas-sterilized polycarbonate filter (containing 10-µm pores) against a sterile parafilm backing resting against a clean glass support plate. Tape all four sides of the filter with the parafilm backing to the glass plate so that a rectangle is formed. Then chill to 4°C inside a plastic sterilized bag (see **Note 2**).
2. In a tissue culture cabinet with the airflow switched off, deliver 1 mL of 2 mg/mL diluted Matrigel or other extracellular matrix solutions evenly across one edge of the chilled polycarbonate filter resting against the parafilm backing and glass support (see **Notes 3** and **4**).
3. With an ethanol-wiped 8-mm glass rod held horizontally and equal hand pressure on both ends, evenly draw the cold Matrigel or other extracellular matrix solution across the entire chilled filter in one quick, continuous motion. It can be seen macroscopically if the entire filter has been coated by visualizing a light pink hue across the filter. Until the procedure feels comfortable, the coating technique can be tested by staining the coated filter with Coomassie brilliant blue (R-250) and then destaining and examining the staining pattern. Specifically, place the coated membrane in a staining solution of 0.25% Coomassie brilliant blue R-250–25% isopropanol–10% acetic acid for 5 min, then transfer the membrane to a dish containing 10% methanol–10% acetic acid in water and gently shake. Replace the wash at 0.5-h intervals until the wash remains clear. A uniformly coated membrane will appear uniformly purple with no change in shading or hue throughout the membrane.
4. Allow the freshly coated filter to air-dry in the tissue culture cabinet with the air supply switched on.
5. While the matrix-coated filter is drying, fill the lower wells (**Fig. 1F**) of the MICS chamber with DMEM or equivalent medium containing 1X Mito+. Make sure the medium completely fills each well and that there are no bubbles present after this procedure (see **Notes 5** and **6**).
6. Carefully excise the dried matrix-coated filter and place over the lower wells of the MICS chamber (with the coated surface facing upward) and make sure there are no bubbles present in the medium of the lower wells after this procedure.
7. Gently place the upper well plate of the MICS chamber over the matrix-coated filter so that it lines up appropriately with the lower well plate.
8. Following the alignment, gently but firmly secure the upper well plate to the lower well plate (with the matrix-coated filter in between) by tightening strategically located screws that connect the upper and lower well plates.
9. Place a sterilized stainless steel pin in each port (**Fig. 1D**).
10. Add 1.0 mL (precisely) of medium containing 1X Mito+ to each upper well (**Fig. 1E**) (see **Notes 5** and **6**).

11. Into each upper well introduce aseptically no more than 2×10^5 dissociated tumor cells in 200 µL or less (*see* **Note 3**).
12. Place the MICS chamber onto a clean plastic lid (that would normally cover a 6-well plastic dish) and also cover the chamber with an additional plastic lid.
13. Place the MICS chamber with top and bottom lids into a plastic bag (unsealed for CO_2/O_2 exchange) then into a 37°C tissue culture incubator with 5% CO_2 for 24–48 h.

3.2. Sampling Post-Invasive Tumor Cells

After permitting the cells to invade through the matrix-coated filter in the MICS chamber for 24–48 h, the following procedure is followed for the quantification of tumor cell invasion. Because the invasive cells are generally found attached to the undersurface of the matrix-coated filter, the procedure described below outlines how to remove the lower well medium plus the invasive cells attached to the filter.

1. Remove the sterile plastic bag containing the MICS chamber from the incubator and carefully examine all the components. After removing the bag, note the volume of medium in the upper and lower wells to ensure there was no leaking during the incubation period.
2. Number the polypropylene culture tubes from 1 to 12 corresponding to the 12 out of 14 wells in the MICS chamber which contain side-sampling ports. (Two inner wells do not contain these ports.) Place each tube in an ice bucket containing crushed ice.
3. Remove the top plastic lid from the MICS chamber and then carefully discard the upper well medium for each well using a glass pipet with suction bulb or gentle vacuum suction.
4. Use a clean Pasteur pipet for each designated lower well that corresponds to a numbered polypropylene tube on ice. Remove the port pin (**Fig. 1D**) and then collect the lower well medium from each well and place the contents of each lower well into the designated polypropylene tube on ice. Save each pipet in the corresponding tube. If trypsin–EDTA was used, add 150 µL of serum to each tube to inactive the trypsin.
5. Using a 10-mL plastic syringe filled with 2 mM Na$_2$-EDTA in PBS or 0.25% trypsin–EDTA in PBS capped with an 18-gauge needle, fill each lower well with the EDTA solution until it flows from each air vent, taking special care to remove all trapped bubbles.
6. Place the MICS chamber containing EDTA solution in the lower wells back into the previously used plastic bag and incubate at 37°C in 5% CO_2 for 20 min.
7. Subsequently, remove the MICS chamber from the incubator and use each designated pipet (resting in the corresponding polypropylene tubes) to remove the EDTA solution from each lower well by gentle trituration. Place this solution which now contains the invasive tumor cells back into the designated polypropylene tube containing the original medium sample on ice (to inactivate the EDTA).

8. After sampling all wells and placing the respective tubes on ice, soak a precut polycarbonate filter (with 3-μm pores) in polylysine (1 mg/mL of H_2O) for 5 min. This will enhance tumor cell attachment to the filter during the next collection-by-filtration step.

9. Place the polylysine-coated filter inside the Minifold apparatus containing a filter backing. Reassemble the filtration apparatus so that it is tightly fitted on all sides and attach it to filtration tubing attached to a vacuum outlet.

10. Gently pipet the contents of each polypropylene tube onto the filter in the Minifold. Each well in the Minifold will correspond to a sample well from the MICS. By gentle filtration, the tumor cells in the medium–EDTA samples of each polypropylene tube will be attached to the polylysine-coated filter.

11. After all samples have been loaded, turn the vacuum off, dismantle the Minifold, and place the polylysine-coated filter containing the invasive tumor cells onto a filter paper saturated with methanol, cell side up, within a covered Petri dish for 5 min.

12. Using the LeukoStat staining kit and forceps, submerge the filter in a malachite green methanol solution for 5–10 s, place in Eosin stain for 30 s, followed by Wright's stain for 40 s, and dip in fresh H_2O until the filter is cleared of background staining.

13. Allow the filter to air-dry on a lab tissue. After drying, place the filter on a clean glass microscope slide and view under a microscope (using a ×25 objective lens) to ensure that the tumor cells are stained appropriately. If the staining is acceptable, add three drops of clean immersion oil to the filter and place a 24 × 60 mm glass cover slip over the filter to complete the mounting procedure. The slides can then be stored horizontally indefinitely.

3.3. Quantifying Tumor Cell Invasion

The invasive cells on the mounted filter can easily be counted using a standard light microscope and a ×25 or ×40 dry objective lens. All the cells in each well or in 6–10 selected high power fields within each well can be counted (*see* **Note 3**). The following formula can then be applied for determining percentage invasion:

$$\frac{\text{Total number of invading cells from lower well sample}}{\text{Total number of seeded cells in upper well sample}} \times 100$$

Percentage invasion can also be corrected for tumor cell proliferation during the 24–48-h invasion assay by collecting and counting the number of cells attached to the upper surface of the matrix-coated filter from the two wells that do not have side-sampling ports.

3.4. Modification for Collecting and Staining Post-Invasion Tumor Cells

Instead of removing the medium and dissociating the invasive tumor cells from each lower well of the MICS chamber, a simpler, although slightly more cumbersome approach can be taken.

1. After removing the MICS chamber from the sterile plastic bag following the 24–48-h incubation, use a Pasteur pipet to discard the upper well medium.
2. Remove all the screws connecting the upper and lower well plates of the MICS chamber and carefully remove the upper plate while leaving the matrix-coated filter in place resting against the lower well plate.
3. Carefully use a folded lab tissue or cotton swab to wipe clean the upper surface of the matrix-coated filter. Then invert the entire filter (cell side up) onto a solid filter saturated with methanol and continue staining as outlined in **step 3**. Staining the entire MICS filter in this manner can be slightly difficult.
4. After the stained filter has air-dried, cut to fit the glass microscope slides. Generally, only three wells can be fitted per slide. Mount with oil as previously described. Because the cells are randomly distributed in the wells, the entire well must be scored by continuous counting (*see* **Note 3**).

4. Notes

1. Commercially purchased matrix solutions may vary in consistency and in the amount of certain growth factors present from lot to lot. This may affect coating as well as the growth and invasive characteristics of the tumor cells during the invasion assay.
2. Sterility is an important consideration in the preparation of the invasion assay. If the MICS chamber with the polycarbonate filter is slightly contaminated, the invasion data will be compromised during the incubation period.
3. Failure to obtain a uniform coating of the polycarbonate filter with Matrigel or extracellular matrix components could lead to inconsistent invasion data among wells. This can occur if the filter to be coated is not appropriately stretched, or, in the case of Matrigel, the coating solution is not chilled and beings to clump. This procedure constitutes one of the most important aspects of this assay. Also, tumor cell cultures should be used at approximately the same degree of confluence from experiment to experiment to ensure consistent invasion data. If mixed cell types are being tested in each experimental well, it may be desirable to prelabel a specific cell type with a particular nontransferable dye—to better assess relative levels of invasiveness among the different cell populations.
4. Other matrix components, growth factors, or cell types (such as endothelial cells or fibroblasts) can be added to the matrices during the coating procedure. The matrix barrier can also be diluted with medium before coating, although, with each new solution, equal coating of the filter must be ensured.
5. A chemoattraction assay can easily be performed in the MICS chamber by adding specific chemoattractants to each lower well, and then assaying the ability of the cells to respond to specific attractants.
6. Anticancer drugs can be screened in the MICS chamber by pretreating cells with specific drugs and comparing their invasive ability with the appropriate controls. Therefore, to standardize experimental data from chamber to chamber, a range of invasive ability is generally reported or representative data from an experiment may be reported. In the case of drug-testing data, relative values can be reported as a percentage of control and controls should be tested in each experimental chamber.

References

1. Liotta, L. A., Lee, C. W., and Morakis, D. J. (1980) New method of preparing large surfaces of intact human basement membrane for tumor invasion studies. *Cancer Lett.* **11,** 141–152.
2. Liotta, L. A., Rao, C. N., and Wewer, V. M. (1986) Biochemical interactions of tumor cells with the basement membrane. *Annu. Rev. Biochem.* **55,** 1037–1057.
3. Poste, G. (1982) Methods and models for studying tumor invasion, in *Tumor Invasion and Metastasis* (Liotta, L. A. and Hart, I. R., eds.), Martinus Nijhoff, The Hague, Boston, London, pp. 147–172.
4. Schor, S. L., Schor, A. M., Winn, B., and Rushton, G. (1982) The use of three-dimensional collagen gels for the study of tumor cell invasion *in vitro*: experimental parameters influencing cell migration into the gel matrix. *Int. J. Cancer* **29,** 57–62.
5. Kleinman, H. K., McGarvey, M. L., Liotta, L. A., Robey, P. G., Tryggvason, K., and Martin, G. R. (1982) Isolation and characterization of type IV procollagen, laminin, and heparan sulfate proteoglycan from the EHS sarcoma. *Biochemistry* **21,** 6188–6193.
6. Albini, A. (1998) Tumor and endothelial cell invasion of basement membranes. *Pathol. Oncol. Res.* **4,** 230–241.
7. Mareel, M. M., Van Roy, F. M., Ludwine, M. M., Boghaert, E. R., and Bruyneel, E. A. (1987) Qualitative and quantitative analysis of tumor invasion *in vivo* and *in vitro. J. Cell Sci. Suppl.* **8,** 141–163.
8. Pauli, B. U., Arsenis, C., Hohberger, L. H., and Schwartz, D. E. (1986) Connective tissue degradation by invasive rat bladder characterization of type IV procollagen, laminin and heparin sulfate proteoglycan from the EHS sarcoma. *Biochemistry* **21,** 6188–6193.
9. Nicolson, G. L. (1982) Metastatic tumor cell attachment and invasion assay utilizing vascular endothelial cell monolayers. *J. Histochem. Cytochem.* **30,** 214–220.
10. Hart, I. R. and Fidler, I. J. (1978) An *in vitro* quantitative assay for tumor cell invasion. *Cancer Res.* **38,** 3218–3224.
11. Ibayashi, N., Herman, M. M., Boyd, J. C., and Rubenstein, L. J. (1990) Relationship of invasiveness to proliferating activity and to cytoskeletal protein production in human neuroepithelial tumors maintained in an organ culture system: use of human cortex and dura as supporting matrices. *Neurosurgery* **26,** 629–637.
12. Albini, A., Iwamoto, Y., Kleinman, H. J., Martin, G. R., Aaronson, S. A., Kozlowski, J. M., and McEwan, R. N. (1987) A rapid *in vitro* assay for quantitating the invasive potential of tumor cells. *Cancer Research* **47,** 3239–3245.
13. Hendrix, M. J. C., Seftor, E. A., Seftor, R. E. B., and Fidler, I. J. (1987) A simple quantitative assay for studying the invasive potential of high and low human metastatic variants. *Cancer Lett.* **38,** 137–147.
14. Seftor, E. A., Seftor, R. E. B., and Hendrix, M. J. C. (1990) Selection of invasive and metastatic subpopulations from a heterogeneous human melanoma cell line. *BioTechniques* **9,** 324–331.

15. Welch, D. R., Lobl, T. J., Seftor, E. A., Wack, P. J., Aeed, P. A., Yohem, K. H., et al. (1989) Use of the Membrane Invasion Culture System (MICS) as a screen for anti-invasive agents. *Int. J. Cancer* **43,** 449–457.
16. Hendrix, M. J. C., Seftor, E. A., Chu, Y-W., Seftor, R. E. B., Nagle, R. B., McDaniel, K. M., et al. (1992) Coexpression of vimentin and keratins by human melanoma tumor cells: correlation with invasive and metastatic potential. *J. Natl. Cancer Inst.* **84,** 165–174.
17. Seftor, R. E. B., Seftor, E. A., Gehlsen, K. R., Stetler-Stevenson, W. G., Brown, P. D., Ruoslahti, E., and Hendrix, M. J. C. (1992) Role of the $\alpha_v\beta_3$ integrin in human melanoma cell invasion. *Proc. Natl. Acad. Sci. USA* **89,** 1557–1561.
18. Chu, Y-W., Runyan, R. B., Oshima, R. G., and Hendrix, M. J. C. (1993) Expression of complete keratin filaments in mouse L cells augments cell migration and invasion. *Proc. Natl. Acad. Sci. USA* **90,** 4261–4265.
19. Hendrix, M. J. C., Seftor, E. A., Chu, Y-W., Trevor, K. T., and Seftor, R. E. B. (1996) Role of intermediate filaments in migration, invasion and metastatis. *Cancer Metast. Rev.* **15,** 507–525.
20. Hendrix, M. J. C., Seftor, E. A., Seftor, R. E. B., Kirschmann, D. A., Gardner, L. M., Boldt, H. C., et al. (1998) Regulation of uveal melanoma interconverted phenotype by hepatocyte growth factor/scatter factor (HGF/SF). *Am. J. Pathol.* **152,** 855–863.

9

Collagen Invasion Assay

Marc E. Bracke, Tom Boterberg, Erik A. Bruyneel,
and Marc M. Mareel

1. Introduction

Invasion occurs when invasion promoter molecules outbalance the function of invasion suppressors (1). Examples of invasion promoters are cell–matrix adhesion molecules, extracellular proteases, and cell motility factors. In normal tissues, positional stability of the cells is maintained through the counteraction of these invasion promoters by invasion suppressors such as enzyme inhibitors and cell-cell adhesion molecules. Within this context, the interaction of the cancer cells with their surrounding extracellular matrix (ECM) is a determining factor. To study this cell–matrix interaction in vitro, several natural ECM types have initially been applied. Bone (2), salt-extracted cartilage (3), and amnion membrane (4) are examples of devitalized substrata that have been launched in the past to discriminate between invasive and noninvasive cells. Lack of homogeneity of these substrata often made interpretation of invasion difficult, and hampered the reproducibility of those assays (5). To overcome these drawbacks, reconstituted and hence more homogeneous ECMs were developed, and proposed as substrata to test invasiveness. Matrigel (6) (as described in Chapter 7 by Hall and Brooks), and employed also in the assay described in Chapter 8 by Hendrix et al.), Humatrix (7) and collagen type I (8) are today frequently used ECMs in invasion assays. It should, however, be noted that, although these preparations may contain cytokines and growth factors, they are unable to react to the confrontation by cancer cells as a living host tissue does.

The collagen invasion assay is based on the preparation of a layer of gelified collagen type I, on top of which a suspension of test cells is seeded. Invasion of the cells into the gel can be monitored with an inverted microscope. Ideally the stage of the microscope is equipped with a computer-assisted stepping motor,

From: *Methods in Molecular Medicine, vol. 58:*
Metastasis Research Protocols, Vol. 2: Cell Behavior In Vitro and In Vivo
Edited by: S. A. Brooks and U. Schumacher © Humana Press Inc., Totowa, NJ

which allows automated stratified focusing at different levels inside the gel *(9)*. One major advantage of the collagen invasion assay is its feasibility to enumerate the cells at different levels. Eventually this leads to the construction of an invasion depth profile, which is quantitative, and allows statistical analysis.

The interaction of invasive cells with collagen type I is not completely understood. Normal epithelial cells tend to establish a polarized epithelium on top of collagen type I in vitro *(10)*. Invasive cells secrete metalloproteases (MMP-1) able to break the collagen type I fibers at characteristic cleavage points *(11)*, and these cleavage products can act as chemotactic agents inside the gel *(12)*. In this scenario tissue inhibitors of metalloproteases (TIMPs) can moderate cell invasion into the collagen layer *(13)*. Both cell–matrix adhesion molecules (integrins) *(14)* and cell–cell adhesion molecules, such as E-cadherin *(15)*, N-CAM *(16)*, and MUC-1 *(17)* have been shown to affect invasion into the collagen type I gel. Finally, certain cell types induce contraction of the collagen gel *(18)*; the contribution of this phenomenon to invasion is still unclear.

Variations on the collagen invasion have been published. Although most users study invasion into gelified collagen on a plain plastic support, others prefer filters *(19)*. The latter setup allows the selection of invasive variants out of a parental cell population at the lower side of the filter support. Still other authors overlay the collagen gel with basal membrane components (laminin and type IV collagen) before the test cells are seeded. In this way, they try to create an even more realistic invasion barrier for epithelial cancer cells *(20)*.

The collagen invasion assay has not only been used to study invasion of cancer cells, but has also proven to be useful for investigations on the interaction of normal cells with the ECM. Examples of noncancer cells that can invade and communicate within the gel are endothelial cells *(21)* and trophoblast cells *(22)*. Many soluble factors have shown to affect the invasion of cancer cells in the assay, and generally phorbol esters appear to be potent stimulators of invasion into type I collagen gels *(23,24)*.

2. Materials

1. Soluble type I collagen, for example, from Upstate Biotechnology (Lake Placid, NY). It is derived from rat tail, and is dissolved at 3.89 mg/mL in 0.02 *M* acetic acid. Keep sterile and store at 4°C.
2. Minimum essential medium (MEM), concentrated 10-fold (e.g., Gibco BRL, Páisley, Scotland). Store at 4°C.
3. Calcium- and magnesium-free Hank's balanced salt solution (CMF-HBSS): Dissolve in 900 mL of distilled water: 8 g of NaCl, 0.4 g of KCl, 0.06 g of KH_2PO_4, 0.35 g of $NaHCO_3$, 0.112 g of $Na_2HPO_4 \cdot 12H_2O$; adjust pH to 7.4 with 2 *M* NaOH and add distilled water to make 1 L. Sterilize by filtration and store at 4°C.

4. Dulbecco's phosphate-buffered saline (PBS^D): Dissolve in 900 mL of distilled water: 8 g of NaCl, 0.2 g of KCl, 0.2 g of KH$_2$PO$_4$, 1.15 g of Na$_2$HPO$_4$; adjust pH to 7.4 with 2 M NaOH and add distilled water to make 1 L. Sterilize by filtration and store at 4 °C.

5. 0.25 M NaHCO$_3$ solution. Dissolve 2.2 g of NaHCO$_3$ in 100 mL of CMF-HBSS. Sterilize by filtration. Do not sterilize the final solution by heating, as NaHCO$_3$ will tend to decompose as CO$_2$ and H$_2$O. Store at 4°C.

6. 1 M NaOH. Store at 4°C.

7. Culture medium. The type of culture medium depends on the types of cells tested in the assay.

8. Moscona solution: Dissolve in 900 mL of distilled water: 8.0 g of NaCl, 0.3 g of KCl, 0.05 g of Na$_2$HPO$_4$·H$_2$O, 0.025 g of KH$_2$PO$_4$, 1.0 g of NaHCO$_3$, 2.0 g D(+)-glucose (dextrose); adjust the pH to 7.0–7.4 with normal HCl and add distilled water to make 1 L. Sterilize by filtration. Store at –20°C.

9. Trypsin–EDTA solution (e.g., Gibco BRL) consisting of 0.5 g of trypsin and 0.2 g of Na$_4$EDTA per liter of CMF-HBSS. Store at –20°C.

10. Melting ice.

11. Six-well culture plates (e.g., Nunc, Roskilde, Denmark).

12. Incubator at 37°C, gassed with 5% or 10% CO$_2$ in air, and 100% saturated with H$_2$O.

13. Bürker hemocytometer.

14. Inverted microscope (e.g., Wild, Heerbrugg, Switzerland) equipped with an objective ×10 and bright-field optics.

15. Sterile 50-mL Erlenmeyer flask.

16. MCF-7/AZ cells are human mammary adenocarcinoma cells *(25)*. They can be used as noninvasive control cells in the assay (*see* **Note 1**). MCF-7/AZ cells are maintained in a 50:50 mixture of DMEM and Ham's F12 Nutrient Mixture, supplemented with 10% fetal bovine serum (FBS), 100 IU/mL of penicillin, 100 µg/mL of streptomycin and 2 µg/mL of amphotericin B.

17. DHD-FIB cells are rat fibroblasts isolated from a colon carcinoma *(26)*. These cells can be used as invasive control cells (*see* **Note 1**). They are maintained in DMEM, supplemented with 10% FBS, 100 IU/mL of penicillin, 100 µg/mL of streptomycin, and 2 µg/mL of amphotericin B.

3. Method

3.1. Incubation of Test Cells on Top of Collagen

1. Prepare the collagen solution for six wells by mixing the following precooled (at 4°C) components in a sterile 50-mL Erlenmeyer flask on melting ice: 2.1 mL of collagen type I, 0.8 mL of MEM (10X), 4.6 mL of PBS^D, 0.8 mL of 0.25 M NaHCO$_3$ solution (*see* **Note 1**). Add 0.15 mL of 1 M NaOH to make the solution alkaline (*see* **Note 2**). Mix gently by pipetting, avoiding the introduction of air bubbles into the solution. The final solution should look purple due to the phenol red pH indicator showing a pH > 9. Pour 1.25 mL of this solution in the outer wells and 1.35 mL in the middle wells. Let the collagen gelify on a flat surface at 37°C in a water-saturated atmosphere of 10% CO$_2$ in air for at least 30 min. This yields a collagen gel with a (central) thickness in the well of 250 µm.

2. Detach the test cells and the control cells from their plastic substratum by "trypsinization." For a 25-cm^2 cell culture flask, wash the cell culture twice with 3 mL of Moscona solution. Then add 3 mL of trypsin–EDTA solution, remove after a few seconds, and incubate at 37°C for 10–15 min. Further, add 5 mL of culture medium with 10% FBS to inhibit the enzymatic activity of trypsin, suspend well, and count the cell number with a Bürker hemocytometer.

3. Gently transfer 5 mL of a suspension containing 1×10^5 test cells (*see* **Note 3**) in each well coated with the collagen gels (*see* **Note 4**). These cells are suspended and incubated in their proper maintenance medium (supplemented with FBS and, e.g., the products to be tested; *see* **Note 5**).

4. Incubate the cells at 37°C in an appropriate atmosphere of CO_2 in H_2O-saturated air for 24 h (*see* **Fig. 1A–C**).

3.2. Analysis of Invasion

1. Focus an inverted microscope (objective lens ×10) downwards from the medium above the collagen to the top of the gel containing the "superficial cells." This level is defined as the layer where the most upper cells are present. This level serves as a reference for the enumeration of "superficial cells" on the one hand, and for the construction of an invasion depth profile on the other.

2. Count the number of superficial cells present in 10–15 microscope fields. A cell is considered superficial when there are no cells above it, or when it is grouped in a monolayer and within a vertical distance of 10 μm relative to the plane of reference. Single individual cells found deeper than 10 μm are interpreted as cells that have migrated into the gel, and are coined "deep" cells (*see* **step 3**). The first field is always chosen near the center of the well, and consecutive fields are located on a straight line starting from this central field. The surface of the gel is not always completely flat, and therefore when there are superficial cells 10 μm deeper on one side of the microscope field compared to the other side, another field is chosen. Avoid cell counting at the periphery (1 cm) of the well, because here meniscus formation of the collagen can disturb the top level of the gel, and can contain fewer cells due to rolling towards the more central parts. Reject fields containing optical artefacts (e.g., small air bubbles).

3. Traverse the total thickness of the collagen gel from top to bottom in steps of 12.5 μm (*see* the manual for the microscope to know what distance one turn of the fine-focussing knob represents) until the bottom level of the gel is reached (*see* **Note 6**). Count for each plane the number of sharply focussed cells present in 10–15 microscope fields (*see* **Note 7**).

3.3. Calculation of Results

1. Calculate the invasion index for each collagen gel. This index is given by the following cell numbers:

$$(\text{deep cells}) \times 100 \, / \, (\text{deep} + \text{superficial cells})$$

It is expressed as a percentage.

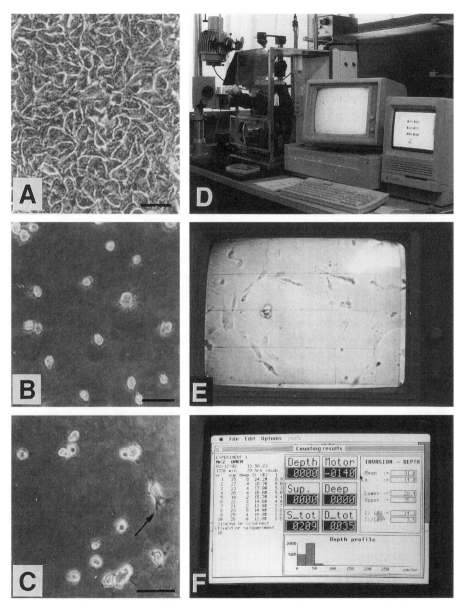

Fig. 1. (A) Confluent monolayer of canine MDCK kidney cells on tissue-culture substratum ready for use in the collagen invasion assay. (B) Top layer of collagen gel with solitary, round-shaped cells after 1 h of incubation. (C) Top layer of collagen gel with invading cells after 24 h of incubation. Some of the cells show cytoplasmatic extensions (arrow) indicating invasive behavior. (D) The computer-assisted inverted microscope. (E) Monitor screen showing invading cells. (F) Window showing invasion index and depth profile. Scale bars = 100 μm.

2. Calculate the mean depth profile plus its standard deviation for each collagen gel. This profile is built up by the serial numbers of deep cells per horizontal gel layer of 250 μm thickness. For statistical comparison within one experiment contingency table (chi-square) analysis is used. For small numbers, Yates continuity correction should be added *(27)*. Differences are considered significant when $p < 0.01$.

3. For statistical comparisons between different experiments, Student's t-test can be applied, provided the number of calculated indexes per group is 3 or higher.

4. Notes

1. Differences between the collagen batches may exist, some of which are even unsuitable for the invasion assay. For this reason invasion indexes obtained with different collagen batches should not be compared with each other. Furthermore, each batch should be tested with an invasive (e.g., DHD-FIB) and a noninvasive (e.g., MCF-7/AZ) cell line before use. The batch is accepted only if the invasion index is higher than 10% and cells are at least 50 μm deep for DHD-FIB and the invasion index is lower than 1% for MCF-7/AZ. It may be necessary to alter the composition described and adapt the collagen concentration to suit the control cells. Using collagen from another company may also help. The control cells should be used in every experiment. Keep in mind that cell characteristics may change during culture. DHD-FIB, for example, tend to change into less invasive cells when they are in culture for several months (about 50 passages).

2. If a precipitate is formed when mixing the products, the solution may be too alkaline. Reduce the amount of NaOH added or reduce its concentration. In our recent experience the assay also works with the collagen made at neutral pH.

3. When working with poorly invasive cells, adding 5×10^5 in stead of 1×10^5 cells per milliliter may be useful to facilitate the assay. Floating cells should be removed prior to analysis of invasion.

4. When working with very invasive cells it may be difficult to discern the top of the collagen gel. Adding some carbon particles will often overcome this problem. The carbon particles will remain on top of the gel and will not invade into the collagen.

5. Always check the osmolality of test products and use them at an isotonic concentration. Hypertonic solutions will dissolve the collagen gel. When treating cells with precious drugs, the end volume of the cell suspension on top of the collagen may be lowered to 1.5 mL.

6. To speed up the analysis of invasion the assay can be automated *(28)* (*see* **Fig. 1D**). The microscope images can be projected onto a video camera (e.g., COHU 4710, San Diego, CA) connected to a monitor (*see* **Fig. 1E**). To control the height of the microscope stage a stepper motor can be used, steered by a computer program (written in our institute by Dr. Luc Vakaet Jr. in McForth, Creative Solutions Inc., Rockville, MD). By pushing the up-and down-arrows of the computer keyboard, the plane of the focus moves accordingly. When a cell is considered sharp on the video monitor, its position is entered in the computer by a keystroke. During counting, the computer program automatically sorts the recorded depth in classes with a width of 25 μm, calculates the invasion index and depth profile for each collagen gel (*see* **Fig. 1F**). The program also contains software for the statistical analysis of the data.

7. To study the dynamics of invasion, time lapse video recordings can be made. The video signal of the camera is recorded on a video recorder (e.g., U-matic VO-5850P, Sony, Tokyo, Japan), controlled by an animation control unit (e.g., EOS AC-580 Electronics, Barry, UK) and time signals (e.g., one pulse every 14 s) are generated by a pulse generator. With this setup two frames are recorded every 14 s. In playback at 25 images/s, cells can thus be seen moving 175 times faster than in reality. During recording the microscope is focussed at a level were superficial cells can still be discerned, but are not in focus (e.g., 40 µm below the reference level). Noninvasive cells will remain out of focus. Invasive cells will gradually come in focus when they reach the plane of interest and go out of focus when they invade deeper into the collagen gel. The video tracks reveal discontinuities in cell motility and in the direction and the sense of cell movements. They also can be used to study shape changes of the cells during invasion into the collagen gel.

References

1. Mareel, M. M., Bracke, M. E., Van Roy, F. M., and de Baetselier, P. (1997) Molecular mechanisms of cancer invasion, in *Encyclopedia of Cancer*, Vol. II, (Bertino, J. R., ed.), Academic Press, San Diego, pp. 1072–1083.
2. Kuettner, K. E., Pauli, B. U., and Soble, L. (1978) Morphological studies on the resistance of cartilage to invasion by osteosarcoma cells *in vitro* and *in vivo*. *Cancer Res.* **38,** 277–287.
3. Pauli, B. U., Memoli, V. A., and Kuettner, K. E. (1981) *In vitro* determination of tumor invasiveness using extracted hyaline cartilage. *Cancer Res.* **41,** 2084–2091.
4. Liotta, L. A., Lee, C. W., and Morakis, D. J. (1980) New method for preparing large surfaces of intact human basement membrane for tumor invasion studies. *Cancer Lett.* **11,** 141–152.
5. Bracke, M. E., Van Cauwenberge, R. M.-L., and Mareel, M. M. (1984) Interaction of malignant cells with salt-extracted cartilage *in vitro*. *Cancer Res.* **44,** 297–304.
6. Albini, A., Iwamoto, Y., Kleinman, H. K., Martin, G. R., Aaronson, S. A., Kozlowski, J. M., and McEwan, R. N. (1987) A rapid *in vitro* assay for quantitating the invasive potential of tumor cells. *Cancer Res.* **47,** 3239–3245.
7. Kedeshian, P., Sternlicht, M. D., Nguyen, M., Shao, Z. M., and Barsky, S. H. (1998) Humatrix, a novel myoepithelial matrical gel with unique biochemical and biological properties. *Cancer Lett.* **123,** 215–226.
8. Schor, S. L., Schor, A. M., Winn, B., and Rushton, G. (1982) The use of three-dimensional collagen gels for the study of tumor cell invasion *in vitro*: experimental parameters influencing cell migration into the gel matrix. *Int. J. Cancer* **29,** 57–62.
9. Vakaet, L. Jr., Vleminckx, K., Van Roy, F., and Mareel, M. (1991) Numerical evaluation of the invasion of closely related cell lines into collagen type I gels. *Invas. Metast.* **11,** 249–260.
10. Docherty, R. J., Forrester, J. V., and Lackie, J. M. (1987) Type I collagen permits invasive behaviour by retinal pigmented epithelial cells *in vitro*. *J. Cell Sci.* **87,** 399–409.
11. Gross, J. and Lapiere, C. M. (1962) Collagenolytic activity in amphibian tissues: a tissue culture assay. *Proc. Natl. Acad. Sci. USA* **48,** 1014–1022.

12. Nabeshima, K., Kataoka, H., and Koono, M. (1986) Enhanced migration of tumor cells in response to collagen degradation products and tumor cell collagenolytic activity. *Invas. Metastas.* **6,** 270–286.

13. Fisher, C., Gilbertson-Beadling, S., Powers, E. A., Petzold, G., Poorman, R., and Mitchell, M. A. (1994) Interstitial collagenase is required for angiogenesis *in vitro. Dev. Biol.* **162,** 499–510.

14. Klein, C. E., Dressel, D., Steinmayer, T., Mauch, C., Eckes, B., Krieg, T., et al. (1991) Integrin α2β1 is upregulated in fibroblasts and highly aggressive melanoma cells in three-dimensional collagen lattices and mediates the reorganization of collagen I fibrils. *J. Cell Biol.* **115,** 1427–1436.

15. Vleminckx, K., Vakaet, L. Jr., Mareel, M., Fiers, W., and Van Roy, F. (1991) Genetic manipulation of E-cadherin expression by epithelial tumor cells reveals an invasion suppressor role. *Cell* **66,** 107–119.

16. Meyer, M. B., Bastholm, L., Nielsen, M. H., Elling, F., Rygaard, J., Chen, W., et al. (1995) Localization of NCAM on MCAM-B-expressing cells with inhibited migration in collagen. *APMIS* **103,** 197–208.

17. Suwa, T., Hinoda, Y., Makiguchi, Y., Takahashi, T., Itoh, F., Adachi, M., et al. (1998) Increased invasiveness of *MUC*1 cDNA-transfected human gastric cancer MKN74 cells. *Int. J. Cancer* **76,** 377–382.

18. Vernon, R. B. and Sage, E. H. (1996) Contraction of fibrillar type I collagen by endothelial cells: a study *in vitro. J. Cell. Biochem.* **60,** 185–197.

19. Mooradian, D. L., McCarthy, J. B., Komanduri, K. V., and Furcht, L. T. (1992) Effects of transforming growth factor-β1 on human pulmonary adenocarcinoma cell adhesion, motility, and invasion *in vitro. J. Natl. Cancer Inst.* **84,** 523–527.

20. Terranova, V. P., Hujanen, E. S., Loeb, D. M., Martin, G. R., Thornburg, L., and Glushko, V. (1986) Use of a reconstituted basement membrane to measure cell invasiveness and select for highly invasive tumor cells. *Proc. Natl. Acad. Sci. USA* **83,** 465–469.

21. Coomber, B. L. (1995) Suramin inhibits C6 glioma-induced angiogenesis *in vitro. J. Cell. Biochem.* **58,** 199–207.

22. Wordinger, R. J., Brun-Zinkernagel, A. M., and Jackson, T. (1991) An ultrastructural study of *in vitro* interaction of guinea-pig and mouse blastocysts with extracellular matrices. *J. Reprod. Fertil.* **93,** 585–587.

23. Komada, N., Nabeshima, K., Koita, H., Kataoka, H., Muraoka, K., and Koone, M. (1993) Characteristics of a metastatic variant to the liver of human rectal adenocarcinoma cell line RCM-1. *Invas. Metast.* **13,** 38–49.

24. Willems, J., Bruyneel, E., Noè, V., Slegers, H., Zwijsen, A., Mège, R.-M., and Mareel, M. (1995) Cadherin-dependent cell aggregation is affected by decapeptide derived from rat extracellular super-oxide dismutase. *FEBS Lett.* **363,** 289–292.

25. Bracke, M. E., Van Larebeke, N. A., Vyncke, B. M., and Mareel, M. M. (1991) Retinoic acid modulates both invasion and plasma membrane ruffling of MCF-7 human mammary carcinoma cells *in vitro. Br. J. Cancer* **63,** 867–872.

26. Dimanche-Boitrel, M. T., Vakaet, L. Jr., Pujuguet, P., Chauffert, B., Martin, M. S., Hammann, A., et al. (1994) *In vivo* and *in vitro* invasiveness of a rat colon cancer cell line maintaining E-cadherin expression. An enhancing role of tumor-associated myofibroblasts. *Int. J. Cancer* **56,** 512–521.
27. Wallenstein, S. (1997) A non-iterative accurate asymptotic confidence interval for the difference between proportions. *Stat. Med.* **16,** 1329–1336.
28. Vakaet, L., Jr. (1991) Studie van het invasieve phenotype in collageen *in vitro*. Doctoral thesis, Ghent University, Ghent, Belgium, p. 72.

10

Chick Heart Invasion Assay

Marc E. Bracke, Tom Boterberg, and Marc M. Mareel

1. Introduction

Tumors are microecosystems in which a continuous cross-talk between cancer cells and host cells decides on the invasive behavior of the tumor cell population as a whole *(1)*. Both compartments secrete activating and inhibitory factors that modulate activities such as cell–extracellular matrix (ECM) interaction, cell–cell adhesion, remodeling of the ECM, and cell motility. For this reason, confrontations of cancer cells with a living normal host tissue in organ culture have been introduced by several groups: Wolff and Schneider in France *(2)*, Easty and Easty in the United Kingdom *(3)*, and Schleich in Germany *(4)*. Embryonic chick heart fragments in organ culture maintain many histological features of their tissue of origin: They are composed of myocytes, fibroblasts, and endothelial cells, and their ECM contains fibronectin, laminin, and several collagen types. Moreover, the fragments remain contractile, and this activity allows the monitoring of their functional integrity during organ culture.

Typically, the assay is based on the confrontation of precultured heart fragments (PHF) with aggregates of test cells. Both spheroidal partners with a standardized diameter are brought together as pairs on a semisolid substratum, until their mutual attachment is firm enough to allow transfer to a liquid medium for further culture in suspension *(5)*. After various incubation periods, ranging from a few days to several weeks, the cultures are fixed for histological processing. Complete serial sectioning of the confronting culture is essential for a histological reconstruction of the interaction between the PHF and the test cells. Noninvasive test cells essentially leave the PHF intact: They grow at one pole or surround the host tissue. Less frequently they are engulfed by the PHF. Invasive cancer cells, however, show progressive occupation and destruction of the heart tissue. In many instances selective immunohistochemistry of heart and test cells is helpful to assess the

From: *Methods in Molecular Medicine, vol. 58:*
Metastasis Research Protocols, Vol. 2: Cell Behavior In Vitro and In Vivo
Edited by: S. A. Brooks and U. Schumacher © Humana Press Inc., Totowa, NJ

distribution of both partners in the sections. Generally, the interaction is described in accordance with a semiquantitative scale *(6)*, but computer-assisted automated image analysis systems have been developed *(7,8)*. The latter setups are meant to provide quantitative information on invasion.

Many variations on the chick heart invasion assay have been applied success-fully in invasion studies. These variations concern the origin of the host tissue, the presentation of the confronting test cells, and the incubation conditions. Heart fragments from species other than chick *(9)*, and other tissues such as liver *(10)*, lung *(11)*, and brain *(12)* have been described. Instead of aggregates, biopsy specimens *(13)*, monolayer fragments *(14)*, and cell suspensions *(15)* have been confronted with PHF in organ culture. Suspension cultures can sometimes be replaced by static cultures on top of a semisolid substratum *(15)*, and serum-free confrontations have been shown to be feasible with some types of test cells *(16)*.

The assay has been instrumental in distinguishing between invasive and noninvasive cell variants, often derived from the same tumor. Such variants of the human cancer cell lines MCF-7 (mammary) and HCT-8 (colonic) have proven to be useful tools to study mechanisms of invasion *(17,18)*. Further, we use the assay to screen for potentially antiinvasive agents *(19,20)*. Here, the proximity of the chick heart assay, including a living host tissue, to the situa-tion in vivo clearly adds to its relevance. It should, however, be admitted that the assay fails to encompass all the elements of the microecosystem present in natural tumors, where, for example, immunological factors can influence the invasive behavior of the cancer cells. At least in one study the absence of such factors in the assay has led to conflicting results between the outcomes of the chick heart assay *(21)* and those of an animal model *(22)*.

2. Materials

2.1. Confronting Culture

1. Moscona solution: Dissolve in 900 mL of distilled water: 8.0 g of NaCl, 0.3 g of KCl, 0.05 g of $Na_2HPO_4 \cdot H_2O$, 0.025 g of KH_2PO_4, 1.0 g of $NaHCO_3$, 2.0 g of D(+)-glucose (dextrose); adjust the pH to 7.0–7.4 with 1 *M* HCl and add distilled water to make 1 L. Sterilize by filtration. Store at –20°C. All filtrations are done with 0.22-µm filters.
2. Physiological salt solution (e.g. Ringer's salt solution: Dissolve in 900 mL of distilled water: 8.6 g of NaCl, 330 mg of $CaCl_2 \cdot 2H_2O$, 300 mg of KCl; adjust pH to 7.4 with NaOH and add distilled water to make 1 L. Sterilize by filtration and store at 4°C).
3. Semisolid agar medium: Dissolve 200 mg of Bacto-agar (Difco, Detroit, MI) in 15 mL of Ringer's salt solution by boiling 3×. Cool the suspension to 40°C and add 7.5 mL of Ringer's salt solution/egg white (1:1) and 7.5 mL of fetal bovine serum.
4. Culture medium (e.g., Eagle's minimum essential medium [EMEM] with 10% fetal bovine serum decomplemented by heating at 56°C for 60 min).

5. 70% Ethanol in water.
6. Paraffin wax.
7. Gyrotory shaker (e.g., New Brunswick Scientific Co., New Brunswick, NJ).
8. Erlenmeyer flasks (50 mL and 5 mL) with stoppers containing an inlet and outlet for gas supply.
9. Glass Pasteur pipets.
10. Glass Petri dishes (diameter = 35 mm).
11. Microdissection (iridectomy) scissors.
12. Ophthalmological enucleation spoon.
13. Stainless steel needles.
14. Blunt and sharp forceps.
15. Macroscope equipped with calibrated ocular grid (e.g., Wild, Heerbrugg, Switzerland).
16. Gas supply (5% or 10% CO_2 in air, depending on the type of culture medium).
17. Embryological watch glasses with sealed lid *(23)* containing semisolid agar medium.
18. Small pieces (about 5 × 5 mm) of filter paper (e.g., Schleicher and Schuell, Dassel, Germany).
19. Paraffin-melting apparatus.

2.2. Histology

2.2.1. Routine Histology

1. Bouin–Hollande fixation solution: Dissolve 2.5 g of cupric acetate (neutral) in 100 mL of single distilled water and slowly add 4.0 g of picric acid. After filtration of the solution through a paper filter, add 10 mL of formalin and 1 mL of acetic acid. Mix 9 parts of this solution with 1 part of a saturated mercuric chloride solution in single-distilled water. This solution contains several toxic substances. Formalin is toxic by inhalation, in contact with skin, and if swallowed. Acetic acid is corrosive for mouth and intestinal tract after ingestion. Picric acid is allergenic and explosive when rapidly heated or by percussion. Mercuric chloride is highly corrosive to mucous membranes and nephrotoxic. Wear protective clothing and gloves for preparing Bouin–Hollande's solution, and handle it in a well-ventilated area remote from fire.
2. Ethanol 100%, 96%, and 70% in water.
3. Elmer's glue tissue adhesive (Ortho Diagnostics, Beerse, Belgium).
4. Eosin 0.1% w/v in water.
5. Harris' hematoxylin (e.g., Accustain®, Sigma, St. Louis, MO).
6. Lugol: 0.5% w/v I_2 in single-distilled water.
7. 0.1 *M* HCl.
8. Isopropanol.
9. Mounting medium (e.g., Fluoromount, Gurr, BDH, Poole, UK).
10. Sodium thiosulfate (5% w/v in water).
11. Mercuric chloride crystals.
12. Xylene. As a benzene derivative xylene may be toxic after inhalation and should be handled in well-ventilated areas only.

2.2.2. Immunohistochemistry

1. Tris-HCl buffer: Dissolve 60 g of Tris base (Tris-[hydroxymethyl]-aminomethane) in 800 mL of distilled water. Bring to pH 7.6 with 6 M HCl (about 65 mL). Add distilled water to make 1 L. Dilute 10X with distilled water before use.
2. Tris-buffered saline (TBS): Dissolve 6.0 g of Tris base and 45.0 g of NaCl in 4.5 L of distilled water. Bring to pH 7.6 with HCl 1 M (about 42 mL). Add distilled water to make 5 L.
3. Tris-BSA 0.1% buffer: Dissolve 12.1 g of Tris base and 45.0 g of NaCl in 4.5 L of distilled water. Bring to pH 8.2 with HCl 1 M (about 42 mL). Add 5.0 g of bovine serum albumin (BSA) and 6.5 g of NaN_3. Add distilled water to make 5 L. NaN_3 is a highly toxic product. Contact with acids liberates very toxic gasses. Wear gloves and avoid ingestion by all means. NaN_3 forms very sensitive explosive compounds with copper, lead and other metals. Flush sinks with copious amounts of water.
4. BSA.
5. Primary antiserum: rabbit anti-chick heart (*see* **Note 1**) *(14)*.
6. Normal goat serum.
7. Secondary antiserum: goat antirabbit.
8. Peroxidase–antiperoxidase complex.
9. Diaminobenzidine. Because benzidine and its salts have been declared as carcinogens, gloves should be worn when handling this substance.

2.2.3. Materials

1. Microtome for paraffin sectioning.
2. Microscope equipped with objective lens ×10 and ×40.
3. Capsules for paraffin embedding.
4. Glass slides and coverslips.
5. High-humidity chamber.
6. Paper towels.
7. Rocking table (e.g., REAX 3, Heidolph, Germany).

3. Methods

3.1. Confronting Culture

3.1.1. Preparation of Precultured Heart Fragments

1. Incubate a fertilized chick egg at 37°C for 9 d. The incubation should be finished 4 d before the start of the confronting culture is planned.
2. Disinfect the shell with 70% ethanol in water. Carry out all further manipulations in a tissue culture cabinet using sterile solutions and materials. Open the shell at the embryonic pole using blunt forceps.
3. Take out the embryo by holding the neck with an enucleation spoon (*see* **Fig. 1A**). Place the embryo in a Petri dish containing Ringer's salt solution. Open the ventral thoracic skin, remove the sternum and dissect out the heart with microdissection scissors (*see* **Fig. 1B**).
4. Transfer the heart to a glass Petri dish containing culture medium. Use a macroscope to remove the atria and associated vessels. Tear off the pericardium from the ventricles with a pair of sharp forceps.

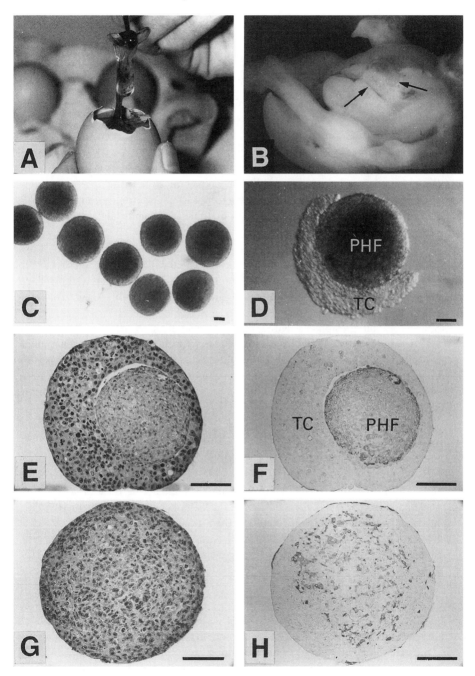

Fig. 1. (**A**) Removal of the chick embryo from the egg by holding its neck with an enucleation spoon. (**B**) Chick embryo with open thorax, showing the heart (arrows) ready for further dissection. (**C**) Embryonic chick heart fragments precultured for 4 d, and selected for a diameter of 0.4 mm *(continued)*.

5. Make incisions into the ventricles, and remove the blood by gently shaking.
6. Transfer the ventricles into another Petri dish containing fresh culture medium. Using a macroscope with a calibrated ocular grid, cut the ventricles into pieces of approx 0.4 mm diameter by means of microdissection scissors. One heart can yield about 100 fragments.
7. Rotate the Petri dish gently to drive all myocard fragments to the center of the disk. Remove all *corpora aliena* with a needle and discard.
8. Transfer the heart fragments to a 50-mL Erlenmeyer flask containing 2–3 mL culture medium using a glass Pasteur pipet.
9. Gas the flask(s) with a mixture of 5% CO_2 in air via the stoppers and incubate the flask(s) on a Gyrotory shaker at 37°C at 70 rpm for 24 h.
10. Transfer the heart fragments (incubated for 24 h) and their culture medium to a Petri dish. Discard *corpora aliena*, necrotic (dark) fragments, and conglomerates of heart fragments with a needle.
11. Incubate the remaining heart fragments in another 50-mL Erlenmeyer flask containing 6 mL of culture medium as described in **step 9** for another 60 h. During this incubation period, the fragments will become spherical. They consist of a core of myoblasts and a thin layer of fibroblastic cells at the periphery (*see* **Note 2**).
12. Select spheroidal fragments with a thin, homogeneous layer of fibroblastic cells and a diameter of 0.4 mm by means of a macroscope and needles. One chick heart will yield about 20 suitable precultured heart fragments (PHFs). Transfer these PHFs, many of which will contract rhythmically at 37°C, to another Petri dish containing fresh culture medium. These PHFs are ready for confrontation with test cells (*see* **Fig. 1C**).

3.1.2. Preparation of Spheroidal Test Cell Aggregates

1. Prepare 6 mL of a suspension containing 1×10^5 test cells/mL in their appropriate culture medium in a 50-mL Erlenmeyer flask. This should be done 3 d before the start of the confronting culture is planned. Incubate the flask on a Gyrotory shaker at 37°C at 70 rpm for 3 d. Gas the flasks with a mixture of 5% or 10% CO_2 in air, depending on the type of culture medium used.
2. View the aggregates under a macroscope equipped with a calibrated ocular grid. Select with a needle spheroidal cell aggregates with a diameter of 0.2 mm (*see* **Note 2**).

Fig. 1. (*continued from previous page*) (**D**) Confrontation of test cells (TC) with a precultured heart fragment (PHF) after incubation on top of a semisolid agar medium for 24 h. (**E,F**) Histological sections of a confronting culture of noninvasive TC and PHF after an incubation period of 8 d in suspension. Staining with hematoxylin eosin (E) or an immunohistochemical method to reveal chick heart antigens (F). (**G,H**) Sections of a confronting culture of invasive TC and PHF after 4 d. Staining with hematoxylin eosin (G) and immunohistochemically for chick heart (H). All scale bars = 100 µm.

3.1.3. Confrontation of Test Cells with PHF

1. Use Pasteur pipets to transfer eight selected PHFs (diameter = 0.4 mm) and eight spheroidal cell aggregates (diameter = 0.2 mm) in a minimal amount of culture medium to an embryological watch glass containing semisolid agar medium.
2. Move individual pairs of PHFs and aggregates with a needle, until they make contact with each other. Aspirate excess medium with a small piece of filter paper.
3. Seal the lid of the watch glass with paraffin, and incubate at 37°C for 4–24 h, dependent on the adhesive properties of the test cells (*see* **Fig. 1D**).
4. Immerse the confronting pairs with prewarmed (37°C) culture medium, and transfer each individual pair with a Pasteur pipet into a 5-mL Erlenmeyer flask containing 1.5 mL of culture medium (*see* **Note 2**).
5. Incubate the flasks on a Gyrotory shaker at 120 rpm and at 37°C. The flasks are gassed with 5% or 10% CO_2 in air, depending on the type of culture medium used. To avoid concentration of the media, moisture the gasses by leading them through two supplementary 5-mL Erlenmeyer flasks filled with 2 mL of Ringer's salt solution. Refresh the culture medium every 8 d.

3.2. Histology

3.2.1. Routine Histology

1. Fix the individual cultures after several days or weeks of incubation as follows. First, transfer the cultures to Ringer's salt solution for a few seconds to remove serum proteins. Next, immerse them in Bouin–Hollande's fixation solution for approx 2 h. Further, rinse the cultures 3× in distilled water before incubating them in water for 2 h to remove as much of the fixation solution as possible. Finally, transfer the cultures to 70% ethanol in water. The fixed cultures can be kept in this solution for a number of days (*see* **Note 1**).
2. Dehydrate the cultures by transferring sequentially to 96% ethanol in water, 100% ethanol or isopropanol, and xylene for 2 h each. Transfer each culture to a separate glass coverslip with a minimal amount of xylene, place the coverslip on the bottom of capsules for paraffin embedding, and cover the fixed material with liquid paraffin wax at 56°C. Incubate at 56°C for 24 h, then cool the embedded material to room temperature.
3. Remove the capsule and the coverslip, and cut out a paraffin block that contains the fixed culture.
4. Make 8-μm thick paraffin sections of the entire confronting pair using a microtome, and collect all sections on three alternating microscope glass slides that have been pretreated with Elmer's glue tissue adhesive as a sticking agent (*see* **Note 2**).
5. Remove the paraffin from one slide by immersing twice in xylene for 10 min.
6. Rehydrate the slides by immersion for 10 s in the following solutions: xylene–ethanol (1:1), 100% ethanol, 96% ethanol in water, 70% ethanol in water, and finally distilled water.
7. Dissolve mercuric chloride crystals by immersion in Lugol solution for 10 s.
8. Clear the sections with 5% w/v sodium thiosulfate in water for 10 s. Then wash the slides thoroughly in distilled water.

9. Incubate the slides in Harris' hematoxylin for 2 min and submerge them briefly in 0.1 *M* HCl. Then wash in running tap water for 10 min.
10. Incubate in eosin 0.1% w/v in water for 1 min.
11. Dehydrate via brief submersion in the following series of solutions: distilled water, 70% ethanol, 96% ethanol, 100% ethanol (twice), xylene–ethanol (1:1) and, finally, xylene.
12. Mount the slides with, for example, Fluoromount. Let the mounting medium harden at 56°C for 24 h.

3.2.2. Immunohistochemistry

1. Follow **steps 1–8** of **Subheading 2.2.1**.
2. Dip the slides in TBS or Tris–0.1% BSA buffer and wipe off excess fluid around the sections using a paper towel.
3. Apply normal goat serum diluted 1:20 in TBS (or 5% BSA in Tris–0.1% BSA buffer) for 30 min in a high-humidity chamber. Then remove excess fluid with a paper towel.
4. Apply the primary antiserum diluted in Tris–0.1% BSA supplemented with 1% normal goat serum for at least 2 h in a high-humidity chamber. The optimal dilution of the primary antiserum should be determined empirically.
5. Wash the slides twice in Tris–0.1% BSA on a rocking table for 5–10 min.
6. Remove excess fluid by means of paper towel and apply goat antirabbit antiserum in excess (e.g., 1:20 in TBS) for at least 1 h in a high-humidity chamber.
7. Wash twice with TBS on a rocking table for 5–10 min.
8. Remove excess fluid by means of paper towel. Apply the peroxidase–antiperoxidase complex diluted 1:250 in TBS supplemented with normal goat serum for at least 1 h in a high-humidity chamber. The dilution of the complex depends on the batch.
9. Wash the slides with TBS and transfer to Tris-HCl buffer, pH 7.6.
10. Transfer the slides to a Tris-HCl buffer containing 0.25 g/L of diaminobenzidine and 0.01% H_2O_2 for a few minutes and stop the incubation when the chick heart is stained. Check regularly under the microscope.
11. Transfer the slides to Tris-HCl for 10 min and then to distilled water.
12. Follow **steps 11** and **12** of **Subheading 3.2.1**.

3.2.3. Histological Evaluation

Invasion is defined as the progressive occupation of the PHF by the confronting test cells. Microscopic analysis of all consecutive sections from a confronting culture allows the reconstruction of the interaction between the test cell aggregate and the PHF in three dimensions (*see* **Note 2**).

The observation of different patterns of interaction has led to the following scale:

Grade 0: Only PHF is found. No confronting cells can be observed.
Grade I: The confronting test cells are attached to the PHF, and do not occupy the heart tissue, even not the outermost fibroblastic cell layers (*see* **Fig. 1E,F**).
Grade IIa: Occupation of the PHF is limited to the outer fibroblast-like and myoblast cell layers.

Grade IIb: The PHF has surrounded the cell aggregate without signs of occupation.
Grade III: The confronting cells have occupied the PHF, but have left more than half of the original amount of heart tissue intact.
Grade IV: The confronting cells have occupied more than half of the original volume of the PHF (*see* **Fig. 1G,H**).

Grades I and II are observed with noninvasive cell populations, while grade III an IV are typical of invasion. To evaluate progression with time, histological analysis should be done on confronting cultures fixed after different incubation periods (*see* **Note 3**).

4. Notes

1. Immunohistochemistry can be applied not only to detect chick heart antigens. With the use of specific antibodies the technique described for chick heart antigens can be applied to other antigens of the cultures as well. For optimal results different fixation methods should be tried out and/or the sections may require enzyme treatment before application of the primary antiserum. One example is incubation with 0.05% trypsin in 0.05 M Tris-HCl buffer at pH 7.8. Different periods of enzymatic pretreatment (e.g., 15, 30, and 60 min) should be tried at 37°C. For antigens that are easily destroyed during fixation, cryosectioning of the cultures can offer an alternative for immunohistochemical analysis. For this, wash the living cultures first with Ringer's salt solution to remove serum proteins. Then add one drop of embedding medium (Reichert-Jung, Nussloch, Germany) to the precooled (–16°C) specimen holder of the cryomicrotome. Embed the confronting culture in the top of this drop before it is completely frozen (the culture can be easily transferred via the edge of a glass coverslip). Then cool the culture to –16°C. Cut 6-µm-thick frozen sections, and collect them on gelatin-coated glass slides. Fix the slides in acetone at 4°C for 10 min before storage at 4°C.

2. A number of problems can occur during the various steps of the assay. During the preparation of PHFs, the fragments may not stay in suspension, but adhere to the vessel wall, which can be overcome by increasing the volume of the culture medium. If the number of PHF is too low and their size too big, however, one should try to diminish the culture medium volume. During the preparation of cell aggregates, failure of the test cells to aggregate is sometimes due to temperature running out of control or to microbial infection, but inability to aggregate may also be an intrinsic characteristic of the cells. During attachment of the aggregates to PHF poor adhesion may be overcome by extending the incubation period on top of the semisolid agar medium or by removing more fluid culture medium around the cultures by means of absorbing filter paper. Check also for microbial contamination. Difficulties during sectioning may be due to disintegration of the paraffin blocks: this occurs when the storage period of the blocks has been too long (melt the paraffin once again). When sectioning artefacts occur, the integrity of the microtome knife and the absence of *corpora aliena* in the fixed cultures should be checked. Necrotic areas in the cultures are signs of poor culture condi-

tions. If these areas are restricted to the center of the cultures, one should suspect the volume of the confrontations being too large. However, more generalized necrosis points toward inappropriate pH control, microbial contamination, or a fixation artefact. Finally, when the sections appear too dark, the immersion period in hematoxylin was too long, or the sections were too thick (>8 μm).

3. When cultures are treated with potentially anti-invasive agents, toxicity tests should be performed. Survival of the cells can be measured by the number of cultures that are able to grow out on tissue culture plastic after explantation without the treating agent. For this confronting cultures are transferred to 24-well tissue culture multidishes. After washing with 1 mL of Moscona's solution, and subsequently with 0.03% w/v EDTA in Moscona's solution, the cultures are treated with 200 μL of trypsin-EDTA (0.05 to 0.2% w/v in Puck's saline A) at 37°C for 20 min. Then 1 mL of culture medium is added for further incubation (change 500 μL of the medium every 6 h). All wells are inspected daily for cell outgrowth from the explants using an inverted microscope (×40). Divide the number of outgrowing cultures by the total number of explanted cultures to obtain an index of survival of the confronting cultures. Compare the results of drug-treated cultures with solvent-treated ones.

4. To assess the effect of potentially anti-invasive agents on cell growth, a procedure for measuring the growth of the confronting cultures can be followed. First, make black and white photographs of the cultures just before fixation, using a macroscope equipped with a photocamera (objective lens ×50). Then, view the negatives with a magnification apparatus and measure in mm the larger *(a)* and smaller *(b)* diameter of the culture on a projection ×6.5. Finally, calculate the approximate volume *(V)* in mm^3 via the formula *(24)*.

$$V = 0.4 \times a \times b^2$$

Calculate the growth of the culture by comparing this final volume with the combined volumes of PHF and cell aggregate at the start of the confrontation.

References

1. Mareel, M. M., Bracke, M. E., Van Roy, F. M., and de Baetselier, P. (1997) Molecular mechanisms of cancer invasion, in *Encyclopedia of Cancer*, Vol. II (Bertino, J. R., ed.), Academic Press, San Diego, pp. 1072–1083.
2. Wolff, E. and Schneider, N. (1957) La transplantation prolongée d'un sarcome de souris sur des organes embryonnaires de poulet cultivés *in vitro. C.R.S. Soc. Biol. (Paris)* **151,** 1291–1292.
3. Easty, G. C. and Easty, D. M. (1963) An organ culture system for the examination of tumor invasion. *Nature* **199,** 1104–1105.
4. Schleich, A. B., Frick, M., and Mayer, A. (1976) Patterns of invasive growth *in vitro*. Human decidua graviditatis confronted with established human cell lines and primary human explants. *J. Natl. Cancer Inst.* **56,** 221–237.
5. Mareel, M., Kint, J., and Meyvisch, C. (1979) Methods of study of the invasion of malignant C3H mouse fibroblasts into embryonic chick heart *in vitro. Virchows Arch. B Cell Pathol.* **30,** 95–111.

6. Mareel, M. M., Bracke, M. E., and Storme, G. A. (1985) Mechanisms of tumor spread: a brief overview, in *Cancer Campaign, vol. 9-The Cancer Patient*, (Grundmann, E., ed.), Gustav Fischer Verlag and Stuttgart, New York, pp. 59–64.

7. De Neve, W. J., Storme, G. A., De Bruyne, G. K. and Mareel, M.M. (1985) An image analysis system for the quantitation of invasion *in vitro. Clin. Exp. Metast.* **3,** 87–101.

8. Smolle, J., Helige, C., Soyer, H.-P., Hoedl, S., Popper, H., Stettner, H., et al. (1990) Quantitative evaluation of melanoma cell invasion in three-dimensional confrontation cultures *in vitro* using automated image analysis. *J. Invest. Dermatol.* **94,** 114–119.

9. McKinnell, R. G., Bruyneel, E. A., Mareel, M. M., Seppanen, E. D., and Mekala, P. R. (1986) Invasion *in vitro* by explants of Lucke renal carcinoma cocultured with normal tissue is temperature dependent. *Clin. Exp. Metast.* **4,** 237–243.

10. Wanson, J. C., de Ridder, L., and Mosselmans, R. (1981) Invasion of hyperplastic nodule cells from diethylnitrosamine treated cells. *Cancer Res.* **41,** 5162–5175.

11. Mareel, M. M., Bruyneel, E. A., Dragonetti, C. H., De Bruyne, G. K., Van Cauwenberge, R. M.-L., Smets, L. A., and Van Rooy, H. (1984) Effect of temperature on invasion of MO4 mouse fibrosarcoma cells in organ culture. *Clin. Exp. Metast.* **2,** 107–125.

12. Laerum, O. D., Steinsvag, S., and Bjerkvig, R. (1985) Cell and tissue culture of the central nervous system: recent developments and current applications. *Acta Neurol. Scand.* **72,** 529–549.

13. Schroyens, W., Mareel, M. M., and Dragonetti, C. (1983) *In vitro* invasiveness of human bladder cancer from cell lines and biopsy specimens. *Clin. Exp. Metast.* **1,** 153–162.

14. Mareel, M. M., De Bruyne, G. K., Vandesande, F., and Dragonetti, C. (1981) Immunohistochemical study of embryonic chick heart invaded by malignant cells in three-dimensional culture. *Invas. Metast.* **1,** 195–204.

15. Bjerkvig, R., Laerum, O. D., and Mella, O. (1986) Glioma cell interactions with fetal rat brain aggregates *in vitro* and with brain tissue *in vivo. Cancer Res.* **46,** 4071–4079.

16. Bracke, M. E., De Mets, M., Van Cauwenberge, R. M.-L., Vakaet, L. Jr., De Bruyne, G. K., and Mareel, M. M. (1986) Confrontation of an invasive (MO_4) and a non-invasive (MDCK) cell line with embryonic chick heart fragments in serum-free culture media. *In Vitro* **22,** 508–514.

17. Bracke, M. E., Van Larebeke, N. A., Vyncke, B. M., and Mareel, M. M. (1991) Retinoic acid modulates both invasion and plasma membrane ruffling of MCF-7 human mammary carcinoma cells *in vitro. Br. J. Cancer* **63,** 867–872.

18. Vermeulen, S. J., Bruyneel, E. A., Bracke, M. E., De Bruyne, G. K., Vennekens, K.M., Vleminckx, K. L., et al. (1995) Transition from the noninvasive to the invasive phenotype and loss of α-catenin in human colon cancer cells. *Cancer Res.* **55,** 4722–4728.

19. Parmar, V. S., Jain, R., Sharma, S. K., Vardhan, A., Jha, A., Taneja, P., et al. (1994) Anti-invasive activity of 3,7-dimethoxyflavone *in vitro. J. Pharmaceut. Sci.* **83,** 1217–1221.

20. Parmar, V. S., Bracke, M. E., Philippé, J., Wengel, J., Jain, S. C., Olsen, C. E., et al. (1997) Anti-invasive activity of alkaloids and polyphenolics *in vitro*. *Bioorg. Med. Chem.* **5,** 1609–1619.
21. Bracke, M. E., Bruyneel, E. A., Vermeulen, S. J., Vennekens, K., Van Marck, V., and Mareel, M. M. (1994) Citrus flavonoid effect on tumor invasion and metastasis. *Food Technol.* **48,** 121–124.
22. Bracke, M. E., Depypere, H. T., Boterberg, T., Van Marck, V. L., Vennekens, K. M., Vanluchene, E., et al. (1999) The influence of tangeretin on tamoxifen's therapeutic benefit in mammary cancer. *J. Natl. Cancer Inst.* **91,** 354–359.
23. Gaillard, P.J. (1951) Organ culture technique using embryologic watch glasses, in *Methods in Medical Research*, Vol. 4, Visser, M. B. (ed)., Year Book Publishers, Chicago, p. 241.
24. Attia, M. A. M. and Weiss, D. W. (1966) Immunology of spontaneous mammary carcinomas in mice. V. Acquired tumor resistance and enhancement in strain A mice infected with mammary tumor virus. *Cancer Res.* **26,** 1787–1800.

11

Adhesion of Tumor Cells to Matrices and Endothelium

G. Ed Rainger

1. Introduction

Cell adhesion is a process fundamental to tumor metastasis. Egress of cells from tumors and their entry into secondary tissues requires the regulated adhesion that underlies the process of cell migration. Thus, adhesion molecules must bind and release counter-receptors on the adhesive substrate in a controlled manner that permits locomotion *(1–3)*. These same molecules must also interact in a complex manner with the intracellular actin cytoskeleton that is the motor for migration *(1–3)*. In addition, it is now clear that there are interactions between adhesive counter receptors that do not mediate primary attachment to a substrate or support migration but are used to sample the adhesive microenvironment. Integration of "adhesive" signals with those from growth factors and cytokines may be used to regulate the pathophysiological responses of cells *(1,4,5)*.

The integrin family of heterodimeric glycoproteins supports the majority of intercellular and cell–matrix interactions that mediate firm adhesion and migration. They possess numerous ligands that can be separated broadly into two groups, the immunoglobulin supergene family of intracellular adhesion molecules expressed on the membranes of counter-adhesive cells (e.g., intercellular adhesion molecule 1 [ICAM-1]) and elements of the extracellular matrix that form the structural scaffolding of tissues (e.g., collagen[s], fibronectin, vitronectin, etc.) *(6)*. The precise adhesive repertoire of each integrin molecule is specific to the combination of α- and β-subunits that compose its structure, and most heterodimeric combinations can recognize more than one ligand *(6)*. To date, at least 16 α-subunits and 8 β-subunits have been identified, although only about 20 α and β combinations have so far been demonstrated on cell membranes *(6)*. Cells express a number of different integrin molecules simultaneously and can rapidly change their spectrum of

From: *Methods in Molecular Medicine, vol. 58:*
Metastasis Research Protocols, Vol. 2: Cell Behavior In Vitro and In Vivo
Edited by: S. A. Brooks and U. Schumacher © Humana Press Inc., Totowa, NJ

integrin expression, for instance by mobilizing internal granule stores in a dynamic fashion. A further degree of complexity is introduced to integrin-mediated adhesion when one considers that cells not only can turn integrins "on" and "off" (a process fundamental to dynamic migration where cells must engage new ligand at the front while releasing ligand at the back of the cell) but may also be able to regulate integrins in a fashion that allows them to recognize specific ligands by changing the activation state of the molecule in response to chemical or physical cues in the environment *(7–9)*.

Clearly not all studies will be designed to scrutinize the integrin-mediated adhesion of tumor cells to the degree of complexity described previously. Indeed, the study of migration *per se* by using migration chambers (which are in effect sophisticated adhesion assays) has been described in Chapters 5 and 8 by Brown and Bicknell and Hendrix et al., respectively. However, it is as well to bear in mind when designing experiments to study the adhesion of tumor cells that adhesion molecules are not a simple molecular glue but can be regulated in a dynamic fashion within the time frame of most assays. In the following chapter, several methodologies are detailed for assessing tumor cell adhesion to matrix proteins and to endothelial cells, including an assay for the adhesion of cells to tissue sections (e.g., sections of primary tumors or secondary target organs). The final method describes a flow-based adhesion assay that models the effects of shear forces generated in the circulation. The specialized adhesion receptors that promote adhesion from flow and their relevance to tumor metastasis are discussed in the introduction to this assay.

2. Materials
2.1. Adhesion to Purified Matrix Elements

1. 96-Well microtiter plate(s) containing immobilized matrix components (*see* **Note 1**).
2. 2×10^5 Test cells/microtiter well.
3. 100 µCi of ^{51}Cr/10^6 cells in RPMI 1640 medium (or equivalent) containing 20 mM 4-(2-hydroxyethyl)-1-piperazineethanesulfonic acid (HEPES).
4. 1% Bovine serum albumin (BSA) in phosphate-buffered saline (PBS), pH 7.4.
5. Wash buffer (e.g., PBS or cell culture medium).
6. 0.5 mol/L NaOH.
7. Gamma counter.

2.2. Adhesion to Endothelium

1. Sterile 15-mm diameter culture plastic coverslips.
2. Sterile 24-well plastic culture plate.
3. 1% Gelatin in PBS, pH 7.4 (sterile).
4. 1×25 cm^2 dish of confluent endothelial cells/24-well culture plate.
5. 2.5 mL of trypsin/EDTA (0.5 U and 180 µg/mL, respectively) in PBS, pH 7.4.
6. Tumor necrosis factor (TNF; 100 U/mL) in endothelial cell culture medium.
7. 5×10^5 Test cells/well of the 24-well plate.

8. 0.1% BSA in PBS, pH 7.4 (PBS–Alb).
9. 1% Glutaraldehyde in PBS.
10. Giemsa's staining solution,
11. Sorensen's buffer, pH 7.2. (This is PBS at pH 7.2.)
12. Microscope slides, coverslips, and mounting medium.
13. Light microscope.

2.3. Adhesion to Tissue Sections

1. 10-mm cubes of tissue, snap frozen in liquid nitrogen.
2. Cryostat.
3. Poly-L-lysine-coated microscope slides (*see* **Note 2**).
4. Acetone.
5. 1×10^5 Test cells/section.
6. Tris-buffered saline, pH 7.4 (TBS: 0.05 M Tris[hydroxymethyl]aminomethane, 0.14 M NaCl; adjust pH with concentrated HCl).
7. TBS, pH 8.2: 0.05 M Tris-HCl, 0.14 M NaCl.
8. 100 µL/section of mouse antihuman CD31 monoclonal antibody (MAb) at 10 µg/mL in TBS, pH 7.4, which will label endothelial cells in the section.
9. 10 µg/mL of a MAb in TBS, pH 7.4, that recognizes a cell specific marker on the adherent cells and that will not interfere with adhesion.
10. 40 µg/mL of affinity-purified goat antimouse antibody immunoglobulins in TBS, pH 7.4.
11. 2 µg/mL of mouse alkaline phosphatase–antialkaline phosphatase MAb (APAAP) in TBS, pH 7.4.
12. 1 mL/section of fast red substrate made just before use (*see* **Note 3**).
13. 1 mL/section of Harris hematoxylin.
14. Distilled water.
15. Microscope slides, coverslips, and mounting medium.
16. Light microscope.

2.4. Adhesion to Endothelium Under Conditions of Flow

1. Sterile 3-aminopropyltriethoxysilane (APES)-coated glass microslides (Camlab, Cambridge, UK) (*see* **Note 4**).
2. 1 mL of 1% gelatin in PBS, pH 7.4.
3. 5 mL of PBS, pH 7.4.
4. 1×25 cm^2 culture flask of confluent endothelial cells/6 microslides.
5. 50 mL of endothelial culture medium.
6. Glass dish for endothelial cell culture in microslides (*see* **Note 5**).
7. Silicone tubing with lumen diameter/wall thickness of 2 mm/0.5 mm and 2 mm/1 mm.
8. Harvard syringe pump (*see* **Note 6**).
9. Electronic microvalve (*see* **Note 7**).
10. Test cells at a concentration of 1×10^6/mL (total volume required will depend upon the wall shear stress selected and therefore the flow rate of the cells; *see* **Note 8**).
11. Videomicroscope with thermostatically controlled temperature box or stage (*see* **Subheading 3.**).

3. Methods

3.1. Adhesion to Purified Matrix Elements

This assay uses a radioactive label preloaded into the cytoplasm of target cells to quantify adhesion. The label is released by lysis of cells adherent to protein immobilized in 96-well microtiter plates. As not all laboratories are equipped to handle radioactive labels, fluorescent markers can be substituted (e.g., 2',7'-*bis*-(2-carboxyethyl)-5-(and 6)-carboxy fluorescein acetoxymethyl ester [BCECF-AM]) and adhesion quantified by fluorimetry. Immunosorbent techniques are also suitable but care must be taken to choose a marker the expression of which is invariable under different experimental regimens. The microtiter plates used in this assay do not permit efficient microscopy; therefore, this assay is unsuitable for the assessment of adhesion by visual counts.

1. Wash unbound matrix components from the wells with PBS.
2. Block unoccupied protein binding sites with 1% BSA for 30 min at 37°C (*see* **Note 9**).
3. Remove unbound albumin and wash once with PBS.
4. Label cells with ^{51}Cr for 1 h at 37°C by pelleting the cells in a centrifuge (400g/5 min) and resuspending in the medium containing 100 µCi of ^{51}Cr (*see* **Subheading 3.**).
5. Wash cells 3× (centrifuge for 5 min at 400g) to remove unincorporated label and resuspend at a final concentration of 2×10^6/mL.
6. Add 2×10^5 test cells/microtiter well (100 µL/well) and incubate for 30 min (*see* **Note 10**) at a constant and reproducible temperature (*see* **Note 11**).
7. Remove nonadherent cells from the wells with three consecutive washes with PBS.
8. Lyse adherent cells with 100 µL of NaOH.
9. Remove supernatant and count radioactive decays in a gamma counter.
10. Calibrate against lysates from known numbers of washed cells or express as a percent of radioactivity from cells in an unwashed well.

3.2. Adhesion to Endothelium

The growth of endothelium on culture plastic coverslips, as described in the current assay, is an ideal format if one intends using microscopy to assess cell adhesion. The microscope objective lens can be brought into close proximity of coverslips removed from culture, stained and mounted on a glass microscope slide. Of course, endothelium can be cultured directly in the wells of a culture plate; however, efficient microscopy is hampered by the architecture of the plate. The use of invert microscopes, which allow one to look through the bottom of the plate up into the cultured cells, can alleviate this problem to some extent; however, plate formats with more than 24 wells (e.g., 48 and 96) are unsuitable for this application because the area of endothelial culture that can be imaged by microscopy is limited by excessive light scatter around the edges of the wells.

1. Prepare confluent monolayers of "resting" EC on the culture plastic coverslips (*see* **Note 12**).
2. After 24 h of culture, remove the medium from the wells and incubate with or without TNF for an appropriate duration (*see* **Note 13**).
3. Remove the TNF and wash the monolayers to remove excess cytokine.
4. Put 5×10^5 test cells into each well and incubate for 30 min (*see* **Note 10**) at 37°C (*see* **Note 11**).
5. Thoroughly wash nonadherent cells from the well with PBS–Alb (2–3 washes).
6. Fix the monolayers in 1% glutaraldehyde for 15 min at room temperature (RT).
7. Dilute Giemsa's stain in Sorensen's buffer at a ratio of 1:5 and filter.
8. Stain coverslips with 1 mL of stain for 5 min. Destain with methanol if necessary.
9. Remove the coverslips from the wells and allow to dry (an additional dip washing step can be inserted here to ensure removal of all nonadherent cells, i.e., dip the coverslips in Sorensen's buffer several times before drying).
10. Mount the plastic coverslip on a microscope slide under a glass coverslip, ensuring that the endothelial monolayer faces the glass coverslip.
11. Using light microscopy count the number of cells adherent to the monolayer in 5–10 fields of view selected at random.

3.3. Adhesion to Tissue Sections

Tissue sections cut from diseased or healthy tissue can provide information on the adhesive environment encountered by tumor cells in vivo. The use of sectioned fixed tissue does, however, restrict the type of information that can be obtained from these types of experiments, for instance, one cannot expect complex interactions between study cells and the substrate (e.g., migration). The following assay was used to compare the adhesion of tumor infiltrating lymphocytes to sections of primary hepatocellular carcinomas and colorectal hepatic metastases *(10)* and is a modification of a protocol first described by Stamper and Woodruff *(11)*. The assay uses immunostaining to highlight lymphocytes and endothelial cells and a counterstain of Mayer's hematoxylin to aid morphological differentiation of the tissue architecture. Clearly tumor cells can substitute for the lymphocytes used in this assay.

1. Cut 10-μm thick sections of the snap-frozen tissue and place onto poly-L-lysine-coated microscope slides. Incubate at RT for 1 h.
2. Fix the sections in acetone for 10 min (at this stage sections can be stored in aluminum foil at –20°C until required).
3. Outline the section with a wax pen, which provides a hydrophobic barrier within which aqueous reagents are retained.
4. Label the test cells with a MAb against a cell specific marker for 30 min at RT and wash twice (centrifuge for 5 min at 400*g*) with TBS, pH 7.4. Resuspend in TBS, pH 7.4, to a final concentration of 1×10^6/mL.
5. To aid visualization label the sections with 100 μL of anti-CD31 MAb for 1 h at RT (this will highlight the endothelium lining the vasculature).

6. Wash excess MAb from the section with TBS, pH 7.4, and add 100 µL of test cell suspension (1×10^5 cells). Incubate for 30 min (*see* **Note 10**) at 37°C (*see* **Note 11**).
7. Tip off the cell suspension and gently wash away nonadherent cells using cold TBS, pH 7.4.
8. Fix the section and adherent cells with acetone.
9. Wash the section in TBS, pH 7.4, and incubate with 100 µL of goat antimouse antibody immunoglobulins for 30 min at RT.
10. Remove unbound goat immunoglobulins with serial washes in TBS, pH 7.4, and incubate section with 100 µL of APAAP MAb for 30 min at RT.
11. Wash the sections twice with TBS, pH 8.2.
12. Apply fast red reagent to the section and incubate for 15 min. A bright pink color should be observed.
13. Stop the color reaction by washing the sections in tap water.
14. Counterstain the section with Harris hematoxylin for 3 min.
15. Wash the sections in distilled water.
16. Mount the sections under coverslips on microscope slides.
17. Using light microscopy count the number of cells adherent to the section in 20 fields of view selected at random. Adhesion to endothelium and extravascular tissues can be readily discriminated at ×200.

3.4. Adhesion to Endothelium Under Conditions of Flow

During metastasis tumor cells are dispersed via the circulation to secondary sites of proliferation. Therefore, one may wish to model tumor cell adhesion to endothelium under the constraints imposed by circulatory flow. Our knowledge of adhesion directly from flow is derived mainly from studies of inflammation and lymphocyte recirculation where leucocytes are recruited from blood by an orchestrated cascade of adhesion and activation that occurs on the surface of microvascular endothelial cells *(12,13)*. For instance, neutrophils utilize selectins (P- and E-selectin on endothelial cells and L-selectin on leucocytes) to initiate capture from flow. Interaction of the selectin molecules with their carbohydrate counter-ligands also supports rolling adhesion and hence causes a marked reduction in cell velocity. Endothelial-borne chemotactic signals then induce immobilization of rolling cells by activating their β2-integrin molecules which in turn bind to IgSF adhesion receptors (e.g., ICAM-1). Onward migration through the endothelial monolayer is supported by integrin–IgSF interaction and regulated by chemotactic agents and surface adhesion receptors such as CD31 *(4,5)*.

It is not clear if one has to invoke a similar paradigm for the adhesion of circulating tumor cells at secondary sites of proliferation. Many tumors demonstrate a degree of tissue specificity during the metastatic process that may correlate with the expression of endothelial and tumor cell adhesion molecules *(14,15)*. In addition, some tumor cells have been demonstrated to bear the sialylated carbohydrates which are ligands for P- and E-selectin, and there is some evidence that these are functionally relevant in vitro *(16,17)*. Alternatively, tumor cells may be efficiently removed from flow by a "passive" mechanical process of entrapment in the microvasculature, a process that has precedent in the recruitment of neutrophils in the lungs where capillary diameters are significantly smaller than in other tissues *(18)*. Subsequent survival of tumor cells would then be dependent upon a suitable stimulatory (e.g., growth factors and cytokines) and adhesive environment for tumor cell migration and replication.

Flow adhesion assays have the great advantage of modeling the physiological milieu of the circulation. However, they are more expensive to set up, technically more demanding, and have a far lower sample throughput than static assays. The flow-based assay that is described later in this section has been used in our own laboratory for investigating the physiological and pathological adhesion of numerous cell types to models of the vessel wall *(5,19–22)* and was first described by Cooke et al. in 1993 *(23)*. It is based around the "microslide," a glass capillary with a rectangular cross section and excellent optical qualities, which is the model vessel **(Fig. 1A)**. One of the lumenal walls of the microslide is coated with adhesive substrate, which in the following example is human umbilical vein endothelial cells **(Fig. 1B)**. The microslide is firmly attached to a glass microscope slide (with superglue) which sits on the stage of a video microscope **(Fig. 1C)**. Using silicone tubing, one end of the microslide is attached to a Harvard syringe pump **(Fig. 1C**; *see* **Note 6)** that pulls either cells or cell-free buffer through the microslide. The choice of perfusate is facilitated by an electronic switching valve, the common outlet of which is attached to the other end of the microslide **(Fig. 1C**; *see* **Note 7)**. Adhesion is viewed directly down the microscope or a video record is made for off-line analysis. Others have used coverslips coated with an adhesive substrate and incorporated within flow chambers for similar purposes; however, as it is beyond the scope of this chapter to review the various formats that have been developed for incorporating flow into adhesion assays, the interested reader is directed toward a comprehensive critique by John Lackie *(24)*.

1. Place 1 cm of 2 mm/0.5 mm silicone tubing halfway onto one end of each APES-coated microslide **(Fig. 1A)**, and using a Gilson pipet perfuse ≅ 60 µL of 1% gelatin into the slide. Incubate for 30 min at 37°C.
2. Remove excess gelatin by perfusing 1 mL of PBS–Alb.
3. Disperse the endothelial cells with trypsin–EDTA (*see* **Note 12**), wash, resuspend in 400 µL of culture medium, and load each microslide with 60 µL of the cell suspension.
4. Culture for 24 h in microslide culture dishes (*see* **Note 5**).
5. Using 2 mm/1 mm silicone tubing connect the microslide into the prewarmed assay as described in the section introduction (a large microscope in a thermostatically controlled Perspex heating box may require up to 2 h to reach 37°C).
6. Equilibrate the microslide with cell free buffer by perfusing for 1 min.

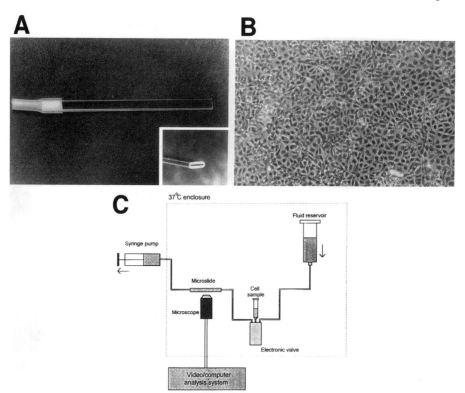

Fig. 1 (**A**) A glass microslide which is the basis of the flow adhesion assay. Microslides are 5 cm long and have a rectangular cross section of 0.3×0.03 cm. They have good optical qualities and support laminar flow of perfused fluids. Silicone tubing for insertion into culture dishes is shown attached on one end of the microslide. (**B**) A confluent monolayer of human umbilical endothelial cells cultured on the lower internal wall of the microslide. (**C**) A schematic representation of the microslide-based flow adhesion assay. The microslide is glued to a glass microscope slide and sits on the stage of a heated videomicroscope (theromostatically controlled at 37°C). One end of the microslide is attached to a Harvard syringe pump using silicone tubing. The pump pulls cells or cell-free buffer through the microslide via silicone tubing attached to an electronic switching valve. The electronic valve allows rapid switching between samples. Adhesion is viewed directly down the microscope or a video record is made for off-line analysis.

7. Switch the electronic valve to perfuse cell suspension for 5 min. A video record can be made from this point.
8. Wash nonadherent cells from the microslide with a 1-min bolus of wash buffer.
9. Make a video record of the adherent cells in 5–10 fields for off-line analysis of adhesion or count adherent cells directly down the microscope. It is essential to make comprehensive video records if complex behavior such as rolling adhesion or migration is to be analyzed (*see* **Note 14**).

4. Notes

1. Matrix proteins such as fibronectin or collagen(s) can be immobilized on tissue culture plastic by incubating at 10 µg/mL for 2 h at 37°C.
2. To coat glass slides with poly-L-lysine, make a solution of 0.01% poly-L-lysine in PBS, pH 7.4. Immerse the slides for 10 min. Remove and store overnight in a dry incubator to "cure."
3. The fast red reagent is mixed just before use and must be used within 20 min. If the reagent turns yellow upon mixing discard it and prepare with fresh components. It is important to use Tris-buffered saline (TBS) in the formulation of the reagent and in all incubation and washing steps of the protocol, as phosphate (e.g., PBS) will interfere with the development of the color reaction.

   To make the reagent, dissolve 10 mg of napthol phosphate in 1 mL of *N,N*-dimethylformamide (use a glass container). Dissolve 50 mg of fast red in 49 mL of 0.05 *M* Tris, pH 8.2. Mix the two solutions and add 50 µL of 1 *M* levamisole. Filter before use.
4. Coating slides with APES provides a silanated substrate that avidly binds the amino-terminus of proteins. This is important in experiments in which endothelium will be exposed to flow, as cells cultured on gelatin bound to uncoated glass do not consistently resist flow generated shear forces. The following protocol can be used to coat large batches of microslides (hundreds), as the process is time consuming and cannot readily be performed before each experiment.

   Immerse the microslides in 50% nitric acid for 12 h. Remove the acid by thoroughly rinsing in water and then wash the microslides several times in anhydrous acetone to remove all residual moisture. Incubate the microslides for 30 s in a 4% solution of APES diluted in anhydrous acetone. Discard the APES and repeat the treatment but incubate in the presence of a molecular sieve (to ensure that the reagent remains anhydrous) for 12 h. Wash the microslides once in anhydrous acetone and then thoroughly wash the microslides with endotoxin-free water. Dry the slides in an incubator and store in a dry place. They will last for several months. Autoclave the slides before use.
5. Once microslides have been seeded with endothelial cells they will require 24-h culture before they can be utilized for experiment. Compared to normal culture regimens the ratio of endothelial surface area to microslide volume is low (there are approx 1.5×10^5 endothelial cells in a total volume of 45 µL) and thus the medium is rapidly depleted of nutrients. To maintain a healthy culture environment the medium in the microslide requires changing every 1–2 h. We have designed glass culture dishes that have glass tubes traversing the wall (**Fig. 2** and **ref. 23**). The microslides, which sit in a reservoir of culture medium, are attached to the tubes with silicone tubing. Silicone tubing attached to the outer end of the tube connects the culture medium reservoir via the microslide to a peristaltic pump that sucks medium to waste. The pump is operated every hour by an electronic timer.
6. To generate nonpulsatile laminar flow it is essential to use a high-quality syringe pump. Peristaltic pumps will not suffice and even syringe pumps at the cheaper end of the market do not generate the smoothness of flow desirable in such a

system. Turbulent or pulsatile flow will ablate a large proportion of adhesion. Harvard syringe pumps are available from Harvard Apparatus Ltd., Fircroft Way, Edenbridge, Kent, TN8 6HE, UK or Harvard Apparatus Ltd., South Natick, MA 01760.

7. The use of a switching device with a small dead volume is important to ensure continuity of flow when switching from cell suspension to wash buffer. The use of manually operated taps is prohibited by the large surges in pressure generated upon switching which can cause detachment of adherent cells. The use of miniature sole-noid valves is recommended as they have a very small dead volume (12 µL) and rapidly switch between ports at the flick of a switch. We routinely use valves manu-factured by The Lee Company Electrofluidic Systems (Lee Products Limited, 3 High Street, Chalfont St. Peter, Gerrards Cross Bucks, SL9 9QE, UK or The Lee Company 2 Pettipaug Rd., P. O. Box 424 Westbrook, CT 06498-0424).

8. The rate at which cells are flowed through the microslide is dependent on the desired wall shear stress. Physiologically, wall shear stresses between 0.1 and 1.0 Pa ($\equiv$ to 1–10 dynes/cm^2) have been demonstrated in post-capillary venules *(25)*, the vessels in which leucocytes are recruited during inflammation. However, adhesion in vitro is rarely observed at wall shear stress above 0.4 Pa, and the majority of adhesive studies utilizing leucocytes are conducted between 0.05 and 0.2 Pa. To calculate the flow rates required for any given wall shear stress apply the relationship:

$$T = \frac{6 \cdot \eta \cdot Q}{w \cdot h^2}$$

where:

T = wall shear stress (Pa)

η = viscosity of perfusing medium (assume this to be $\cong 0.7 \times 10^{-3}$ Pa $\cdot$ s for aqueous buffers at 37°C)

Q = flow rate of the medium (mL/s)

w = width of the microslide (= 0.3 cm)

h = height of the microslide (= 0.03 cm).

9. It is important to block unoccupied protein binding sites to inhibit the nonspecific interaction of cells with tissue culture plastic. One percent albumin efficiently blocks both plastic and glass and is not a ligand for integrins except the $\alpha_M\beta_2$ heterodimer (CD11b/CD18; MAC-1) found on some leucocyte subsets *(5,6)*. Albumin blockade will also inhibit the deposition of soluble proteins such as fibrinogen and fibronectin if serum or plasma is present in the cell suspension medium. Such proteins are suitable ligands for a number of the integrin heterodimers *(6)* and could introduce an element of matrix-independent adhesion.

10. The levels of adhesion will be strongly influenced by the number of cells that contact the matrix or endothelium. Static adhesion assays must be conducted over periods that allow sedimentation of suspended cells onto the adhesive substrate. Thus, although 30–60 min will allow efficient sedimentation such periods may also allow a significant accumulation of the secretory products of adherent cells.

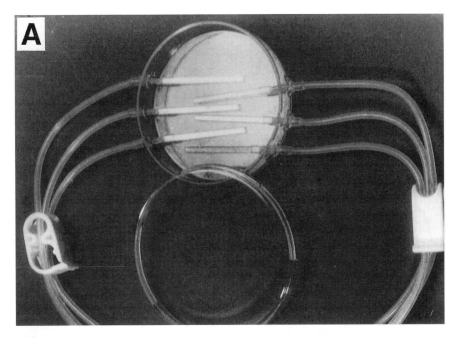

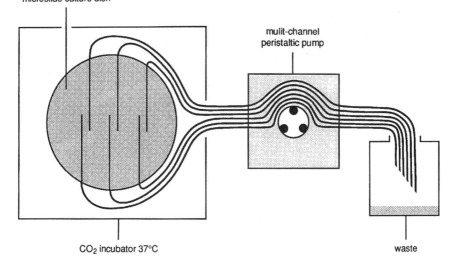

Fig. 2. (**A**) A glass dish for the culture of endothelial cells in microslides *(23)*. Using silicone tubing, each of six microslides is attached to a glass port that traverses the wall of the culture dish. The culture dish is filled with culture medium and this is drawn to waste through the microslide at hourly intervals via silicone tubing running through a peristaltic pump. (**B**) Schematic representation of the glass culture dish and peristaltic pump which support hourly transfusions of fresh culture medium into microslides containing endothelial monolayers.

These have the potential to influence adhesive responses by:
a. modulating the function and/or expression of their own adhesion receptors in an autocrine manner
b. modulating the function and/or expression of the adhesion receptors and chemotactic agents on endothelial cells if these are the adhesive substrate.

11. All of the assays detailed in the current chapter are conducted at 37°C. It is possible to run successful assays at room temperature but there is no physiological basis for doing so. Results from assays conducted at different temperatures may not be directly comparable as the kinetics of the receptor–ligand interactions that support adhesion will be different.

It is possible to run assays at 4°C, the rationale for doing so being that integrin–ligand interactions are ablated at this temperature and other forms of adhesion made apparent. As a generalization, however, this is untrue and the ability or inability to function at 4°C is probably specific to individual integrin molecules (e.g., *26*).

The original Stamper Woodruff assay was conducted at 7°C to maintain the architecture of the tissue sections *(11)*. These assays can, however, be run at 37°C as long as the tissue sections are firmly adherent to glass slides precoated with poly-L lysine.

12. To prepare confluent monolayers of endothelium on plastic coverslips, put a single plastic coverslip into each well of the 24-well plate, ensuring that the surface compatible with cell culture is face up. Add 0.5 mL of gelatin and incubate for 30 min at 37°C. Remove the gelatin and wash once with sterile PBS–Alb. Remove the medium from the endothelial cells and disperse the monolayer with trypsin–EDTA. Once the cells have detached from the dish neutralize the trypsin by the addition of 1 mL of antitrypsin or serum-containing medium. Wash the cells (centrifuge for 5 min at 400g at room temperature) and disperse into 24 mL of culture medium. Add 1 mL of EC suspension to each well and culture at 37°C for 24 h before commencing experiment.

13. Stimulating endothelial cells with cytokines such as TNF induces the expression of various adhesion molecules and chemotactic agents that promote the attachment and activation of adherent cells. This process generally proceeds via the *de novo* transcription and synthesis of the relevant protein(s). While the precise kinetics of expression is specific to individual molecules *(12,13)*, cytokine stimulation of endothelium requires between 1 and 2 h to promote significant surface expression of molecules. Generally 4–24 h periods of stimulation are used.

14. Two parameters for rolling adhesion are routinely analyzed, that is, rolling velocity and the percentage of adherent cells rolling. Rolling velocity is generally invariable throughout the experiment, being largely dependent upon the density of rolling receptor expressed on the substrate, and can thus be measured on a video recorded from any part of the experiment. The percentage of cells rolling, however, may change dramatically over the duration of the experiment and clearly one should assess this parameter at a precisely defined time point. We generally count rolling and stationary adherent cells after the perfusion of the cell bolus and once nonadherent cells have been washed from the assay system with cell-free buffer, that is, in the current example 6 min after first perfusing the cells.

When analyzing migration one may wish to simply count the number of cells that have undergone subendothelial migration. Again, it is important to define a precise time point at which this parameter is measured as it may vary markedly over the duration of the experiment. If one wishes to analyze the migration velocity of individual cells then video records should be made from the start of the experiment. It is also important to remain on the same microscope field for the duration of the experiment to be able to follow the same cell over time. A method for manually tracking cells is described in **ref. 5**. There are also a number of automated tracking systems available on the market.

It is possible to assess the degree of subendothelial migration in such an adhesion system. Generally migrated cells have a large surface area and are phase dark while cells adherent to the apical surface of endothelium are phase bright and less spread. Initially you should verify which are above and below the endothelium using high-power oil immersion microscopy. In our own experiments, we have found that the best method to verify migration of leucocytes is to remove the trypsin-sensitive endothelium along with apically adherent cells, which leaves the more trypsin-resistant migrated cells behind. For example, when investigating the adhesion of purified neutrophils to TNF-stimulated endothelium >95% of the phase-dark cells were indeed migrated and trypsin insensitive (personal communication from Dr. Thin Luu, Department of Physiology, University of Birmingham).

References

1. Matsumoto, K., Ziober, B. L., Yao, C. C., and Cramer, R. H. (1995) Growth-factor regulation of integrin-mediated cell motility. *Cancer Metast. Rev.* **14,** 205–217.
2. Huttenlocher, A., Ginsberg, M., and Horwitz, A. F. (1995) Modulation of cell migration by integrin affinity and cytoskeletal interactions. *Arthr. Rheum.* **38,** 430.
3. Huttenlocher, A., Ginsberg, M. H., and Horwitz, A. F. (1996) Modulation of cell-migration by integrin-mediated cytoskeletal linkages and ligand-binding affinity. *J. Cell Biol.* **134,** 1551–1562.
4. Imhof, B. A., Weerasinghe, D., Brown, E. J., Lindberg, F. P., Hammel, P., Piali, L., Dessing, M., and Gisler, R. (1997) Cross talk between αVβ3 and α4β1 integrins regulates lymphocyte migration on vascular cell adhesion molecule-1. *Eur. J. Immunol.* **27,** 3242–3252.
5. Rainger, G. E., Buckley, C., Simmons, D. L., and Nash, G. B. (1997) Cross-talk between cell adhesion molecules regulates the migration velocity of neutrophils. *Curr. Biol.* **7,** 316–325.
6. Newham, P. and Humphries, M. J. (1996) Integrin adhesion receptors: structure, function and implications for biomedicine. *Mol. Med. Today* **2,** 304–314.
7. Masumoto, A. and Hemler, M. E. (1993) Multiple activation states of VLA-4. Mechanistic differences between adhesion to CS1/fibronectin and to vascular cell adhesion molecule-1. *J. Biol. Chem.* **268,** 228–234.
8. Binnerts, M. E., Vankooyk, Y., Simmons, D. L., and Figdor, C. G. (1994) Distinct binding of T-lymphocytes to ICAM-1, ICAM-2 and ICAM-3 upon activation of LFA-1. *Eur. J. Immunol.* **124,** 2155–2160.

9. Vermotdesroches, C., Wijdenes, J., Valmu, L., Roy, C., Pigott, R., Nartamo, P., and Gahmberg, C. G. (1995) A CD44 monoclonal-antibody differentially regulates CD11a/CD18 binding to intercellular adhesion molecules CD54, CD102 and CD50. *Eur. J. Immunol.* **125,** 2460–2464.

10. Yoong, K. F., McNab, G., Hubscher, S. G., and Adams, D. H. (1998) Vascular adhesion molecule-1 and ICAM-1 support the adhesion of tumor infiltrating lymphocytes to tumor endothelium in human hepatocellular carcinoma. *J. Immunol.* **160,** 3978–3988.

11. Stamper, H. B. and Woodruff, J. J. (1976) Lymphocyte homing into lymph nodes: in vitro demonstration of the selective affinity of recirculating lymphocytes for high-endothelial venules. *J. Exp. Med.* **144,** 828–833.

12. Springer, T. A. (1995) Traffic signals on endothelium for lymphocyte recirculation and leukocyte emigration. *Annu. Rev. Physiol.* **57,** 827–872.

13. Imhof, B. A. and Dunon, D. (1995) Leukocyte migration and adhesion. *Adv. Immunol.* **58,** 345–416.

14. Pauli, B. U., Augustinvoss, H. G., Elsabban, M. E., Johnson, R. C., and Hammer, D. A. (1990) Organ preference of matastasis- the role of endothelial-cell adhesion molecules. *Cancer Metast. Rev.* **9,** 175–189.

15. McCarthy, S. A., Kuzu, I., Gatter, K. C., and Bicknell, R. (1991) Heterogeneity of the endothelial cell and its role in organ preference of tumor-metastasis. *Trends Pharmaceut. Sci.* **12,** 462–467.

16. Stone, J. P. and Wagner, D. D. (1993) P-selectin mediates adhesion of platelets to neuroblastoma and small-cell lung-cancer. *J. Clin. Invest.* **92,** 804–813.

17. Goetz, D. J., Brandley, B. K., and Hammer, D. A. (1996) An E-selectin-IgG chimera supports sialylated dependent adhesion of colon-carcinoma cells under fluid-flow. *Ann. Biomed. Eng.* **24,** 87–98.

18. Lien, D. C., Wagner, W. W., Capen, A. L., Haslett, C., Hensen, W. L., Hoffmeister, J. C., et al. (1987) Physiological neutrophil sequestration in the lung: visual evidence for localisation in capillaries. *J. App. Physiol.* **62,** 1236–1243.

19. Buttrum, S. M., Hatton, R., and Nash, G. B. (1993) Selectin-mediated rolling of neutrophils on immobilised platelets. *Blood* **82,** 1165–1174.

20. Cooke, B. M., Berndt, A. R., Craig, A. G., Newbold, C. I., and Nash, G. B. (1994) Rolling and static adhesion of red blood cells parasitised by *Plasmodium falciparum*: separate roles for ICAM-1, CD36 and thrombospondin. *Br. J. Haematol.* **87,** 162–170.

21. Rainger, G. E., Fisher, A. C., Shearman, C., and Nash, G. B. (1995) Adhesion of flowing neutrophils to cultured endothelial cells after hypoxia and reoxygenation in-vitro. *Am. J. Physiol. (Heart Circ. Physiol.)* **269,** H1398–H1406.

22. Rainger, G. E., Wautier, M. P., Nash, G. B., and Wautier, J. L. (1996) Prolonged E-selectin induction by monocytes potentiates the adhesion of neutrophils to cultured endothelial cells. *Br. J. Haematol.* **92,** 192–199.

23. Cooke, B. M., Usami, S., Perry, I., and Nash, G. B. (1993) A simplified method for culture of endothelial cells and analysis of blood cells under conditions of flow. *Microvasc. Res.* **45,** 33–45.

24. Lackie, J. (1991) Adhesion from Flow, in *Measuring Cell Adhesion,* Curtis, A. S. G. and Lackie, J. M. (eds.), John Wiley and Sons, Chichester, NY, pp. 41–65.

25. Jones, D. A., Smith, C. W., and McIntire, L. V. (1995) Effects of fluid shear stress on leukocyte adhesion to endothelial cells, in *Physiology and Pathophysiology of Leukocyte Adhesion,* Granger, D. N. and Schmid-Schonbein, G. W. (eds.), Oxford Univertsity Press, New York, pp. 148–168.

26. Needham, L. A., Dijk, S., VanPigott, R., Edwards, M., Shepherd, M., Hemingway, I., et al. (1994) Activation dependent and independent VLA-4 binding sites on vascular cell adhesion molecule-1. *Cell Adhes. Commun.* **2,** 87–99.

12

Assessment of Angiogenic Factors

The Chick Chorioallantoic Membrane Assay

Adam Jones, Chisato Fujiyama, Stephen Hague, and Roy Bicknell

1. Introduction

Angiogenesis is the growth of new vessels from existing vessels. It is important in the physiological processes of wound healing, embryogenesis, and the female menstrual cycle and involved in pathologies such as diabetic retinopathy and rheumatoid arthritis (*1*). There is now abundant evidence that tumors are angiogenesis dependent. Unless tumors can stimulate angiogenesis, and generate their own blood supply, they fail to grow larger than 2–3 mm^3. The angiogenic status of a tumor can be assessed directly using immunohistochemistry on pathology sections (*see* Chapter 13 by Kilic and Ergün in this volume and Chapter 7 by Ranieri and Gasparini and Chapter 8 by Turner and Harris in the companion volume) to count the number of blood vessels within a given area (microvessel density [MVD]). MVD is a prognostic indicator in a number of tumors including breast, bladder, and prostate (*2*). Angiogenic capacity can also be measured by assaying the various stimulatory and inhibitory factors that regulate angiogenesis. This can be done either by determining the mRNA level using ribonuclease protection (*see* Chapter 16 by Jones et al. in the companion volume) or the protein by either Western blotting (*see* Chapter 11 by Blancher and Jones in the companion volume) or with one of the commercially available enzyme-linked immunosorbent assay (ELISA) kits. Again, levels of these factors have been shown to be prognostic in a number of tumors.

There is now much interest in antiangiogenic therapy as a therapeutic approach against tumors. This has several theoretical advantages over conventional therapy. First, by targeting the tumor blood supply it may be possible that one treatment, specific to tumor vasculature, can be used against a variety

From: *Methods in Molecular Medicine, vol. 58:*
Metastasis Research Protocols, Vol. 2: Cell Behavior In Vitro and In Vivo
Edited by: S. A. Brooks and U. Schumacher © Humana Press Inc., Totowa, NJ

of different tumor types, rather than more tumor type specific treatment as is the case with most conventional chemotherapy. Second, in antiangiogenesis therapy, because the "target" is the blood vessels, any drug given systemically will gain direct access to its target site, thus avoiding the problem of tissue penetration encountered with conventional chemotherapy. Lastly, as endothelial cells are genetically more stable than tumor cells they are less likely to develop drug resistance to an antiangiogenesis agent, unlike carcinoma cells when treated conventionally *(3)*.

The search is therefore on to find out more about angiogenic stimulators and inhibitors. In vitro this is done by studying endothelial cell proliferation, migration, and tubule formation, all essential steps in new vessel formation. Transfection experiments with specific stimulators/inhibitors have been used in combination with in vitro and in vivo experiments to determine how this modifies tumor behavior *(4)*. Many of these approaches are described in other chapters in this book.

Intermediate between these experimental approaches are those in which various substances can be tested for pro- or antiangiogenic capacity in vivo. These include the rodent sponge model *(5)*, the rabbit cornea *(6)*, and the chick chorioallantoic membrane (CAM) assay. The CAM assay was initially used in the study of embryonic development and later modified to study tumor angiogenesis *(7)*. All work on the same principle that a putative stimulator is placed in a site where subsequent blood vessel growth can be easily quantitated. A positive response is seen as vascular remodelling with vessels growing toward the test substance. In addition, a "haze" may be seen representing increased microvessel sprouting (**Fig. 1**). Alternatively blood vessel growth can be stimulated using known proangiogenic molecules and then various possible antiangiogenic molecules can be tested for their ability to inhibit this. For initial widespread screening, the CAM assay is probably more appropriate than using either rats or rabbits, and this technique will be described here.

The CAM assay involves incubation of fertilized chick eggs for 9 d during which time the CAM is developing. This is followed by exposure of the CAM and application of test substances on collagen plugs or methylcellulose discs. Finally the CAM is removed from the egg, fixed, and analyzed.

2. Materials

1. White fertile chick eggs obtained at d 1–2 postlaying.
2. Egg incubator with rotation ability.
3. Egg lume candling lamp.
4. 70% Ethanol.
5. Microportable dentist's drill with circular rotating blade.
6. Dustoff (Black and Decker).
7. Sterile routine tissue culture medium.

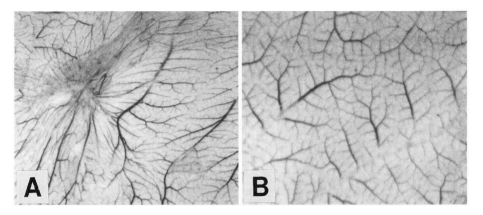

Fig. 1. (**A**) A typical positive response with "spokewheeling" of vessels and an angiogenic "haze" around a test substance. (**B**) A negative response with background vessels only.

8. 25/26-Gauge hypodermic needle.
9. Pasteur pipet.
10. Fine forceps and scissors.
11. Paraffin film.
12. Vitrogen 100 (a type 1 collagen, Collagen Corporation, Palo Alto, CA).
13. 1% Sodium nitroprusside.
14. Phosphate-buffered saline A (PBSA).
15. 10% Buffered formalin
16. Image analyzer and appropriate software.

This is a comprehensive list of equipment; many alternatives can be found to perform the various steps dependent on the availability within the laboratory. All stages take place at room temperature and instruments need to be disinfected with 70% ethanol prior to use.

3. Method

3.1. The CAM Assay

1. White fertile chick eggs obtained on d 1–2 after laying are incubated at 37°C and 60% humidity in an egg incubator with automatic rotation every 30 min for a further 7–8 d (*see* **Notes 1** and **2**).
2. On d 9, the eggs are candled by placing them on an egg lume candling lamp. This illuminates the air sac, usually at the more pointed end, and the embryonic vessels usually at the opposite end. These sites are marked with pencil.
3. In a tissue culture hood the egg is wiped with 70% ethanol.
4. When dry a 1 × 1 mm hole is made into the air sac by making a cross with the dentist's drill rotating head.

5. At the opposite end (usually) a 2×2 mm square window is cut over the embryonic vessels. Here, cut through the egg shell without going through the inner shell membrane underneath.
6. Blow traces of egg shell dust off the egg using "dustoff" or equivalent.
7. Gently lift this cut window off the underlying membrane using fine forceps.
8. Place a drop of sterile medium on this membrane and pierce the membrane through the centre of this drop using a 25/26-gauge hypodermic needle, at a shallow angle to avoid damage to the CAM.
9. Apply gentle suction to the air sac hole at the other end with a Pasteur pipet and rubber sucker. This pulls the CAM away from the shell membrane creating a false air sac.
10. The CAM window can then be enlarged to approx 10×10 mm. Remove the egg shell carefully. It is difficult, but if possible try to cut through the shell separately leaving the underlying shell membrane and then remove this membrane next by cutting it from the edges of the window. This helps to reduce egg dust falling onto the CAM (*see* **Note 3**).
11. Place a collagen plug containing test substance on the CAM. Avoid large vessels, as this will affect subsequent analysis.
12. Cover both exposed holes by wrapping paraffin film soaked in 70% ethanol around the egg.
13. Incubate the eggs, at 37°C and 60% humidity, for a further 3 d without rotation this time.
14. On d 12, peel back/cut back the egg shell to just above where the CAM meets the shell.
15. The angiogenic response can be assessed subjectively at this stage.
16. Add 0.5 mL of 1 % solution of sodium nitroprusside in PBSA to the CAM and leave for 2 min. This causes the vessels to dilate and fill with blood.
17. Add 1.5 mL of 10% buffered formalin for 10 min to fix the CAM.
18. Excise the CAM as close as possible to the shell using fine scissors and forceps and place it in a universal tube with 20 mL of 10% buffered formalin. It can be kept like this for approx 1 wk if necessary prior to quantifying the vessels by image analysis.

3.2. Preparation of Collagen Plug

1. Vitrogen 100 is neutralized to pH 7.4 according to the manufacturer's instructions. (80% Vitrogen + 10% 10X PBSA + 10% 0.1 M NaOH).
2. Keep vitrogen on ice during preparation of plug to prevent premature gel formation.
3. Mix the test substance with vitrogen in a ratio 1:10 (*see* **Note 4**).
4. Add 2 mL of this mixture to 6-well plates and incubate for 2 h at 37°C.
5. Collagen plugs are punched out using a plastic pipet tip cut to 2–3 mm in diameter (*see* **Note 5**).

3.3. Image Analysis

One of the criticisms of the CAM assay is quantification of responses. A subjective interpretation of response can be obtained by simply visualizing the

CAM. More objective responses can be obtained using various image analyzers and software packages. Estimates of angiogenic activity can then be made by measuring total vessel length within a given area around the test substance or total area of blood vessels/ total area around the test substance.

4. Notes

1. It is a good idea to cut the window in the egg, reseal the window using paraffin film, and replace in the incubator, the day before starting the assay. Thus, eggs exhibiting damage or inflammation can be discarded.
2. Incubate the eggs within their egg boxes. This avoids disturbance of the CAM and excessive movement of the collagen plug.
3. If large pieces of shell fall onto the CAM it may be possible to remove these using fine forceps. It is probably best to discard eggs where pieces of shell have fallen onto the CAM and have not been removed very easily, as these eggs may develop false positive responses due to inflammation. As a general rule, it is sensible to allocate 5–10 eggs per sample point required, to allow for technical difficulties. With practise preparation of the eggs becomes rapid, taking only minutes per egg.
4. The assay can be adapted to investigate potential angiogenic inhibitory substances. This can be done by mixing the unknown substance with a fixed concentration of a known angiogenic substance such as basic fibroblast growth factor all within the collagen plug. Alternatively, the CAM could be stimulated first with a collagen plug of basic fibroblast growth factor for 48–72 h. An inhibitory plug then introduced and result assessed 24–48 h later.
5. As an alternative to collagen gel, which can have a tendency to move on the CAM, it is possible to use a methylcellulose disc to introduce test substances. This is done as follows: Prepare a 0.5% w/v methylcellulose solution (Sigma) in distilled water. Autoclave for 30 min, then stir at 4°C for 4 h, having added test substances dissolved to a final concentration per 10 μL. Pipet 10 μL of this methylcellulose/test substance solution onto the top of Teflon rods, fixed end on to a Petri dish. Dry for 4 h in a sterile culture hood and use the discs, thus formed, within 24 h.

References

1. Ferrara, N. and Davis-Smyth, T. D. (1997) The biology of vascular endothelial growth factor. *Endocrinol. Rev.* **10,** 4–25.
2. Gasparini, G. (1997) Prognostic and predictive value of intra-tumoural microvessel density in human solid tumours, in *Tumour Angiogenesis* (Bicknell, R., Lewis, C., and Ferrara, N., eds.), Oxford University Press, Oxford, pp. 29–44.
3. Boehm, T., Folkman, J., Browder, T., and O'Reilly, M. S. (1997) Antiangiogenic therapy of experimental cancer does not induce acquired drug resistance. *Nature* **390,** 404–407.
4. Zhang-H. T., Craft, P., and Scott, P., et al. (1995) Enhancement of tumour growth and vascular density by transfection of vascular endothelial growth factor into MCF-7 cells breast carcinoma cells. *J. Natl. Cancer Inst.* **87,** 213–218.

5. Andrade, S. P., Fan, T. P., and Lewis, G. P. (1987) Quantitative *in vivo* studies on angiogenesis in a rat sponge model. *Br. J. Exp. Pathol.* **68,** 755–766.

6. Gimbrone, M., Cotran, R., Leapman, S., and Folkman, J. (1974) Tumour growth and neovascularization: an experimental model using the rabbit cornea. *J. Natl. Cancer Inst.* **52,** 413–427.

7. Folkman, J. (1995) Tumour angiogenesis. *Adv. Cancer Res.* **43,** 175–203.

13

Methods to Evaluate the Formation and Stabilization of Blood Vessels and Their Role in Tumor Growth and Metastasis

Nerbil Kilic and Süleyman Ergün

1. Introduction

It is becoming more and more clear that angiogenic mechanisms leading to structural formation of blood vessels are very complex, and understanding them depends on studies performed by means of a wide methodological spectrum ranging from molecular biological techniques to morphological analyses *(1–4)*. To study the maturation and stabilization of newly formed blood vessels, processes that include many successive steps, the following aspects and methods are important:

1. Examination of structural components of the vascular wall indicating vascular stabilization by means of light and electron microscopy.
2. Immunohistochemical and immune electron microscopic studies on tissues and cells with improved methods for precise localization of angiogenic factors during vascular maturation.
3. Chemotactic assay on human endothelial cells using the Boyden chamber to test their migration response to angiogenesis activators and inhibitors.
4. Three-dimensional endothelial tube formation assay on collagen gel: an in vitro angiogenesis model.
5. Chorioallantoic membrane (CAM) assay as an easy in vivo angiogenesis assay.

Many of these techniques have already been described in other chapters in this volume. In this chapter, we bring them together to form a comprehensive approach to evaluation of the formation and stabilization of blood vessels and their role in tumor growth and metastasis.

From: *Methods in Molecular Medicine, vol. 58:*
Metastasis Research Protocols, Vol. 2: Cell Behavior In Vitro and In Vivo
Edited by: S. A. Brooks and U. Schumacher © Humana Press Inc., Totowa, NJ

1.1. Examination of Vascular Morphology (see Notes 1 and 2)

The development of the vascular system includes proliferation and migration of endothelial cells, formation of endothelial tubes, construction of basement membrane, integration of peri-endothelial cells into the vascular wall, and differentiation into large blood vessels (**Fig. 1A**) and capillaries (**Fig. 1B**). This process, which can be called vascular stabilization, is also an important parameter for vascular permeability. The evaluation of vascular stability is essential for the assessment of (1) blood vessel maturation, (2) angiogenic potency, and (3) tumor growth and metastasis, which could make it a valuable tool for assessment of tumor malignancy.

In this context, the following structural components of the vascular wall should be studied by light and transmission electron microscopy (TEM) based on semithin (**Fig. 2A,F**) and fine sections (**Fig. 3A,B**):

> Endothelial cell morphology
> Interendothelial junctions
> Basement membrane
> Peri-endothelial cells (pericytes in capillaries, smooth muscles in large blood vessels)

1.2. Immunostaining Methods

The aim of immunostaining cells or tissues is to analyze:

1. The expression of angiogenic factors and their receptors.
2. Differences concerning the expression pattern of these factors between normal and tumor tissues or
3. Between the blood vessels formed by physiologic angiogenesis (uterus, ovary, and placenta) and tumor angiogenesis.
4. Ultrastructural localization of these factors in the vascular wall or in cells by immune electron microscopy.

1.2.1. Immunohistochemistry (see **Notes 3–9**)

Techniques for immunocytochemistry are described in detail in Chapter 2 by Brooks in the companion volume. In comparison to cryosections, immuno-histochemistry on paraffin sections has the advantage that tissue structure is preserved better. Therefore, we prefer the paraffin embedding of tissue pieces if the antibodies are usable also on paraffin sections.

Through a combination of the peroxidase–antiperoxidase (PAP) and the avidin–botin complex (ABC) techniques, peroxidase activity was enhanced *(5)* and developed by means of the nickel–glucose oxidase technique described by Itoh et al. *(6)*, as modified by Záborszky and Léránth *(7)*. This method also allows clear immunostaining of receptors, which is more difficult mainly owing to the low level of expression of such factors, for example, the receptors for vascular endothelial growth factor (VEGF) Flt-1 and KDR *(8,9)*.

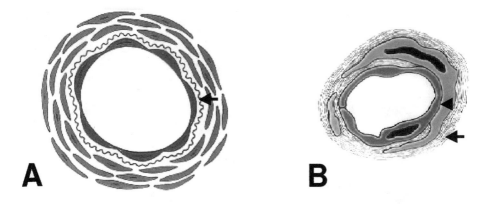

Fig. 1. **(A)** The main structural components of a mature large blood vessel such as several layers of smooth muscle cells, elastica interna (arrow), and endothelial cells. **(B)** Graphical representation of a mature capillary showing typical wall construction with endothelial cells and pericytes that are embedded in the common basal lamina (arrow). Occasionally, endothelial cells and pericytes are in direct contact (arrowhead).

1.2.2. Immune Electron Microscopic Studies (see **Notes 10–13**)

Immunohistochemistry on paraffin sections **(Fig. 4A)** is a good method to localize factors in different tissues and cells but subcellular and ultrastructural localization of these factors is possible only with the immune electron microscopical method. Different techniques are available to perform immune electron microscopy, as described in Polak and Priestley *(10)*. We report here a modified method of postembedding immune electron microscopy and demonstrate the ultrastructural localization of von-Willebrand factor in endothelial cells **(Fig. 4B,C)** as an example. In contrast to the free-floating technique, the antigens are visualized in this method first on semithin sections and observed by light microscopy. Thereafter, these immune-labeled semithin sections can be removed from slides as described in **Fig. 5** and cut further into fine sections for electron microscopy.

1.3. Chemotactic Assay (see **Notes 14–17**)

Endothelial cell migration (chemotaxis) is one of the essential steps of angiogenesis and is stimulated by several angiogenic activators. The chemotactic response of endothelial cells to activators or inhibitors of angiogenesis can be tested in vitro using a Boyden chamber, as described in Chapter 5 by Brown and Bicknell. In this technique, the passage of endothelial cells through a membrane containing pores (here 8 µm in diameter) is a parameter that can be influenced by different factors. This assay is a powerful method to study endothelial chemotaxis and can be performed in 1 d *(11,12)*.

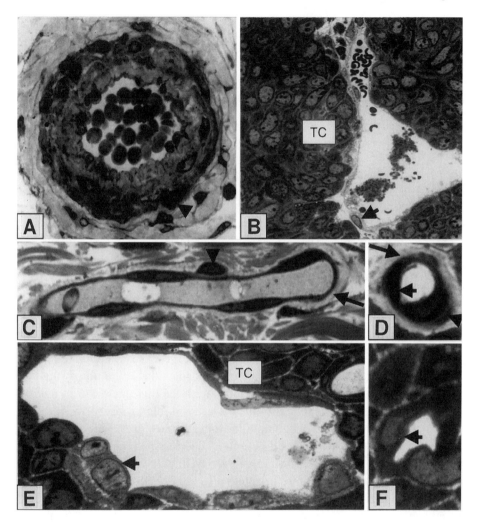

Fig. 2. Structural components of the vascular wall are best recognizable by light microscopically on semithin sections as demonstrated in (A) for a mature large blood vessel and in (B) for a large tumor blood vessel surrounded directly by tumor cells (TC) (×750). Note that in contrast to the normal blood vessel which possesses several layers of smooth muscle cells (arrowhead), the wall of the large tumor vessel demonstrates only endothelial cells (arrow) but lacks smooth muscle cells (×750). Using longitudinal (C and E) (×1500) and/or cross-sections (D and F) (×2500) of capillaries it is possible to observe if they already possess pericytes (arrowhead) and a basement membrane (large arrow). Both kinds of sections reveal that in contrast to normal capillaries (C and D) tumor capillaries (E and F) lack pericytes and basement membrane, and endothelial cells (arrow) of tumor capillaries are roundly shaped (F). These capillaries are surrounded directly by tumor cells (TC).

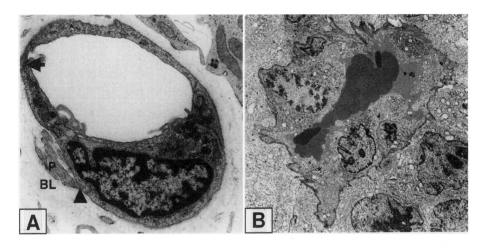

Fig. 3. In addition, to light microscopy on semithin sections electron microscopic studies allow the recognition of further structural characteristics of the normal vascular wall: inter-endothelial junctions (arrow), transcytotic vesicles (*), contact between endothelial cells and basement membrane, presence of partial contact (arrowhead) between endothelial cells and pericytes (P), and finally the structure of basal lamina (BL), which encloses normally endothelial cells as well as pericytes (**A**). Most of these structures apart from transcytotic vesicles are missing or poorly developed in tumor capillaries, especially basement membrane, specialized inter-endothelial junctions, and pericytes (**B**) (×5600).

1.4. Endothelial Tube Formation Assay (see Notes 18–20)

Beside endothelial proliferation and migration endothelial tube formation is a further important process in angiogenesis. During this process, endothelial cells degrade and invade the interstitial extracellular matrix and then form new capillary sprouts. Endothelial tube assay is an in vitro angiogenesis assay in which endothelial cells can be induced by different angiogenic activators to invade a three-dimensional collagen gel and form capillary-like tubular structures *(13,14)*. Usually, the tubes become visible within 2–4 d and then can be held a few days longer by repeated stimulation with angiogenic factors. It is of benefit that the effect of angiogenic inhibitors can also be tested on already induced endothelial tubes.

1.5. Chick Chorioallantoic Membrane Assay (see Notes 21–25)

Chorioallantoic membrane (CAM) assay is an inexpensive and easy in vivo angiogenesis assay and is described in Chapter 12 by Jones et al. In CAM angiogenesis is present until development d 12–13. Therefore, activators or inhibitors of angiogenesis should be applied to CAM in two phases: (1) at d 6 or 7 (in this phase physiologic angiogenesis is still active) and (2) at d 12 or 13

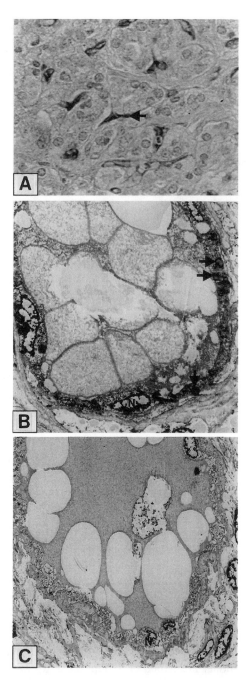

Fig. 4. (A) Usual immunohistochemical staining on paraffin sections, for example, for von-Willebrand factor, using the glucose oxidase method allows the visualization of blood vessels (arrow). This method does not permit exact cellular localization of the

(in these phases the blood vessels are mostly of the quiescent type). It offers the possibility to test the factors of interest in comparison to other known angiogenic or antiangiogenic factors on the same CAM. It is also possible to block the effect of these factors through specific antibodies. A further advantage is that the process can be observed in vivo and photographs taken light microscopically while the experiment is running **(Fig. 7A)**. The observations can be supplemented by further embedding the stimulated areas of CAM in Epon for light and electron microscopy or in paraffin for immunohistochemistry. These methods allow further analyses such as different statistical evaluations. It may also be of interest to know that for this in vivo assay no further security precautions are necessary. One disadvantage may be that the factor of interest does not function in this assay; therefore other more complicated assays such as the cornea pocket assay could become necessary *(15,16)*.

2. Materials

2.1. Examination of Vascular Morphology: Semithin Technique and TEM (see Notes 1 and 2)

1. Phosphate-buffered glutaraldehyde: 5.5% glutaraldehyde, 0.05 M phosphate buffer, pH 7.1–7.4.
2. 1% Osmium tetroxide (OsO_4) in saccharose–phosphate buffer: 2% OsO_4/saccharose–phosphate buffer (1:1).
3. Saccharose-phosphate buffer: 6.84 g of saccharose, 100 mL of 0.2 M phosphate buffer, pH 7.2–7.4.
4. 2% OsO_4 in distilled water (prepare 1 d before use so it will be fully dissolved).
5. Epon 812 (Serva, Heidelberg, Germany).
6. Propylene oxide.
7. DePeX (Merck, Germany).

2.1.1. Fine Sections from Epon-Embedded Tissue Blocks

In addition to the materials given in **Subheading 2.1.**

1. Gelatin capsules.
2. Lead citrate (Merck, Germany) and uranyl acetate (Merck, Germany).
3. Microtome.
4. Copper grids.

---

investigated factors (×450). **(B)** The subcellular localization of von-Willebrand factor (arrows) within endothelial cells by postembedding immune electron microscopy using the glucose oxidase method. Prior to fine sectioning for electron microscopy, tissue pieces were fixed with glutaraldehyde, embedded in Epon, and cut in semithin sections that were used for immunostaining. Note that the dark staining of the nucleus (N) is because of the fixation in osmium tetroxide (OsO_4) and is therefore nonspecific (×3600). **(C)** No specific immunostaining is visible in the control. Also, here the nucleus is nonspecific marked with OsO_4 (×3600).

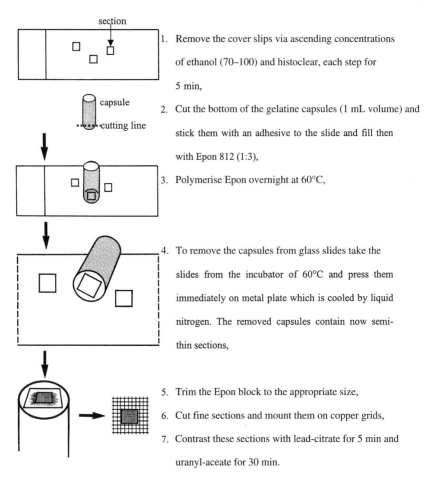

1. Remove the cover slips via ascending concentrations of ethanol (70–100) and histoclear, each step for 5 min,

2. Cut the bottom of the gelatine capsules (1 mL volume) and stick them with an adhesive to the slide and fill then with Epon 812 (1:3),

3. Polymerise Epon overnight at 60°C,

4. To remove the capsules from glass slides take the slides from the incubator of 60°C and press them immediately on metal plate which is cooled by liquid nitrogen. The removed capsules contain now semithin sections,

5. Trim the Epon block to the appropriate size,

6. Cut fine sections and mount them on copper grids,

7. Contrast these sections with lead-citrate for 5 min and uranyl-aceate for 30 min.

Fig. 5. Immune-labeled semithin sections are removed from slides and cut into fine sections for electron microscopy.

2.2. Immunostaining Methods

2.2.1. Immunohistochemistry (see Notes 3–9)

2.2.1.1. FIXATIONS

1. Bouin's solution: 5 mL of glacial acetic acid, 25 mL of 40% formaldehyde, 75 mL 1.2% picric acid (prepare fresh daily).
2. Or 4% paraformaldehyde: 4 g of paraformaldehyde (powder, **cave toxicity**!), 100 mL of phosphate-buffered saline (PBS) on a hotplate until the solution becomes clear, avoid boiling, then let cool down to room temperature. Do not use NaOH or HCl to clear the solution!

2.2.1.2. PARAFFIN-EMBEDDING

1. Fix tissues in Bouin's solution for 12–24 h.

Further procedure for embedding:

2. Place tissue pieces in 80% isopropanol for 60 min at room temperature (RT).
3. 96% Isopropanol for 60 min and for 90 min at RT.
4. 100% Isopropanol for 3 × 60 min and for 3 × 90 min at RT.
5. Paraplast–isopropanol for 120 min at 60°C.
6. Paraplast for 120 min at 60°C.
7. Paraplast for 120 min at 60°C.

2.2.1.3. PRETREATMENT

1. Precoat slides with chrome–gelatine prior to cutting sections: 500 mg of gelatine, 50 mg of chrome–alaune (potassium chrome sulfate), 100 mL of distilled water. Mix the components together and heat to 50°C while stirring the solution. Filter the warm clear solution twice.
2. Cut 5–7 μm thick sections from paraffin blocks and mount them on the precoated slides.
3. Histoclear.
4. Prepare ethanol in concentrations of 100%, 96%, 80%, and 70%.
5. Prepare 1.5% H_2O_2–methanol to block nonspecific peroxidase reaction.

2.2.1.4. SERUM AND ANTIBODIES

1. Normal serum: 2% normal rabbit serum (NRS) or 2% normal swine serum (NSS) are mostly used, but it depends on the species used for production of secondary antibody.
2. Primary antibody: Dilute it in PBS–0.2% bovine serum albumin (BSA) –0.01% NaN_3 if there is no further recommendation from the supplier.
3. Secondary antibody: Dilute in PBS (1:250), commonly antimouse IgG–biotin (produced in rabbit) if monoclonal antibody has been used or antirabbit IgG–biotin (produced in mouse) if polyclonal antibody was applied; again, consider the species in which the primary antibody has been produced.
4. PAP: Dilute in PBS (1:100), cave species (*see* **step 3**).
5. ABC: Dilute in PBS (1:250), mix solution A and B 30 min prior to use.

2.2.1.5. PEROXIDASE ACTIVATION WITH GLUCOSE OXIDASE

1. 30 mL of 0.1 M PBS, pH 7.4.
2. 15 mg of DAB (3,3'-diaminobenzidine tetrahydrochloride) (**warning: hazardous**).
3. 12 mg of ammonium chloride.
4. 600 μL 0.05 M nickel sulfate.
5. 600 μL of 10% β-D-glucose.
6. At the end: 100 μL (=0.12 mg) of glucose oxidase.

2.2.1.6. PEROXIDASE DEVELOPMENT WITH H_2O_2

1. 50 mL of Tris-HCl, pH 7.6.
2. 10 mg DAB (**warning: hazardous**).
3. 0.1 mL v/v H_2O_2 solution, 2.9 mL distilled water.

2.2.1.7. MOUNTING MEDIUM

1. DePeX.

2.2.2. Immune Electron Microscopy (see **Notes 10–13**)

1. 2 g of anhydrous KOH in 10 mL of methanol.
2. 5 mL of propylene oxide.
3. PAP pen.
4. Eppendorf pipet.
5. Epon remover solution (KOH–methanol–propylene oxide).
6. Absorbent paper.
7. 1:1 Methanol–PBS.
8. Moist chamber.
9. 0.2% BSA in PBS + 0.01% Triton X, 0.1% NaN_3.
10. Microcentrifuge.
11. DePeX mounting medium.

2.3. Chemotactic Assay (see **Notes 14–17**)

1. Endothelial cells and medium.
2. Serum-free medium–0.1% BSA: for HUVEC mostly Earle's medium 199 is the basal medium.
3. Chamber apparatus: Boyden chamber (two sides with wells, gasket, screws) (Neuro Probe Inc., Gaithersburg, MD).
4. Filter: Nucleopore polycarbonate membrane (8 μm).
5. Collagen (100 μg/mL): For membrane preparation (1 mg/mL of stock) (Vitrogen 100, Collagen Corp., Fremont, CA).
6. 0.2 N 0.1% Acetic acid: Add 5.75 mL of 17.4 M stock acetic acid to distilled water to form a 500-mL solution.
7. Cotton swabs, Q-tips, forceps.
8. Diff-Quik (Fast green in methanol is used for fixing cells to membrane; eosin is used for staining nuclei; thiazine dye is used to stain cytoplasm) (Dade Behring, Düdingen, Switzerland).

2.4. Endothelial Tube Formation Assay (see **Notes 18–20**)

1. 3.95 mL of distilled water.
2. 1 mL of 10X minimum essential medium (MEM).
3. 100 μL of L-glutamine (store at –20°C prior to use).
4. 100 μL of sodium pyruvate.
5. 4 mL of collagen (Vitrogen 100, Collagen Corp., Fremont, CA).
6. 500 μL of 7.5% sodium bicarbonate.

7. 40 µL of 0.1 *M* sodium hydroxide.
8. Ice, 50-mL tube, 24-well or 48-well cell culture plates.

2.5. CAM Assay (see Notes 21–25)

1. Plastic box for the eggs.
2. Chick eggs (Valo, Lohmann, Cuxhaven, Germany).
3. Mesh tissue (2 × 2 and 4 × 4 mm) (Tetko cat. no. 3-300/50, Rüschlikon, Switzerland).
4. Collagen (Vitrogen 100).

3. Methods

3.1. Examination of Vascular Morphology (see also Subheadings 1.1. and 2.1.)

1. Tissue should be cut in 2 × 2 mm pieces to obtain optimal fixation results in phosphate-buffered glutaraldehyde (5.5 %) for 12 h.
2. This is followed by further fixation in 2% OsO_4/saccharose–phosphate buffer (1:1) at 4°C for 2 h.
3. Next, the tissue is dehydrated in ethanol with ascending concentrations for 15 min each such as 35%, 50%, 70%, 96% and 3× in 100% ethanol.
4. The tissue should be incubated with propylene oxide for 2.5 h at 37°C.
5. Afterwards, the tissue pieces have to be incubated with propylene oxide–Epon (1:1) for 1h at 37°C.
6. The samples are subsequently incubated in propylene oxide–Epon (1:3) for 12 h (or overnight) at 37°C in closed tubes.
7. To ensure polymerization the Epon samples should be kept first at 37°C for 5–10 h, second at 45°C for 12 h, and finally at 60°C for 12–24 h.
8. Prior to the cutting of sections the edges of these blocks should be trimmed to the appropriate size.
   These Epon blocks serve as the basis for:
   a. semithin sections (0.5–2 µm thick) for light microscopic studies and
   b. fine (ultrathin) sections (70–90 nm) for electron microscopic examinations.

3.1.1. Semithin Section Technique (see Note 1)

Semithin sections (0.5–2 mm) from the tissue blocks made via a microtome should be stained with toluidine blue–pyronine, mounted on glass slides, and covered with coverslips using DePeX (Merck, Germany).

Toluidine blue–pyronine staining procedure *(17)*:

Dilution:
1. 1% toluidine blue (Chroma, Köngen, Germany) in 1% borax (dinatrium-tetraborat-10 hydrat) (Merck, Darmstadt, Germany).
2. 1% Pyronine G (Merck, Darmstadt, Germany) in distilled water.

Mix both solutions in the proportion toluidine blue–pyronine G (7:3).

1. Prior to use staining solution should be filtered.
2. Sections should be stained for 2–10 min at 80°C.

3. Then the sections should be transferred to glass slides that have been heated in incubator before use.
4. Sections should be covered with glass coverslips mounted via DePeX. Stained sections should be kept in darkness because of bleaching.

3.1.2. Transmission Electron Microscopy (TEM) (see **Note 2**)

Fine sections from Epon-embedded tissue blocks:

1. Fine sections (ca. 70–90 nm) from tissue blocks embedded in Epon 812 (*see* **Subheading 3.1.**) cut with microtome should be mounted on the copper grids.
2. The sections should be contrasted with lead citrate for 5 min.
3. The sections should then be contrasted with uranyl acetate for 30 min.

In comparison to light microscopy, electron microscopic examination of these fine sections allows the detailed study of:

1. Endothelial cell morphology (flattened or roundly shaped).
2. Inter-endothelial junctions (closed or open and which type of junctions).
3. The constitution of basal lamina (existence of lamina densa and peri-vascular connective tissue).
4. The contact between the endothelial tubes and the basal lamina.
5. The existence of peri-endothelial cells (pericytes in capillaries, smooth muscle cells in large blood vessels).
6. If these cells are partly in touch with endothelial cells and are integrated in the common basal lamina.

In many cases it is of particular interest to perform electron microscopic studies on microvessels that have been observed by light microscopy on semithin sections. To this aim, the procedure shown in **Fig. 5** should be applied.

1. Remove the coverslips via ascending concentrations of ethanol (70–100%) and Histoclear, each step for 5 min.
2. Cut the bottom of gelatin capsules (1 mL volume) and attach them to the slide with an adhesive and fill then with Epon 812 (1:3).
3. Allow to polymerize in Epon overnight at 60°C.
4. To remove the capsules from glass slides take the slides from the incubator of 60°C and press them immediately on a metal plate that is cooled by liquid nitrogen. The removed capsules now contain semithin sections.
5. Trim the Epon block to the appropriate size.
6. Cut fine sections and mount them on copper grids.
7. Contrast these sections with lead citrate for 5 min and uranyl acetate for 30 min.

3.2. Immunostaining Methods

(see also Subheadings 1.2. and 2.2.)

3.2.1. Immunohistochemistry (see **Notes 3–9**)

3.2.1.1. INDIRECT IMMUNOHISTOCHEMISTRY (THREE-STEP PROCEDURE)

1. Pretreatment:

a. Place paraffin wax-embedded sections in Histoclear for 2 × 5 min, then take through descending concentrations of ethanol (100%, 95%, 70%) for 5 min each.
b. Wash afterwards with distilled water for 5 min and then place in PBS for 15 min.
c. If necessary, block endogenous peroxidase by incubating sections in 1.5% H_2O_2 in methanol for 30 min before rehydrating in descending ethanol. This is particularly important when using polyclonal antibodies.
d. To block the nonspecific binding of secondary antibody, the sections should be incubated with 2% normal serum (dissolved in PBS) of that species that has been used for production of secondary antibody for 30 min. Mostly it is normal rabbit serum (NRS) if the primary antibody is monoclonal and normal swine serum (NSS) if it is polyclonal.

2. Primary antibody:
   a. Next, remove the serum by shaking the slides briefly and drying the area around the section without touching it.
   b. Then apply the solution with primary antibody on the section in the desired dilution. It is advisable to take three different dilutions of primary antibody when using it for the first time to test in which dilution the antibody gives the best immunoreaction.
   c. Let the sections incubate with antibody overnight at 4°C. In some cases, particularly when studying receptors the incubation time can be prolonged to 48 h.

3. Secondary antibody:
   a. On the second day, wash sections in PBS 3× for 10 min.
   b. Incubate them for 60 min with biotinylated secondary antibody (mostly IgG-biotin, for species *see* **step 1d**).
   c. Afterwards, wash sections in PBS 2× for 10 min.

4. Peroxidase antiperoxidase (PAP):
   a. Next, apply PAP (of adequate species) in a working dilution of 1:100 to the sections and wait for 30 min.
   b. Wash again in PBS for 2× for 10 min.

5. Avidin–biotin complex (ABC):
   a. Incubate the sections with prepared ABC solution for 30 min.
   b. Wash again in PBS for 1× for 10 min.

6. Development of immunoreaction:
   a. After further washing in PBS for 10 min, visualize the immunoreaction using the nickel-enhanced glucose oxidase technique.
   b. Dissolve 15 mg of DAB in 30 mL of PBS, then add 12 mg of ammoniumchloride, 600 µL of nickel sulfate, and 600 µL of β-D-glucose.
   c. Lastly, add 600 µL of glucose oxidase to the solution shortly before incubation of the sections contained in it.
   d. To obtain best visualization of the antigen observe the color development under the microscope.
   e. Stop the immunoreaction at the latest after 30 min by removing the development solution and washing with PBS (3× for 5 min).
   f. If counterstaining is needed stain the sections in Calcium Red for 1–2 min.
   g. Dehydrate the sections in ascending ethanol concentrations.
   h. Apply coverslips using DePeX.

Note: In comparison to this three-step procedure, the two-step technique is performed without the PAP step.

3.2.1.2. METHOD FOR DIRECT IMMUNOHISTOCHEMISTRY

Direct immunohistochemistry using biotin-labeled first antibody makes it possible to shorten the time.

1. The steps from pretreatment until the application of the primary antibody are the same as described in the indirect immunohistochemistry protocol.
2. Wash the sections in PBS for 2× for 10 min.
3. Then continue with the ABC step (as described previously).

3.2.2. Double-Staining

1. For double staining with two different primary antibodies, visualize the first immunostaining using the nickel-enhanced glucose oxidase technique of peroxidase development.
2. After this first staining, treat the sections again with the appropriate normal serum for 30 min.
3. Next, incubate with the second primary antibody for 24 h.
4. Develop the second immunoreaction using DAB–H_2O_2. Usually this staining is terminated after 10 min.
5. Follow the protocol described above in **Subheading 3.2.1.1., step 6e–h**.
6. The order of labeling will give a black color for the first and a brown color for the second antigen.

3.2.3. Immunohistochemistry on Cells

1. For immunohistochemistry on endothelial cells the cells should be grown on chamber slides, preferably on glass slides.
2. Fix cells in 4% paraformaldehyde for 15 min.
3. Wash with PBS 3× for 10 min.
4. Proceed with applying normal serum on the cells for 30 min.
5. Add primary antibody for 24 h.
6. Continue with the protocol for indirect immunohistochemistry.

The dehydration step in ascending ethanol series at the end is necessary so the mounting medium will adhere to the slide. In contrast, rehydration in descending alcohol series at the beginning is only for deparaffinization of paraffin sections.

3.2.4. Immune Electron Microscopy (see **Notes 10–13**)

Epon remover solution:

1. Dissolve 2 g of anhydrous KOH in 10 mL of methanol. The reaction is exothermic but it is necessary to apply some heat from a hotplate—**take care not to boil the methanol!**

2. While the KOH–methanol is still warm add 5 mL of propylene oxide. Use immediately while still warm.

Incubation on Epon sections:

1. The protocol begins with semithin Epon sections (0.5–1 μm thick) on glass slides (for further description *see* **Subheading 3.1.2.**). Dry at room temperature. With a wax pen, draw a circle around each section to contain the drops of solutions.
2. With an Eppendorf pipet drop Epon remover solution (KOH–methanol–propylene oxide) onto each slide for 2.5 min. The slides should be placed on absorbent paper (Lab mat) for this purpose.
3. Wash in 1:1 methanol–PBS for 3 min, then wash in PBS for 2 × 5 min.
4. For incubation, the slides are placed on a dampened double thickness paper towel. They should be covered to reduce evaporation. The resulting apparatus is referred to as a "moist chamber."
5. Block on a drop of 0.2% BSA in PBS + 0.01% Triton X, 0.1% NaN_3 for 10–20 min.
6. Incubate with 20 μL of primary antibody for 1 h (room temperature) to overnight (at 4°C). The concentration of antibody and incubation time are variable depending on the antibody used. Dilute the antibody in the 0.2% BSA blocking solution described previously. Microcentrifuge at 20,000*g* for 1 min prior to use.
7. Wash in PBS for 3× for 5 min.
8. Incubate with secondary antibody for 45 (or 30) min.
9. Wash in PBS for 3× for 5 min.
10. Development of immunoreaction should be performed as described in **Subheading 3.2.**
11. Put a drop of DePeX mounting medium over a part of labeled sections and carefully place a coverslip on the slide for light microscopic observation.
12. For electron microscopic studies, these immune-labeled sections should be reembedded in Epon as described in **Subheading 3.1.2.**

3.3. Chemotactic Assay (see also Subheadings 1.3., 2.3., and Notes 14–17)

1. Preparing the filter:
   a. Make 100 mL of collagen solution: 3.6 mL of Vitrogen 100 in 0.2 *M* acetic acid.
   b. Submerge the membrane completely in collagen solution.
   c. Incubate the membrane overnight (at least 4 h) at 37°C.
   d. The next day rinse wet membrane several times with serum-free medium/BSA using a Pasteur pipet. Avoid any bubbles and dirt on the membrane!
   e. Place wet membrane on slide and let it dry.
2. Setup for assay:
   a. Prepare a protocol containing concentration of cells used, of chemotactic agents, date and time of experiment, and a chamber letter.
   b. Prepare proteins in desired doses, 100 μL of each solution. The proteins should be dissolved in serum-free medium containing 0.5% BSA.
3. Harvesting the cells:
   a. Aspirate media and wash cells once with PBS.

   b. Trypsinate cells as usual.
   c. Bring up in media containing FCS.
   d. Take 20 μL of well mixed cell suspension to count cells using a Neubauer
       counting chamber and calculate how much of the cell suspension is needed:
       final concentrations of 300,000 cells/mL or 15,000 cells/well are necessary.
   e. Centrifuge cells for 5–7 min by 1600g.
   f. Aspirate supernatant and resuspend pellet in 10 mL of serum-free medium–BSA.
   g. Centrifuge again.
   h. Resuspend pellet this time in 5 mL of serum-free medium/0.1% BSA.
4. Preparing the wells:
   a. Choose an orientation in which order the chemotactic agents should be added
       to the bottom chamber. Add approx 30 μL of each agent to each well and each
       agent should be added in three wells.
   b. Place the filter as recommended by the supplier. Once the filter is in place,
       press down lightly on the frame to ensure that it adhers to the lower plate.
   c. Mount the gasket on the upper chamber and close the top plate and press
       firmly on it as you turn the knobs about one-third turn clockwise to seal the
       plates together.
   d. Allow to equilibrate in 5% CO_2 incubator (37°C) for several hours (for
       HUVECs usually 5 h; for microvascular endothelial cells 6 h).
5. Disassembling of chamber and staining filter:
   a. Remove the chamber from the incubator.
   b. Open the chamber gently and remove the filter carefully.
   c. Place filter (filter side up) for several minutes in Diff-Quick fixative and stain
       the cells first with eosin and then with thiazide dye each for 2–3 min.
   d. Clear immediately the nonmigrated cells from the top of the filter using a wet
       Q-tip and then let the filter dry.
   e. Count migrated cells using a light microscope: three areas of defined size
       should be counted in each well of the filter and the data should be entered in
       the chamber letter. For each agent the mean value of three wells should be
       calculated and visualized statistically.

3.4. Endothelial Tube Formation Assay
(see also Subheadings 1.4., 2.4., and Notes 18–20)

   Preparation of three-dimensional collagen gel:

1. All materials should be kept on ice under a laminar flow hood. Maintain sterility!
2. It is important to follow the sequence noted in **Subheading 2.4.** and to work quickly!
3. Use a 50-mL tube for preparing the gel. This makes it easier for further handling
   and keeping it sterile.
4. Mix gently after adding each component to the suspension (*see* **Subheading 2.4.**).
   All components will amount to 10 mL of gel.
5. After adding sodium hydroxide, pipet exactly 400 μL of the mixture quickly into
   a 24-well or 180 μL of gel in each well of a 48-well (tissue culture dishes)
   microplate. Avoid any bubbles.

Collagen gel invasion assay:

1. Endothelial cells should be seeded onto collagen gels at $2.5-5 \times 10^4$ cells/well in 300 µL of full medium.
2. Reduce the concentration of fetal calf serum (FCS) to 2% on the second or third day when the cells reach subconfluence to confluence and add then the compounds.
3. If necessary medium and compounds can be renewed every 2–3 d.

Quantification of invasion:

1. It is possible to quantify endothelial cell invasion by photographing three selected fields by phase-contrast microscopy **(Fig. 6A)**.
2. It is possible to measure invasion by determining the total additive length of all cellular structures that have formed cell cords or tubes *(18)*.

Processing for light and electron microscopy:

1. To this aim collagen gels should be fixed with 5.5% glutaraldehyde for at least 20 min but this fixation time can be prolonged to many weeks.
2. The gels then need to be removed from the wells. The border of the gels should be separated by a knife and then they should be aspirated very gently with a pipet and placed again in the 5.5% glutaraldehyde fixative for 12 h or longer.
3. These are postfixed in 1% osmium tetroxide (OsO_4) in saccharose–phosphate buffer: 2% OsO_4/saccharose–phosphate buffer (1:1).
4. The gels are stained *en bloc* with 2.5% uranyl acetate in ethanol.
5. They are not dehydrated through graded ethanol (75%, 95%, 100%).
6. The gels are then embedded in Epon 812 in flat molds.
7. Semithin sections (0.5–1 µm thick) are cut with ultramicrotome.
8. The sections are stained with 1% toluidine blue.

Also thin (80 nm thick) sections can be made from Epon blocks (*see* proceeding protocol) for electron microscopic analyses.

With light microscopy of semithin sections one can visualize the penetration of endothelial cells into the gel and capillary-like tube formation after stimulation of the cells with angiogenic factors **(Fig. 6B)** while in the control most of the endothelial cells lie on the gel surface and do not form tubes.

3.5. Chick CAM Assay (see also Subheadings 1.5., 2.5., and Notes 21–25)

The assay involves: preparation of the eggs, preparation of the mesh, placing the meshes containing the factors, and analysis.

1. Clean the eggs with 70% ethanol and work under the laminar flow hood. Open a window in the egg shell with sterile forceps with thick ends beginning from the concave end of the egg over the bubble. Avoid disruption of the egg membrane. In the second step, use new sterile forceps with thin ends to remove the membrane. Be careful not to damage the yolk with the embryo. Then place the eggs into the plastic box.

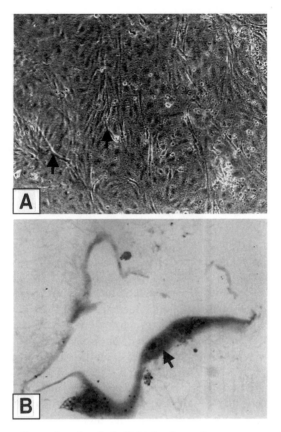

Fig. 6. (**A**) Three-dimensional endothelial tube formation assay on collagen gel. After stimulation with VEGF part of the cells are organized in endothelial tubes (arrows) (×100). (**B**) Conclusive evidence for capillary-like endothelial tube formation (arrow) can be obtained only in semithin sections of the gels (×750).

2. Mesh tissue should be cut into squares of 4×4 and 2×2 mm size and autoclaved prior to use. Neutralize 2 mL of type I collagen (Vitrogen 100) with 200 µL of 10× PBS and 40 µL of 0.1 N NaOH. Keep the neutralized Vitrogen on ice to avoid polymerization. Prepare a suspension by mixing the peptides with the neutralized Vitrogen. Pipet 20 µL of the suspension onto a 4×4 mm mesh and allow it to polymerize at 37°C. It is possible to apply another 2×2 mm mesh square onto the first to complete the sandwich.
3. Place the meshes with the polymerized mixture onto the CAM between two large vascular branches, preferably in the periphery. Ideally, three meshes should be used in each egg.
4. Angiogenic effects can be observed best after 48 h of stimulation of the CAM. There are many possibilities to measure and analyze capillary sprouting. Using the macroscope allows observation and documentation of the development of

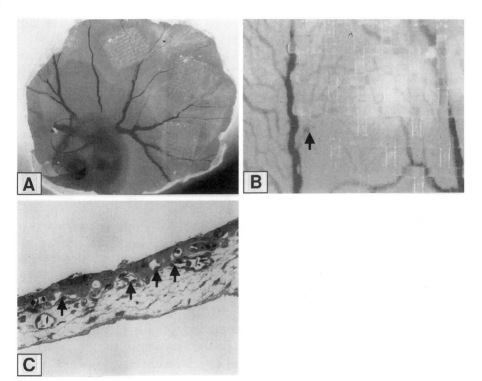

Fig. 7. Chick CAM assay. (**A**) Overview of blood vessels with the meshes in place that were used for application of angiogenic factors (×2). (**B**) Higher magnification reveals high density of brush-like vessels (arrow) after stimulation with VEGF for 48 h adjacent to and beneath the mesh (×25). (**C**) The meshes are important not only for application of factors but also for further analyses such as removal of the stimulated area and its light microscopical study using semithin sections. These semithin sections allow quantification of vascular density. This semithin section of a stimulated area of (**B**) shows also high density of blood vessels, particularly in the epithelial layer (arrows) (×650).

branch-like vessels (**Fig. 7B**). In addition, it is very useful to recover the meshes from the CAM after 48 h, fix them in glutaraldehyde, and process for light microscopical examination (**Fig. 7C**).

4. Notes

4.1. Examination of Vascular Morphology

4.1.1. Semithin Section Technique

1. The light microscopic evaluation of such sections is easy and allows the observation of cellular construction of blood vessel wall and perivascular tissues *(19)*. The wall of normal large blood vessels is composed of endothelial cells, several layers of smooth muscle cells and peri-vascular connective tissue (**Fig. 2A**). Such a construction of the

vascular wall is absent in large tumor blood vessels (**Fig. 2B**) in which smooth muscle cell layers are lacking or are poorly developed (**Fig. 2B**). Particularly, use of the ×100 objective lens permits assessment of the relationship between several components of the vascular wall such as the form of endothelial cells and the presence of basement membrane and peri-endothelial cells (pericytes in capillaries or smooth muscle cells in large blood vessels) (**Fig. 2C–F**). This is especially important for the observation of capillaries. The semithin technique allows identification of structural differences between normal (**Fig. 2C,D**) and tumor capillaries (**Fig. 2E–F**). As shown in **Fig. 2E–F** in tumor capillaries the endothelial cell are organized very loose owing to the lack of basement membrane and pericytes. This is important for tumor metastasis because the passage of tumor cells through such nonstabilized vascular wall is more easily achieved than through the normal blood vessels wall. With this technique, it is possible to evaluate if and how high the part of tumor blood vessels is that demonstrates such a nonstabilized vascular wall. Our studies on different tumor tissues revealed that in highly malignant tumors the majority of blood vessels are of the nonstabilized type and that there are region-specific differences within tumor tissues.

a. A weaker staining in the section center compared to the marginal zones is mostly caused by bad fixation of the tissue block. This is often the case when tissue pieces are too large.
b. For the evaluation of structural components it is important to handle the tissue pieces very carefully to avoid structural damages prior to fixation.
c. Spotted staining of sections mostly occurs when the staining solution has not been filtered.
d. Take care not to trap air bubbles under the coverslip when mounting it on the section.

4.1.2. Transmission Electron Microscopy (TEM)

2. In addition to light microscopic observation on semithin sections, electron microscopic analyses are appropriate to visualize interendothelial contact zones and to make clear if periendothelial cells are integrated in the basal lamina and if they have contact to endothelial cells, as shown for a normal capillary in **Fig. 3A**. Endothelial cells of newly formed blood vessels without basal lamina are mostly roundly shaped and there no specialized inter-endothelial contact zones are recognizable (**Fig. 3B**). In these cases there are also no peri-endothelial cells integrated in the vascular wall. The construction of a basal lamina is one of the main steps indicating vascular maturation. Successively, the recruitment of peri-endothelial cells and the formation of closed inter-endothelial contacts lead to a flattened shape of endothelial cells and mark the stabilization of the vascular wall. The further differentiation into large and small blood vessels is a process induced by different hydrostatic pressures and depends on the requirement of vascular permeability.
   Furthermore, it should be considered that pericytes (peri-endothelial cells in capillaries) do not form a closed layer around the endothelial tube and therefore

often only their processes are visible in cross-sections through vascular wall. Per definitionem, only those peri-endothelial cells are called pericytes that are integrated in the common basal lamina with endothelial cells.

   a. Collect waste of osmium, propylene oxide and Epon separately!

   b. Avoid air bubbles during placement of the gelatine capsule on the section; the whole semithin section should be covered by Epon. Otherwise the section can be damaged.

   c. Trim the new Epon block so that usable fine sections can be made as fast as possible. Consider that from a semithin section a maximum of 9–11 fine sections can be made.

4.2. Immunostaining Methods

4.2.1. Immunohistochemistry

3. Depending on the use of monoclonal or polyclonal antibody appropriate serum, second and third antibodies should be used. Often, anti-monoclonal antibodies are obtained from rabbit immunized against mouse and polyclonal antibodies from swine immunized against rabbit.

4. The following controls should be performed:

   a. Conduct preabsorption with the respective peptide.

   b. Replace the primary, secondary, or tertiary antibodies with PBS.

   c. Visualize only the peroxidase.

   d. Instead of the primary antisera, incubate sections with normal rabbit serum in concentrations ranging between 0.1% and 0.01%.

5. **DAB is toxic!** Store DAB in the dark to avoid the loss of its activity. Consider that it takes time until DAB is fully dissolved in PBS.

6. The mounting of sections using DePeX should be performed under the fume hood because the intensive smell causes headaches.

7. No immunoreaction:

   a. Primary antibody titer is incorrect: prepare different concentrations of the antibody and incubate the immunoreaction under the microscope for longer time.

   b. Primary antibody may not be useable for paraffin-embedded sections: if no usable primary antibody is available, perform immunohistochemistry on cryosections.

8. Strong background reaction:

   a. In general: The incubation time may be too long if primary antibody or secondary reagent could be too concentrated, if the wrong blocking serum has been used, if sections are too thick (sections should be at maximum 10 μm thick).

   b. Nonspecific staining in endothelial cells: Cationic conjugate of rabbit-Fab fragments and horseradish peroxidase type VI may react with the anionic parts of endothelial cytoplasm. Therefore, avoid horseradish peroxidase type VI.

   c. In erythrocytes, granulocytes, and monocytes (histiocytes) the (immuno) reaction is based on the endogenous peroxidase activity.

   d. For suppression use 1.5% H_2O_2–methanol for 30 min after the 100% ethanol step.

9. Other problems:

   a. Poor adhesion of the section to the slide causes poor morphology. Therefore,

use chrome-gelatine-precoated slides and place freshly cut sections overnight in an incubator to let them dry.
b. Cells are fixed on plastic slides. Avoid dehydration in ethanol and histoclear. Replace DePeX with gelatine to mount coverslips on the slides.

4.2.2. Immune Electron Microscopic Studies

10. It is very important that the semithin sections on the slides are as smooth as possible to avoid artificial background staining.
11. Use sections of different thickness depending on substances investigated: for small substances use 2 µm thick sections and for large molecules or for receptors sections of approx 4–7 µm thickness are of advantage.
12. Take care that the sections are small and can be removed from the slides entirely.
13. Avoid air bubbles during the reembedding process.

4.3. Chemotactic Assay

14. Use gloves and do not touch chamber apparatus with your fingers (lipids on your fingers are good stimulants for cell migration).
15. If no or few cells on the filter are visible:
    a. Incubation time was too short.
    b. The number of the cells was too small.
    c. There was no contact between sample solutions and the filter.
    d. Wells were not sufficiently cleaned.
16. If there are no significant differences between cell number in wells:
    a. The migrated cells were erroneously wiped from the filter.
    b. The incubation time was too long.
17. Other warnings:
    a. Make sure a slight meniscus is formed when agents are added.
    b. Be careful of air bubbles.

4.4. Endothelial Tube Formation Assay

18. The cell density on the collagen gel should be handled differentially: Human microvascular endothelial cells should be seeded onto the collagen gel at a high density (approximately confluent) whereas human umbilical vein endothelial cells can be seeded subconfluent.
19. Do not touch the gel with the pipet when placing the cells onto the gel or during application of angiogenic agents.
20. Do not cut the gels in pieces before fixation in glutaraldehyde or in Bouin's solution; otherwise the tubes can be damaged.

4.5. Chick CAM Assay

21. Do not touch the CAM during the opening process and do not use eggs undergoing bleeding.
22. Apply the meshes very gently to the CAM to avoid microinjury of blood vessels.
23. Do not place the meshes near the chick embryo.

24. To avoid a fast polymerization of collagen mix under the hood keep it on ice.
25. Another possibility is to crack the egg shells in a glass Petri dish to gain space for inserting the meshes. In this method, however, the loss of eggs is much higher than by breaking a window in the shell.

Acknowledgments

The authors are grateful to M. Böge, A. Salewski, S. Schlemmheit, and V. Hess for their laboratory assistance. We thank Dr. J. Weil and Dr. K. Lamszus and M. Ericsson (Harvard Medical School, Boston) for their technical advice. We also thank S. Harneit for editing the English text and M. Lück for graphic work.

References

1. Hanahan, D. and Folkman, J. (1996) Patterns and emerging mechanisms of the angiogenic switch during tumorigenesis. *Cell* **86,** 353–364.
2. Folkman, J. and D'Amore, P. A. (1996) Blood vessel formation: what is its molecular basis? *Cell* **87,** 1153–1155.
3. Hanahan, D. (1997) Signaling vascular morphogenesis and maintenance. *Science* **277,** 48–50.
4. Ergün, S., Kilic, N., Ziegler, G., Hansen, A., Nollan, P., Götze, J., et al. (2000) CEA-related cell adhesion molecule 1: A potent angiogenic factor and a major effector of vascular endothelial growth factor. *Mol. Cell* **5,** 311–320.
5. Davidoff, M. S. and Schulze, W. (1990) Combination of the peroxidase anti-peroxidase (PAP) and avidin–biotin–peroxidase complex (ABC) techniques: an amplification alternative in immunocytochemical staining. *Histochemistry* **93,** 531–536.
6. Itoh, Z., Akiva, K., Nakamura, S., Miguno, M., Nakamura, Y., and Sugimoto, T. (1979) Application of coupled oxidation reaction to electron microscopic demonstration of horseradish peroxidase : cobalt glucose oxidase method. *Brain Res.* **75,** 341–346.
7. Záborszky, L. and Léránth, C. (1985) Simultaneous ultrastructural demonstration of retrogradely transported horseradish peroxidase and choline acetyltransferase immunoreactivity. *Histochemistry* **82,** 529–537.
8. Ergün, S., Kilic, N., Fiedler, W., and Mukhopadhyay, A. K. (1997) Vascular endothelial growth factor and its receptors in normal human testicular tissue. *Mol. Cell. Endocrinol.* **131,** 9–20.
9. Ergün, S., Luttmer, W., Fiedler, W., and Holstein, A. F. (1998) Functional expression and localization of vascular endothelial growth factor and its receptors in the human epididymis. *Biol. Reprod.* **58,** 160–168.
10. Polak, J. M. and Priestley, J. V. (1992) *Electron Microscopic Immunocytochemistry. Principles and Practice.* (Polak, J. M. and Priestley, J. V., eds.), Oxford University Press, Oxford.
11. Zetter, B. R. (1987) Assay of capillary endothelial cell migration. *Methods Enzymol.* **147,** 135–44.
12. Schmidt, N. O., Westphal, M., Hagel, C., Ergün, S., Stavrou, D., Rosen, I. M., and Lamszus, K. (1999) Levels of vascular endothelial growth factor, hepatocyte

growth factor/scatter factor and basic fibroblast growth factor in human gliomas and their relation to angiogenesis. *Int. J. Cancer (Pred. Oncol.)* **84,** 10–18.

13. Montesano, R., Orci, L., and Vassali, P. (1983) In vitro rapid organization of endothelial cells into capillary-like networks is promoted by collagen matrices. *J. Cell. Biol.* **97,** 1648–1652.

14. Montesano, R. and Pepper, M. S. (1996) Three-dimensional in vitro assay of endothelial cell invasion and capillary tube morphogenesis. In Little, C. and Sage, H. (eds.), *Vascular Morphogenesis*, Birkhauser, Boston.

15. Iruela-Arispe, M. L., Lane, T. F., Redmond, D., O´Reilly, M., Bolender, R. P., Kavanagh, T. J., and Sage, E. H. (1995) Expression of SPARC during development of the chicken chorioallantoic membrane: evidence for regulated proteolysis in vivo. *Mol. Biol. Cell* **6,** 327–343.

16. Klagsbrun, M., Knighton, D., and Folkman, J. (1976) Tumor angiogenesis activity in cells grown in tissue culture. *Cancer Res.* **36,** 110–114.

17. Holstein, A. F. and Wulfhekel, U. (1971) Die Semidünnschnitt-Technik als Grundlage für eine cytologische Beurteilung der Spermatogenese des Menschen. *Andrologia* **3,** 65–69.

18. Pepper, N. S., Ferrara, N., Orci, L., and Montesano, R. (1992) Potent synergism between vascular endothelial growth factor and basic fibroblast growth factor in the induction of angiogenesis in vitro. *Biochem. Biophys. Res. Commun.* **189,** 824–831.

19. Ergün, S., Davidoff, M. S., and Holstein, A. F. (1996) Capillaries in the lamina propria of human seminiferous tubules are partly fenestrated. *Cell Tissue Res.* **286,** 93–102.

14

Galectin-3 Binding and Metastasis

Pratima Nangia-Makker, Yuichiro Honjo, and Avraham Raz

1. Introduction

Galectin-3 (gal-3) is a member of a growing family of carbohydrate-binding proteins. It consists of two functional domains: an amino-(N)-terminal domain, which is cleavable by collagenases and is responsible for dimerization as well as secretion of the protein, and a carboxy-(C)-terminal domain with affinity for carbohydrates containing *N*-acetylactosamine residues. Gal-3 is present in the nucleus, the cytoplasm, and also the extracellular matrix of many normal and neoplastic cell types. However, an array of reports show an up-regulation of this protein in transformed and metastatic cell lines *(1,2)*. Moreover, in many human carcinomas, an increased expression of gal-3 correlates with progressive tumor stages *(3–6)*.

Several lines of analysis have demonstrated that the galectins participate in cell–cell and cell–matrix interactions by recognizing and binding complementary glycoconjugates and thereby play a crucial role in normal and pathological processes. Elevated expression of the protein is associated with an increased capacity for anchorage-independent growth, homotypic aggregation, and tumor cell lung colonization *(7–9)*. In this chapter we describe the method of purification of gal-3 from transformed *E. coli* and some of the commonly used functional assays for gal-3 binding. These functions of gal-3 are dependent on its carbohydrate binding properties and therefore can be inhibited by specific disaccharide inhibitor, namely lactose.

To analyze the binding of gal-3 to its receptors, the most commonly used protocol involves labeling the protein either by biotin or by ^{125}I *(10,11)*. We have discussed the biotinylation protocol because of its relative simplicity and avoidance of radioactive reagents. After binding of biotin-labeled protein to the cell surface receptors, the binding efficiency can be measured in terms of color development by using a substrate chromogen mixture.

From: *Methods in Molecular Medicine, vol. 58:*
Metastasis Research Protocols, Vol. 2: Cell Behavior In Vitro and In Vivo
Edited by: S. A. Brooks and U. Schumacher © Humana Press Inc., Totowa, NJ

Laminin, fibronectin, or collagen type IV are the extracellular matrix (ECM) proteins with affinity for gal-3 *(12)*. In **Subheading 3.2.1.**, we describe the assay for binding of the cell surface proteins to ECM ligands. Because a number of surface proteins can bind to a ligand, this is generally performed as an indirect assay with a number of cell lines varying in their gal-3 expression that are derived from the same origin.

It has been presumed that tumor cell surface lectins might play a role in cellular interactions in vivo that are important for the formation of emboli and for the arrest of circulating tumor cells *(13)*. Homotypic aggregation is an assay that reflects on the formation of tumor cell emboli in circulation. This assay is performed using asialofetuin, which is a glycoprotein possessing several branched oligosaccharide side chains with terminal nonreducing galactosyl residues. It binds to the lectins present on the cell surface of tumor cells and induces homotypic aggregation by serving as a crosslinking bridge between adjacent cells *(14)*.

One in vitro property of tumorigenic cells is their ability to grow progressively in semisolid medium, which indicates an autonomy from growth regulatory mechanisms *(15)*. Anchorage-independent growth is an assay in which the cells are seeded on soft agar and allowed to grow. The cells that divide and form colonies over a period of 10–15 d usually exhibit a higher metastatic potential in in vivo studies *(6)*.

2. Materials

2.1. Purification of Gal-3

1. LB broth: 1% Tryptone, 0.5% yeast, 1% NaCl, 10 mM MgCl$_2$, pH 7.5.
2. Gal-3 expressing bacterial clone: *E. coli* transformed with a suitable vector containing cDNA encoding the human gal-3 transcript.
3. Ampicillin: 1% Ampicillin. Ampicillin stock should be stored at –20°C.
4. Lysis buffer: 150 mM NaCl; 1% Nonidet P-40 (NP-40), 0.5% deoxycholate (DOC), 0.1% sodium dodecyl sulfate (SDS), 50 mM Tris-Tris-HCl, pH 8.0; 0.1% leupeptin; 1 mM phenylmethylsulfonyl fluoride (PMSF). Leupeptin and PMSF stocks should be stored at –20°C and added prior to use.
5. Isopropyl-β-D-thiogalactopyranoside (IPTG): 0.1 M IPTG.
6. Phosphate buffer: 8 mM Na$_2$HPO$_4$, 2 mM NaH$_2$PO$_4$, 1 mM MgSO$_4$, 1 mM PMSF, 0.2% NaN$_3$, 5 mM dithiothreitol (DTT) (pH 7.2). PMSF and DTT should be added just prior to use.
7. Elution buffer: phosphate buffer containing 0.3 M lactose.
8. 3-(*N*-Morpholino)propane sulfonic acid (MOPS) buffer: 0.5 M, pH 7.5.
9. Asialofetuin column: Prepare as follows and store at 4°C.

2.2. Preparation of Asialofetuin

1. Dissolve 100 mg of fetuin in 40 mL of 0.025 N H$_2$SO$_4$.
2. Incubate the solution at 80°C for 1 h.
3. Dialyze against 40 L of distilled H$_2$O to remove the SO$_4$ ions.

4. Lyophilize overnight and resuspend in 13 mL of water.
5. To make sure that the fetuin is converted into asialofetuin, run it on a reducing SDS-polyacrylamide gel. Fetuin runs at ~66 kDa, whereas asialofetuin runs a little lower (*see* **Note 1**).

2.3. Preparing Asialofetuin Column

1. Dissolve asialofetuin in 0.5 *M* MOPS buffer at a concentration of 10 mg/mL.
2. Take 5 mL of affigel-15 (Bio-Rad cat. no. 153-6051) slurry and wash with 15 vol of cold deionized water, less than 20 min before the coupling reaction.
3. For the coupling reaction combine 4 mL of 10 mg/mL cold asialofetuin–buffer solution with 4 mL of affigel-15. Mix at 4°C for 2 h.
4. Centrifuge the slurry, pour off the supernatant, and resuspend in deionized water. Add 1 *M* ethanolamine, pH 8.0, at 0.1 mL/mL of mixture to block the unreacted sites. Agitate gently at 4°C for 1 h.
5. Pack a column with the slurry, leave overnight in a cold room, and wash with 0.1 *M* MOPS buffer until eluent is free of protein.
6. Equilibrate column in 10 m*M* phosphate buffer containing 0.2% sodium azide (*see* **Note 2**).

2.4. Binding of Gal-3 to Cell Surface Receptors

1. Recombinant gal-3.
2. EZ-link, Sufo-NHS-Biotinylation Kit (Pierce, IL).
3. Substrate chromogen mixture (prepared immediately before use): Dissolve 0.5 mg/mL of ABTS 2,2'-azino-thiazoline sulfonic acid (ABTS) in 0.1 *M* citrate buffer, pH 4.2, containing 0.03% hydrogen peroxide. Alternatively, ABTS substrate kit for HRP (Zymed Laboratories, Inc., CA) can be used.
4. Lactose: 1 *M* in distilled H_2O.
5. 96-Well microtiter plates.
6. Enzyme-linked immunosorbent assay (ELISA) plate reader.

2.5. Binding of Gal-3 to Soluble ECM Proteins

1. 96-Well microtiter plates.
2. Engelbreth-Holm-Swarm (EHS) laminin or human placenta laminin:100 µg/mL, store at –20°C.
3. Collagen type IV: 100 µg/mL, store at –20°C.
4. Fibronectin: 100 µg/mL, store at –20°C.
5. Phosphate-buffered saline (PBS).
6. Bovine serum albumin (BSA): 30% in distilled water; store at 4°C.
7. Alamar blue (Biosource International).
8. ELISA Plate reader.

2.6. Homotypic Aggregation

1. EDTA: 0.02% in $Ca^{+2}Mg^{+2}$ free (CMF)-PBS.
2. Asialofetuin: As described in **Subheading 2.1.**
3. Formaldehyde.

4. Trypan blue: 0.4% in normal saline.
5. Glass tubes coated with Sigmacote (Sigma Chemical): Pour 1 mL of Sigmacote in the glass tube and rotate the tube, so that the entire area inside the tube is covered with Sigmacote. Let it dry and wash the excess with distilled water.
6. Orbital shaker.
7. Hemocytometer.

2.7. Anchorage Independent Growth

1. Complete medium: Appropriate medium with 10% fetal bovine serum (FBS).
2. 1% Agar solution: Add 1 g of sea-plaque agarose in 10 mL of distilled H_2O and autoclave. Cool down to 45°C and add 90 mL of complete medium and mix well. Agar solution in medium can be stored at 45°C for 2–3 d.
3. 2.5% Glutaraldehyde.
4. 6-Well plates.

3. Methods
3.1. Isolation of Recombinant Gal-3

1. Inoculate 10 mL of LB broth containing 100 µg/mL of ampicillin with gal-3 expressing bacterial clone.
2. Incubate overnight at 37°C with constant shaking at 225 rpm.
3. Use the overnight bacterial culture to inoculate fresh 10×200 mL of LB containing 100 µg/mL of ampicillin.
4. Incubate for 3 h at 37°C with shaking at 225 rpm (*see* **Note 3**).
5. Add ampicillin again and 2.5 mL of IPTG stock to induce the protein synthesis. It is important to add more ampicillin to allow only the resistant bacteria to grow.
6. Incubate for 4 h at 37°C with shaking at 225 rpm.
7. Transfer the contents to centrifuge bottles and centrifuge for 15 min at 1000*g* at 4°C.
8. Discard the supernatant and resuspend pellet containing the bacteria in 20 mL of PBS, combine into one bottle, and centrifuge for 15 min at 1000*g* at 4°C .
9. Discard the supernatant and store pellet at –70°C overnight. The pellet can be stored for up to 1 wk without losing the protein yield.
10. Resuspend pellet in 80 mL of ice-cold lysis buffer.
11. Disrupt the cells with a probe type sonicator using multiple short bursts at maximum intensity for 4×30 s on ice. Do not sonicate for more than 30 s at one time; otherwise the temperature of the lysate will increase and degrade some of the proteins. In between the strokes, cool the lysate on ice.
12. Centrifuge the lysate for 20 min at 18,000*g* and save the supernatant. The rest of the steps are performed in a cold room.
13. Equilibrate the asialofetuin column with three bed volumes of phosphate buffer.
14. Load the supernatant from **step 13**. Allow the supernatant to flow through the column at the rate of 10–12 drops per minute.
15. Wash the column with three bed volumes of phosphate buffer.
16. Elute the protein with 15 mL of elution buffer in 1-mL fractions.
17. Wash the column with three bed volumes of phosphate buffer. The column can be reused if stored properly at 4°C.

18. Measure the protein content of the samples collected from **step 16** by using standard protein estimation methods. Pool samples containing the protein and dialyze against PBS until all lactose is removed from the samples. The purified protein can be stored at –70°C (*see* **Notes 4–7**).

3.2. Binding of Gal-3 to Cell Surface Receptors

1. Isolate recombinant gal-3 as described in **Subheading 3.1.**

3.2.1. Biotinylation of Gal-3

1. Dissolve 2 mg of protein in 1 mL of PBS solution and calculate the number of millimoles dissolved using the following formula:

$$\frac{\text{mg of protein}}{\text{MW of protein}} \quad = \quad \text{mmol of protein}$$

2. Dissolve 2 mg of sulfo–NHS–biotin in 100 µL of distilled water and add 30 µL of this solution to the protein solution to give 20-fold molar excess over gal-3.
3. Incubate on ice for 2 h for biotinylation of gal-3 to be completed.
4. To remove excess salt from the protein, equilibrate the 10-mL desalting column with 30 mL of PBS and apply the protein sample. Allow the sample to permeate the gel. Add buffer to the column in 1-ml aliquots and collect 1-ml fractions of the purified eluent protein in separate test tubes.
5. Monitor protein content in the tubes by absorbance at 280 nm and pool fractions containing protein (*see* **Note 8**).

3.2.2. Binding of Gal-3 to the Receptors

1. Plate cells in a 96-Well plate at a density of 1×10^4 cells per well and incubate overnight.
2. Adjust the concentration of biotinylated gal-3 ranging from 0 to 20 µL/50 µL.
3. Remove medium from the cells.
4. Add fresh medium containing 0.5% fetal calf serum (FCS) and add 50 µL of biotin-labeled gal-3 at different concentrations (*see* **Note 9**).
5. Incubate the plates for 2 h at 37°C.
6. Wash 3× with PBS to remove unbound proteins.
7. Add a 1:1000 dilution of horseadish peroxidase (HRP)-conjugated streptavidin–avidin complex to the wells. The HRP-conjugated complex binds to biotin-labeled gal-3. Incubate for 30 min at room temperature.
8. Wash with PBS 3× to remove unbound complex.
9. Color development is obtained by the addition of 100 µL of substrate chromogen mixture. Incubate for 1 min (*see* **Note 10**).
10. Measure optical density (OD) at 405 nm.

3.3. Binding of Gal-3 to ECM

1. Coat the 96-well microtiter plates with serially diluted (0–10 µg) EHS laminin, collagen type IV, or fibronectin.

2. Incubate the plates for 1 h at 37°C or at 4°C overnight to dry the ECM protein (*see* **Note 11**).
3. Block the nonspecific sites in the wells by incubating with sterile 1% BSA in PBS for 1 h at 37°C.
4. Wash wells with sterile PBS 3× to remove extra proteins.
5. Trypsinize the cells and seed at 4×10^4 cells per well.
6. Allow the cells to adhere to the plates for 15 min to 24 h. This time can be varied according to the requirement of the experiment.
7. Wash off the nonadherent cells with medium. Repeat twice (*see* **Note 12**).
8. To count the number of cells attached to the ECM proteins, add 200 µL of medium and a 1:10 dilution of Alamar blue. The live cells create a reducing environment that changes the color of dye from blue to pink.
9. Incubate for 3–4 h at room temperature.
10. Read absorbance at 570 nm.

3.4. Homotypic Aggregation

1. Detach the cells from monolayer with 0.02% EDTA in CMF-PBS. Use of trypsin is avoided because it may interfere with the surface proteins.
2. Suspend at 1×10^6 cells per ml in CMF-PBS with or without 20 µg/mL asialofetuin.
3. Place 0.5-mL aliquots in siliconized glass tubes. Agitate at 80 rpm for 60 min at 37°C.
4. Terminate the aggregation by fixing the cells with 1% formaldehyde in CMF-PBS.
5. Count the number of single cells by hemacytometer (*see* **Notes 13–15**) **(Fig.1)**.
6. Calculate % aggregation by $(1 - Nt/Nc) \times 100$, where Nc is the number of single cells in control and Nt is the number of single cells in the presence of test compound.

3.5. Anchorage-Independent Growth

1. Pour 2 mL of 1% agar solution into 6-well plates.
2. Allow it to solidify at room temperature for 15–20 min. Transfer to 4°C for 2 h. Plates can be wrapped with parafilm and stored at 4°C for about 2 wk.
3. Suspend 500 or 1000 cells in 1 mL of complete medium. Immediately add 1 mL of 1% agar solution. Mix and pour gently on the plates (*see* **Note 13**).
4. Let the cell-containing top layer solidify at room temperature for 15 min and 2 h at 4°C.
5. Transfer to 37°C in a CO_2 incubator for overnight.
6. Next morning, add 1 mL of complete medium, and allow the colonies to grow for 2 wk. Medium should be changed 2× per week (*see* **Note 16**).
7. Fix colonies with 2.5% glutaraldehyde and compare the number and size of the colonies **(Fig. 2)**.

4. Notes

1. In the dialyzed form, asialofetuin can be stored at 4°C for months.
2. The binding efficiency of asailofetuin in the column can be determined by calculating the protein content in the flow through.

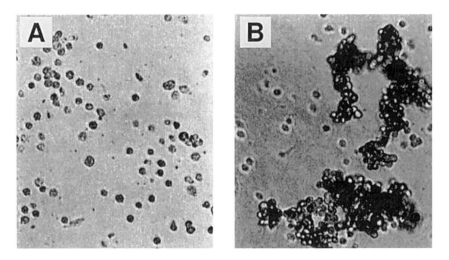

Fig. 1. Homotypic aggregation of Hs852 cells in the absence (**A**) or presence (**B**) of asialofetuin.

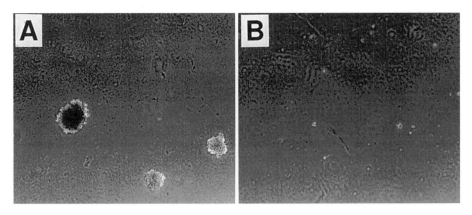

Fig. 2. Soft agar colony formation by a metastatic (MDA-MB-435) (**A**) and nontumorigenic (BT-549) (**B**) breast cancer cell line.

3. After **step 5**, determine the OD at 600 nm. It should be 0.5.
4. The normal yield of gal-3 from 1 L of bacterial culture varies from 1–5 mg. If the yield is too low, we suggest going through **Notes 5–7**.
5. After **step 13**, resuspend the pellet in fresh lysis buffer (20 mL/tube) and repeat sonication and centrifugation, again saving the supernatant.
6. After **step 15**, save the flowthrough and reload onto the column.
7. At no stage let the column dry, because it will reduce the binding efficiency.
8. Store biotinylated protein at 4°C until ready for use. The protein can be stored under these conditions for 1 wk.

9. In some wells 50–100 m*M* lactose can be added along with the protein for specific inhibitory studies.
10. The biotin–streptavidin complex cleaves H_2O_2 which is coupled to the oxidation of substrate ABTS, giving a green end product.
11. Make sure to keep the plates in a horizontal position, so that there is a uniform coating on the well.
12. The wells should be washed thoroughly to remove the unbound protein. However, the washes should be gentle so the cells remain unaffected.
13. Make sure that the cells are a single-cell suspension after detaching from monolayers.
14. It is important to siliconize the glass tubes in which aggregation is performed so cells do not adhere to the glass.
15. The aggregates are usually very fragile and can be disrupted by harsh pipetting.
16. The agarose layers should be allowed to gel completely to prevent the sliding of the top layer or passage of the cells to the bottom of the plates.

Acknowledgment

This work was supported in part by NIH Grant RO1-CA46120.

References

1. Raz, A. and Lotan, R. (1987) Endogenous galactoside-binding lectins: a new class of functional tumor cell surface molecules related to metastasis. *Cancer Metast. Rev.* **6,** 433–452.
2. Raz, A., Zhu, D., Hogan, V., Shah, N., Raz, T., Karkash, R., et al. (1990) Evidence for the role of 34-kDa galactoside-binding lectin in transformation and metastasis. *Int. J. Cancer* **46,** 871–877.
3. Lotan, R., Ito, H., Yasui, W., Yokozaki, H., Lotan, D., and Tahara, E. (1994) Expression of a 31 kDa lactose-binding lectin in normal human gastric mucosa and in primary and metastatic gastric carcinomas. *Int. J. Cancer* **56,** 474–480.
4. Bresalier, R. S., Mazurek, N., Sternberg, L. R., Byrd, J. C., Yunker, C. K., Nangia-Makker, P., and Raz, A. (1998) Metastasis of human colon cancer is altered by modifying expression of the beta galactoside-binding protein galectin-3. *Gastroenterology* **115,** 287–296.
5. Xu, X.-C., El-Nagger, A., and Lotan, R. (1995) Differential expression of galectin-1 and galectin-3 in thyroid tumors: potential diagnostic implications. *Am. J. Pathol.* **147,** 815–822.
6. Nangia-Makker, P., Thompson, E. W., Hogan, C., Ochieng, J., and Raz, A. (1995) Induction of tumorigenicity by gal-3 in a non-tumorigenic human breast carcinoma cell line. *Int. J. Oncol.* **7,** 1079–1087.
7. Lotan, R., Lotan, D., and Raz, A. (1985) Inhibition of tumor cell colony formation in culture by a monoclonal antibody to endogenous lectin. *Cancer Res.* **45,** 4349–4353.
8. Meromsky, L., Lotan, R., and Raz, A. (1986) Implications of endogenous tumor cell surface lectins as mediators of cellular interactions and lung colonization. *Cancer Res.* **46,** 5270–5275.
9. Lotan, R. and Raz, A. (1988) Endogenous lectins as mediators of tumor cell adhesion. *J. Cell. Biochem.* **37,** 107–117.

10. Raz, A., Meromsky, L., Zvibel, I., and Lotan, L. (1987) Transformation-related changes in the expression of endogenous cell lectins. *Int. J. Cancer* **39,** 353–360.
11. Dong, S. and Hughes, R. C. (1997) Macrophage surface glycoproteins binding to galectin-3 (Mac2-antigen). *Glycoconj. J.* **14,** 267–274.
12. Warfield, P. R., Nangia-Makker, P., Raz, A., and Ochieng, J. (1997) Adhesion of human breast carcinoma to extracellular matrix proteins is modulated by galectin-3. *Invas. Metast.* **17,** 101–112.
13. Lotan, R. and Raz, A. (1983) Low colony formation in vivo and culture as exhibited by metastatic melanoma cells selected for reduced homotypic aggregation. *Cancer Res.* **43,** 2088–2093.
14. Inohara, H. and Raz, A. (1994) Effects of natural complex carbohydrate (citrus pectin) on murine melanoma cell properies related to galectin-3 functions. *Glycoconj. J.* **11,** 527–532.
15. Cifone, M. A. and Fidler, I. J. (1980) Correlation of patterns of anchorage-independent growth with in vivo behavior of cells from a murine fibrosarcoma. *Proc. Natl. Acad. Sci. USA* **77,** 1039–1043.

III

ANIMAL MODELS OF METASTASIS

15

Basic Principles for the Study of Metastasis Using Animal Models

Suzanne A. Eccles

1. Introduction: Why Do We Need In Vivo Metastasis Models?

Metastasis is the most devastating aspect of cancer, and the major reason for treatment failure. It is perhaps surprising, therefore, that it is only relatively recently that a wide variety of clinically relevant metastasis models have become generally available. For more than 20 years, the mainstays of cancer research were a handful of transplanted rodent tumors. A few of these (most notably B16F10 and Lewis lung carcinoma) were used as metastasis models, generally by injecting the cells intravenously to give lung colonies. The cancer research community and pharmaceutical industry could be criticized for coming up with few if any new drugs effective against solid tumor metastases. Yet is this surprising when for many years the "NCI screen" consisted of mouse ascites tumors? These are localized, "liquid" tumors, where drug access is direct and blood supply irrelevant, a poor model for solid deposits in a multiplicity of body compartments with varying vascular architecture and function. Such assays are more likely to produce drugs effective against leukemias (*1*).

This primary screen was dropped in favor of panels of human tumor cell lines grown in monolayer culture in vitro and exposed to drugs for short periods. This is possibly an appropriate strategy for simple cytotoxic agents, but random screening for antimitotic drugs has given way to development of new agents directed at novel molecular targets that drive the malignant phenotype. It is now recognized that drugs that do not have a direct DNA-damaging effect may require much longer exposure to cells to exert their effects. There is also a growing appreciation of the importance of the microenvironment, and the need to test new drugs in the appropriate cellular context. For example, inhibitors of certain signal transduction elements (e.g., *ras* farnesyltransferase) are poorly active in

From: *Methods in Molecular Medicine, vol. 58:*
Metastasis Research Protocols, Vol. 2: Cell Behavior In Vitro and In Vivo
Edited by: S. A. Brooks and U. Schumacher © Humana Press Inc., Totowa, NJ

"2D" (monolayer) cultures and only accurately assessible in 3D or "nonattached" cell proliferation assays *(2,3)*. Similarly, many drugs have an antiangiogenic component that can greatly increase their efficacy in vivo *(4)*. Such properties are not detectable in in vitro assays or "hollow fiber" in vivo tumor assays.

Drug resistance (including relative expression of multidrug resistance markers) varies with site of tumor growth *(5,6)*, and an interesting "community effect" whereby resistance (independent of drug access) is induced in tumor spheroids has recently been described *(7)*. These observations show that monolayer cultures are likely to be unrealistically sensitive to cytotoxic drugs compared with solid tumor metastases. In contrast, some important potential targets for therapy (e.g., epidermal growth factor receptor [EGFR]) are upregulated in metastasis *(8,9)* — and indeed contribute directly to the invasive and angiogenic phenotype *(10,11)*; hence, assaying potential inhibitors in vitro or against primary xenograft tumors may underestimate efficacy against metastases.

Until recently, there was little encouragement for the use of metastatic tumors in drug discovery initiatives, where the imperative was high-throughput screening, and such models were considered cumbersome, expensive, and difficult *(12)*. Nevertheless, the exclusive use of reductionist assays can be more "expensive" in the long run if they fail to identify agents that are effective against metastases. The poor predictability of many of the tumor cell lines in current use was elegantly demonstrated in a study by Freije et al., who asked the deceptively simple question: "Do any of the current anticancer drugs in clinical use show any selectivity for metastatic cells?" They used cells with low nm23 (which in several tumor types is associated with the metastatic phenotype), and tested a wide variety of drugs using the COMPARE computer algorithm. The clear outcome was that none of the 171 standard cytotoxic agents showed any selectivity for these cells *(13)*. Nevertheless, it was possible to identify 40 new agents in the NCI repository of 30,000 compounds with the desired selectivity for metastatic cells, suggesting that such a strategy is viable.

More effective therapeutics will emerge from a better understanding of the key differences between normal cells and metastatic cancer cells—cell proliferation (the original target for chemotherapeutic agents) does not give us that differential. Because tumor progression involves further genetic changes, an appreciation of those molecules that are misregulated in metastases will provide more opportunities for effectively targeting disseminated disease. For example, it is clear that the c-*erb*B oncogenes are overexpressed in cancers with high metastatic potential, and data show that their activation upregulates many components of the metastatic phenotype, including cell motility, invasion, protease production, and angiogenesis. Also, such cells are more likely to be refractory to conventional therapy. These observations not only explain some of the failures of current drugs, but also provide new, validated, molecular targets for intervention *(14–16)*.

It has been claimed that the systems for identifying new drugs are faulty, and animal models have been criticized for failing to predict efficacy in humans *(1)*. I believe this does not invalidate the use of experimental models, but eloquently illustrates that the *wrong* (often simple "ectopic" nonmetastatic xenograft) models may be of limited value. Similar criticisms have been leveled at the failure of preclinical testing to identify the teratogenic activity of thalidomide; again this could be reinterpreted to indicate that if the *right* tests had been done (as they have since), the correct result would have been obtained. Well-chosen models will lead to a greater understanding of the molecular bases of metastasis, and hence to the development of more effective therapies. The challenges faced by a tumor cell as it leaves the primary site and ultimately settles and proliferates at a secondary site are (at the cellular and molecular level) likely to be very similar in mice and men. Our task is to identify these basic requirements and design experiments appropriate for testing new agents. These will vary depending on the target and which component of the metastatic cascade is involved. This section of the book will guide the reader through some of the recent developments in in vivo modeling. However, no model is perfect, and further refinements and advances will come only if sufficient investment is made to rigorously assess their predictive value *(17)*.

2. Choice of System: What Are We Modeling?

Often, a metastasis model is used for a study simply because it is available within a department and the group is familiar with it. It may, however, be ideal for some studies but not others. A better strategy would be to evaluate exactly what properties are required from the model for the hypothesis under test and select as appropriate from all available sources. Every model has strengths and weaknesses—no single human cancer could serve as a model for all, so it is unrealistic to expect one or a few animal tumors to do so. Sometimes simple in vitro systems that mimic a particular aspect of metastasis (motility, protease secretion) are sufficient to test a hypothesis; usually at least some further in vivo assays are required. If the question relates to the process of metastasis itself, then ideally systems that closely mirror the clinical condition (in terms of incidence and distribution of metastases) are preferable. If the aim is to compare drugs for efficacy against minimal residual disease, then it may matter less whether they originated from a primary tumor or from a syringe.

3. "Experimental" vs Spontaneous Metastasis

There has been a great deal of discussion of the relative merits of "spontaneous" vs "experimental" (i.e., intravenously induced) metastasis. There is no doubt that the two are not equivalent, but the latter can be very useful if precise quantitation is required. For example, we found that uptake of monoclonal antibodies recognizing tumor antigens was critically dependent on tumor site, size, and total tumor burden. To compare the relative efficacy of antibodies, we needed to control these variables to a far greater degree than would have been possible with spontaneous dissemination from a primary site; hence, we studied antibody localization in tumor colonies produced in lung or liver following injection of cells into the appropriate vein *(18)*. In addition, in this instance using rat tumor models enabled us to compare peripheral vs intrahepatic arterial administration of antibody, to dissect tumors individually, and gain a great deal of information that would not have been technically feasible in the mouse. This has also proved valuable in showing (in a rat mammary carcinoma model) that matrix metalloproteinase (MMP) inhibitors can have both an anti-invasive action (demonstrated by reduced lung colony number) and an antiangiogenic activity (manifest in reduced growth rate of tumors postextravasation). However, in this case efficacy was confirmed in a spontaneous metastasis model, which also enabled us to test effects on lymphatic metastasis *(19)*.

On the other hand, some early work studying anticoagulants as therapy against metastatic disease may have given misleading results in lung colony assays, as it is now known that the bolus injection of trypsinized cells has very different hemodynamic consequences than the slow release of metastasising cells. Many "spontaneous" metastasis assays utilize the footpad or spleen, and although such techniques in many cases lead to a high incidence of metastases in popliteal lymph nodes and liver respectively, the tumor cells almost certainly are forced directly into the vasculature by mechanical pressures. These techniques are therefore more suited to therapeutic interventions rather than to studies of basic mechanisms of metastasis.

4. Hosts

In the chapters that follow, the relative merits of a variety of syngeneic, xenogeneic, transplantable, and transgenic systems are described. In some experiments, it may be important for there to be a functional immune system; in others, if targeting a human tumor antigen, xenografts will be required. It must be recognized that not only is the immune system defective in congenitally immune-deprived animals, but also there are examples of specific cytokines and other molecular mediators that do not "communicate" across species. This may be one of the reasons why xenografts do not in general metastasise as readily as syngeneic tumors *(20,21)*. Also, with the increasing interest in antiangiogenic therapies, there is a further limitation that however many tumor systems are tested for their sensitivity, the vasculature is always identical—the mouse host. A further important consideration is the health and well-being of the animals we use; notes on animal welfare are given at the end of this chapter.

5. When Is a Metastasis Not a Metastasis?

There are two opposing problems here that deserve to be aired. First, we have the situation where it is difficult to determine (particularly in the face of gross tumor burden) whether a tumor is a true *metastasis* (i.e., by definition—a secondary deposit at a distant site, disseminated in the blood or lymph) or simply an extension. For example, tumors in the peritoneal cavity may seed and spread into the visceral organs, they may even invade deep within the tissues, but I would argue that unless the cells escape the confines of the peritoneum and localize in a site (such as the lung) that is not in direct contiguity with the original site, they have only demonstrated invasive (not metastatic) potential. Similarly, when tumors are grown superficially, they may invade across the peritoneal wall and again spread to the viscera. "Kissing metastases" (not metastases at all) may occur when tumor in the liver, for example, spreads to the kidney by direct contact.

Perhaps an addendum to this is that not all lumps and lesions are metastases. Care should be taken to confirm by histology (and identification of specific markers if possible) that any suspicious lesions are indeed identical in type to the primary tumor. Some athymic and severe combined immune-deficient (SCID) mice are prone to lymphoreticular neoplasms that often present as nodules in the groin and axilla; these are easily mistaken on superficial examination for lymph node metastases. Similarly, early experiments with *N*-methyl-nitrosourea (NMU)-induced rat mammary tumors (and the same may apply to transgenic strains) yielded lung tumors. These were identified as metastases when in fact in some cases they were second primary tumors due to the systemic effects of the carcinogen.

This may be seen as semantics, but it could well be that different molecular mechanisms are required for local extension/invasion and true metastasis. It is likely that opportunistic spread will not be genetically defined, whereas acquisition of a true metastatic phenotype should depend on the activation (or deactivation) of specific genes involved in tumor cell dissemination or its control.

With the increasing sophistication of molecular methods of detection of tumor cells and genetic "tagging" we are often faced (both in the laboratory and the clinic) with the task of identifying (for example) a "polymerase-chain reaction (PCR) positive" tissue sample, or single cancer cells in blood or bone marrow. In some cases (e.g., breast cancer) it is possible to sample regional nodes during surgery to test for the presence of disseminated cells. However, detection depends upon either histological examination of a limited number of sections, which may miss small tumor deposits, or genetic techniques such as PCR or reverse-transcriptase-PCR (RT-PCR) which (at least with some primers) may give false-positive results *(22)*. In the latter case, all we may have to go on is the presence of an "abnormal" genetic sequence—perhaps an oncogene, or tumor marker gene.

We have explored the use of human "Alu" sequences as a sensitive and quantitative indicator of the presence of human tumor cells in the lungs of nude mice following intravenous injection (based on methods described by Weisberg et al. *[23]*). There was a direct correlation between the numbers of cells injected and the "signal" detected. However, we found that even when we injected killed tumor cells intravenously, the lungs remain "PCR-positive" for several weeks (unpublished observations). Clearly, this technique would have limitations for assessing the effects of therapy, at least in short-term assays. These results suggest that genetic material from dead cells can persist for longer than one would imagine, perhaps taken up by macrophages, or otherwise protected from complete degradation. The implication is that a positive PCR signal cannot be assumed to indicate the presence of viable, clonogenic tumor cells. Similarly, when single viable tumor cells or small clumps are detected, there is no way of knowing whether they are capable of growth into a gross metastasis. Elegant work by Pantel showed that colorectal cancer patients could harbor cytokeratin- and c-*erb*B-2 oncogene–positive cells in their bone marrow, yet such patients do not develop metastases at this site *(24)*.

We also need to consider the use of genetically tagged cells, for example, using GFP—eloquently championed in Chapter 24 by Rocha et al. and Chapter 25 by Hoffman—which is revolutionising the detection of micrometastases and dormant cells in experimental models. These depend upon the introduction of prokaryotic or invertebrate genes into mammalian cells, and it is important to keep in mind that not only the genes themselves, but also the selection and cloning procedures employed may either influence or inadvertently select certain cellular phenotypes. It is possible that in some tumor–host combinations, recognition of the bacterial gene product may occur. Cells may lose their "tag" during in vivo growth so that counting only positive lesions might underestimate the total number *(25)*. Caution in the interpretation of "molecular" quantitation of micrometastases is therefore advised, and it is always essential to check that introduction of the label does not alter cell behavior in vivo by independent means.

6. Troubleshooting

If metastasis journals had a problem page, one of the most common questions would be: "Why doesn't Dr. Xs 'metastatic' cell line work in my lab?" This is a very common and underreported problem. The following is basic and common-sense advice for novices:

1. *Always* to obtain cell lines from a reputable source and ensure that they are mycoplasma-free, ideally using a highly sensitive PCR-based assay rather than relying on staining techniques. Cells will not "perform" if they are unhealthy, and even *nu/nu* mice can recognize and eradicate infected cells.

2. Follow *to the letter* instructions from the sender regarding the cells' handling, growth, maintenance, subculturing, and in vivo use, however unusual they may seem. This is likely to be based on years of experience and one ignores it at one's risk. Culture media, supplements, and degree of confluency at harvest *do* matter.

3. Take account of the host animal strain. "C57bl" mice, for instance, may be genetically distinct in different colonies, and both tumors and animals can undergo genetic "drift," rendering them imperfectly syngeneic. It is also clear that different strains of *nu/nu* mice have are more or less "permissive" of metastasis. NCr and Balb/C athymic are generally considered acceptable. SCID mice (particularly NOD/SCID) or beige/nude/SCID mice may sometimes give better results than *nu/nu*, but this must be tested for each cell line and is not a universal panacea *(26)*.

4. Check the health of the animals and the conditions of their environment. Any low-grade infection can influence responses to tumors, and even diet, chlorination levels in water, temperature, and humidity or the stress of a noisy environment can affect the development of metastases.

5. Do not be impatient. Sometimes the first metastasis can take longer to manifest than expected. Although animal maintenance costs are an issue, it may be more economical to wait a few more weeks than to abort the experiment and start again. The judicious use of "tagged" cells may expedite detection and isolation of disseminated cells for further rounds of selection to increase incidence and reproducibility.

6. Use animals of the correct sex (obvious for hormone-responsive tumors, but ideally should also be matched to that of the tumor for nonendocrine tumors in case of sex-linked effects and endocrine regulation of molecules involved in metastasis, e.g., angiogenic factors).

7. Use the correct orthotopic site, as it is now well established that this gives the best opportunity for cells to express their metastatic phenotype. However, many highly malignant (especially syngeneic) tumors will readily metastasize from almost any site.

8. A detailed and authoritative review of practicalities and techniques for in vivo metastasis assays has been produced by Welch *(27)*.

7. Ethics and Animal Care

Although many articles have been published describing the practicalities of establishing and running metastasis models, ethical considerations and care of the animals are rarely addressed. Most countries have regulations of some kind, but there is little if any consistency in their standards or implementation. In the United Kingdom, the general welfare of laboratory animals and the performance of regulated procedures are covered by the Animals (Scientific Procedures) Act (1986). These are administered by the Home Office and all experimental procedures require specific authority via Project licenses and Personal Licenses. However, there are few publications specifically relating to the care of experimental animals with cancers, let alone those that develop metastases. Also, as there has recently been a dramatic increase in the numbers and types of novel models available (e.g., transgenic and "gene knockout" animals, orthotopic systems, etc.) most guidelines are out of date and often inadequate. Unfortunately, in the absence of strict, universally applied and enforceable laws, images of animals overburdened with massive infiltrating tumors (often erroneously claimed to be "metastases") are all too common in the scientific literature. Basic general principles of animal care can be found in the *UKCCCR Guidelines for the Welfare of Animals in Experimental Neoplasia (28)* and similar publications *(29–31)*. In addition, the introduction of local ethical review processes should increase awareness of the importance of these issues in all our institutions.

Research workers in the United Kingdom have ethical and legal responsibilities to consider the "three Rs"—reduction, refinement, and replacement—when designing their experiments. In vitro alternatives should be used where feasible, and should always precede in vivo experimentation. This is a particularly difficult issue in metastasis research, because, by its very nature, the process depends on subtle interactions between tumor and host cells, dynamics of blood and lymphatic circulation, and both positive and negative microenvironmental influences. Certain aspects of the metastatic cascade can be mimicked in vitro (e.g., tumor cell interactions with stromal components, motility, invasion) and useful "intermediates" have been devised in the use of chick heart (*see* Chapter 10 by Bracke et al.) and human amnion. Nevertheless, all such systems need to be validated to show that principles that emerge, or drugs that are active in such screens, do translate into the "real" in vivo pathological process.

Once a metastasis model has been chosen, it is imperative that all experimentalists and husbandry personnel understand the probable course of the disease in the animals. If a new model is being introduced or developed, pilot studies in small numbers of animals will be necessary to gain experience of its biological properties. Detailed records should be kept so that reproducibility (or otherwise) of latency, distribution, and incidence of metastasis can be tracked. Clearly, symptoms will differ depending on whether the animal is predicted to develop metastases in lung, liver, brain, or other sites. The onset of symptoms can be sudden, and may be missed (or mistaken for other causes) if the tumor behavior is not explained to staff and relevant information on probable time course and outcomes provided. "Intentional death" is not an acceptable endpoint, and the use of "survival curves" (except where animals are humanely killed when symptomatic) should be actively discouraged.

Many organ colonization assays (e.g., lung colonies following tumor cell inoculation into a peripheral vein; liver colonies after tumor cell inoculation into a mesenteric vein) can provide a more easily controlled, surrogate "metastasis" assay suitable for certain applications. Once a model is fully characterized, animals can be humanely killed well before the tumors cause any symptoms, at which time both numbers and sizes of individual colonies can be readily quantified. At later times, colonies may become confluent, and in addition to the increased probability of interfering with organ function, tumor burden can then only be crudely assessed by organ weight or other indirect means. This can be highly inaccurate owing to the development of areas of necrosis, infarction, or inflammation *(27)*.

"Care Plans" can be very useful in a busy Unit where different metastasis models are run concurrently. These should clearly state the contact details of the experimentalist (plus deputy in case unavailable), details of the tumor, site of implantation or inoculation, expected signs of metastatic disease (e.g., shortness of breath, palpable axillary nodes, abdominal swelling, weight loss, etc.) and the course of action to be taken in each case. Animals at risk of developing metastases should be checked at least once daily. There should in all cases be clear guidelines as to the maximum permissible size of any superficial tumors, and details of experimental endpoints. In some metastasis models, the primary tumor (whether in subcutaneous or mammary fat pad sites, spleen, etc.) may be left *in situ*. Although in most cases the probability of detecting metastatic disease increases with the growth period (or size) of the primary tumor, it is unethical to allow these tumors to reach excessive sizes simply to maximize the "yield" of metastases. What is more, such practices increase the risk of confusing direct extension of tumor into organs with true (blood or lymph borne) distant metastasis. It is discouraging to note that in some instances, tumor burdens of up to 50% of the weight of the mouse have been recorded in such assays. A maximum of 5–10% should not be exceeded. If the primary tumor is removed after a certain period, to allow time for any disseminated cells to develop into metastases (a more clinically relevant model) there may be a risk of local recurrence. This will also need "flagging" in the Care Plan, and recurrences should be recorded (and ideally animals excluded from analysis) as they can influence metastatic incidence. Excision of tumors at a relatively small size (e.g., for subcutaneous tumors <10 mm mean diameter in mice, 15 mm in rats) with a reasonably wide margin should minimize this problem.

References

1. Gura, T. (1997) Systems for identifying new drugs are often faulty. *Science* **278,** 1041–1042.
2. Zent, R., Ailenberg, M., and Silverman, M. (1998) Tyrosine kinase signalling pathways of rat mesangial cells in 3-dimensional cultures: response to fetal bovine serum and platelet-derived growth factor BB. *Exp. Cell Res.* **240,** 134–143.
3. Rak, J., Mitsuhashi, Y., Erdos, V., et al. (1995) Massive programmed cell death in intestinal epithelial cells induced by three-dimensional growth conditions: suppression by mutant c-H-*ras* oncogene expression. *J. Cell. Biol.* **131,** 1587–1598.
4. Kohl, N. E., Wilson, F. R., Mossier, S. D., et al. (1994) Protein farnesyltransferase inhibitors block the growth of ras-independent tumors in nude mice. *Proc. Natl. Acad Sci USA* **91,** 9141–9145.

5. Wilmanns, C., Fan, D., O'Brian, C. A., Bucana, C. D., and Fidler, I. J. (1992) Orthotopic and ectopic organ environments differentially influence the sensitivity of murine colon carcinoma cells to doxorubicin and 5-fluorouracil. *Int J. Cancer* **52,** 98–104.

6. Dong, Z., Radinsky, R., Fan, D., et al. (1994) Organ-specific modulation of steady-state mdr gene expression and drug resistance in murine colon cancer cells. *J. Natl. Cancer Inst.* **86,** 913–920.

7. St Croix, B., Rak, J. W., Kapitain, S., et al. (1996) Reversal by hyaluronidase of adhesion-dependent multicellular drug resistance in mammary carcinoma cells. *J. Natl. Cancer Inst.* **88,** 1285–1296.

8. Radinsky, R. (1995) Molecular mechanisms for organ-specific colon carcinoma metastasis. *Eur. J. Cancer* **31A,** 1091–1095.

9. Eccles, S., Modjtahedi, H., Court, W., Titley, J., Box, G., and Dean, C. J. (1996) Preclinical studies with human tumor xenografts using rat monoclonal antibodies directed against the epidermal growth factor receptor, in *EGF Receptor in Tumor Growth and Progression*, Lichtner, R. B. and Harkins, R. N. (eds.), Springer-Verlag, Berlin.

10. O-charoenrat, P., Modjtahedi, H., Rhys-Evans, P., Court, W., Box, G., and Eccles, S. (2000) Epidermal growth factor-like ligands differentially upregulate matrix metalloproteinase-9 in head and neck squamous carcinoma cells. *Cancer Res.* **60,** 1121–1128.

11. Petit, A., Rak, J., and Hung, M-C. (1997) Neutralizing antibodies against EGFR and erbB-2/neu receptor tyrosine kinases down-regulate vascular endothelial growth factor production by tumor cells in vitro and in vivo. *Am. J. Pathol.* **151,** 1523–1530.

12. Lane, D. (1998) The promise of molecular oncology. *Lancet* **351**(Suppl. 2), SII17–20.

13. Freije, J. M. P., Lawrence, J., Hollingshead, M. G., et al. (1997) Identification of compounds with preferential inhibitory activity against low-Nm-23 expressing breast carcinoma and melanoma cell lines. *Nature Med.* **3,** 395–400.

14. Eccles, S. A., Court, W. J., Box, G. A., Dean, C. J., Melton, R. G., and Springer, C. J. (1994) Regression of established breast carcinoma xenografts with antibody-directed enzyme prodrug therapy against c-erbB2 p185. *Cancer Res.* **54,** 5171–5177.

15. Eccles, S. A., Modjtahedi, H., Court, W., Sandle, J., and Dean, C. J. (1995) Significance of the c-erbB family of receptor tyrosine kinase in metastatic cancer and their potential as targets for immunotherapy. *Invas. Metast.* **14,** 337–348.

16. Eccles, S. (1998) c-*erb*B-2 as a target for immunotherapy. *Exp. Opin. Invest. Drugs* **7,** 1879–1896.

17. Kerbel, R. S. (1999) What is the optimal rodent model for anti-tumor drug testing? *Cancer Metast. Rev.* **17,** 301–304.

18. Eccles, S. A., Purvies, H. P., Styles, J. M., Hobbs, S. M., and Dean, C. J. (1988) Potential of monoclonal antibodies for localisation and treatment of disseminated disease: studies in syngeneic rat tumor systems. *Adv. Exp. Med. Biol.* **233,** 329–339.

19. Eccles, S. A., Box, G. M., Court, W. J., Bone, E. A., Thomas, W., and Brown, P. D. (1996). Control of lymphatic and hematogenous metastasis of a rat mammary carcinoma by the matrix metalloproteinase inhibitor batimastat (BB-94). *Cancer Res.* **56,** 2815–2822.

20. Eccles, S. A. (1983) Differentiation and neoplasia. Invasion and metastasis: experimental systems. *J. Pathol.* **141**, 333–353.
21. Barnett, S. C. and Eccles, S. A. (1984) Studies of mammary carcinoma metastasis in a mouse model system I. Derivation and characterisation of cells with different metastatic properties during tumor progression in vivo. *Clin. Exp. Metast.* **2**, 15–36.
22. Bostick, P., et al. (1998) Limitations of specific reverse-transcriptase polymerase chain reaction markers in the detection of metastases in the lymph nodes and blood of cancer patients. *J. Clin. Oncol.* **16**, 2632–2640.
23. Weisberg, T., Cahill, B. K., and Vary, C. P. H. (1996) Non-radioisotopic detection of human xenogeneic DNA in a mouse transplantation model. *Mol. Cell Probes* **10**, 139–146.
24. Pantel, K., Schlimok, G., Braun, S., et al. (1993) Differential expression of proliferation-associated molecules in individual micrometastatic carcinoma cells. *J. Natl. Cancer Inst.* **85**, 1419–1423.
25. Fujimaki, T., Ellis, L. M., Bucana, C. D., Radinsky, R., Price, J. E., and Fidler, I. J. (1993) Simultaneous radiolabel, genetic tagging and proliferation assays to study the organ distribution and fate of metastatic cells. *Int. J. Oncol.* **2**, 895–901.
26. Garafalo, A., Chirivi, R. G. S., Scanziani, E., Mayo, J. G., Vecchi, A., and Giavazzi, R. (1993) Comparative study on the metastatic behaviour of human tumors in nude, beige/nude/Xid and severe combined immune-deficient mice. *Invas. Metast.* **13**, 82–91.
27. Welch, D. W. (1997) Technical considerations for studying cancer metastasis *in vivo. Clin. Exp. Metast.* **15**, 272–306.
28. *UKCCCR Guidelines for the Welfare of Animals in Experimental Neoplasia*, 2nd ed., 1997.
29. Balls, M. (1994) Replacement of animal procedures: alternatives in research, education and testing. *Lab. Anim.* **28**, 193–211.
30. Festing, M. F. W. (1994) reduction of animal use: experimental design and quality of experiments. *Lab. Anim.* **28**, 212–221.
31. Schiffer, S. P. (1997) Animal welfare and colony management in cancer research. *Breast Cancer Res. Treat.* **46**, 313–331.

16

The Chick Embryo Metastasis Model

Eric Petitclerc and Peter C. Brooks

1. Introduction

1.1. Clinical Implication of Tumor Cell Metastasis

The growth and dissemination of malignant tumors continues to have a devastating impact on people throughout the United States and the rest of the world. In fact, it is estimated that well over a half a million new cases of cancer will be diagnosed per year *(1)*. The most commonly used clinical approaches to treat cancer include surgical removal of the primary tumor, chemotherapy, and radiation, all of which have varying degrees of success. Importantly, a major obstacle contributing to the failure of treatment in many cases involves the metastatic dissemination of tumor cells from the primary tumor mass to distant sites. While some progress has been achieved in understanding the complex biochemical and molecular mechanisms regulating tumor invasion, much remains to be learned.

1.2. Metastatic Cascade

The metastatic cascade involves a series of cellular events that are linked both temporally and spatially *(2–5)*. Malignant cells must complete all the individual steps within the cascade to successfully establish secondary tumor foci **(Fig. 1)**. Interestingly, studies have indicated that only a small percentage of malignant cells possess the required characteristics for the establishment of metastases *(6,7)*. In general, metastasis begins by an initial change in cell–cell adhesive interactions which allows dissociation of tumor cells from the primary tumor mass. This is followed by local invasion and migration into the proteolytically modified interstitial matrix. During hematagenous metastasis, the tumor cells undergo a process called intravasation by which they gain access to the host circulation. Next, the tumor cells must evade host immune

From: *Methods in Molecular Medicine, vol. 58:*
Metastasis Research Protocols, Vol. 2: Cell Behavior In Vitro and In Vivo
Edited by: S. A. Brooks and U. Schumacher © Humana Press Inc., Totowa, NJ

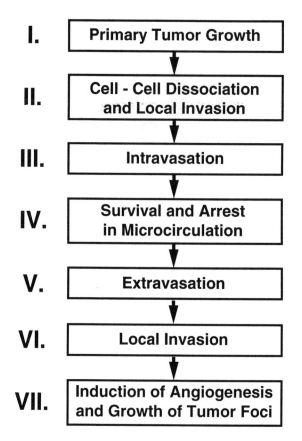

Fig. 1. General steps in tumor metastasis. Tumor cell metastasis is a complex series of events that involve the coordination of a number of cellular and biochemical processes. For the successful establishment of a secondary metastatic tumor foci, the tumor cells must traverse all the steps that compose the metastatic cascade.

surveillance and survive the physical shear forces found within the circulation. Eventually, the tumor cells arrest in the microvasculature and undergo extravasation and leave the circulation. This is followed by local invasion and the establishment of secondary metastatic foci. Finally, for these small metastatic deposits to grow and expand beyond a minimal size, they must induce angiogenesis to provide blood vessels for their continued growth and survival.

1.3. Molecular Regulators of Metastasis

Because understanding the mechanisms regulating tumor metastasis is of particular clinical importance, a great deal of effort has been focused on identifying molecules that may regulate this process. It is important to point out that the molecules discussed in the following paragraphs are only a small fraction of factors thought to regulate tumor invasion and are discussed only to illustrate the variety and complexity of metastasis regulating molecules. In this regard, studies have identified families of molecules that regulate metastasis including growth factors and their receptors, cell adhesion molecules, proteolytic enzymes, and extracellular matrix (ECM) components *(2–7)*. Some of the more widely studied growth factors that have been implicated in tumor metastasis include transforming growth factors-α and -β (TGF-α and -β), epidermal growth factor (EGF), vascular endothelial growth factor (VEGF), insulin, insulin-like growth factor-1 (IGF-1), and a number of interleukins, to name just a few *(8–12)*. These molecules and their receptors may impact tumor metastasis in a variety of ways including regulating tumor and endothelial cell proliferation *(8–12)*. In addition, they may also modulate the expression and activity of cell adhesion molecules, which in turn can regulate adhesive and migratory activity *(8–13)*. These molecules can also influence the expression and activity of proteolytic enzymes known to facilitate ECM remodeling *(8–13)*. Finally, these growth factors may regulate the synthesis of ECM components such as collagen, fibronectin, and laminin, all critical regulators of cellular invasion *(8–13)*.

A second family of molecules shown to facilitate tumor metastasis include cell adhesion receptors. At least four distinct families have been implicated in metastasis including integrins, cadherins, selectins, and the immunoglobulin (Ig) supergene family *(14–20)*. In general, caderins, selectins, and Ig family members function predominantly in regulating cell–cell interactions, whereas members of the integrin family typically promote cell–ECM interactions *(14)*. These molecules promote cell–cell and cell–ECM interactions, which in turn regulate a diverse set of processes such as tumor cell proliferation, differentiation, apoptosis, adhesion, migration, and invasion *(21–23)*.

A third category of molecules that contribute to tumor metastasis include proteolytic enzymes. Proteases from at least four distinct families including serine, cysteine, aspartate, and metalloproteases have been implicated in the metastatic cascade *(24–26)*. The activity of these molecules helps to create a permissive microenvironment into which malignant tumor cells can invade, migrate, survive, and proliferate *(24–26)*. This permissive microenvironment can be created by these enzymes in a number of ways such as breaking down restrictive ECM barriers, thus facilitating local invasion *(24–26)*. In addition, these enzymes may proteolytically release matrix sequestered growth factors, thereby contributing to tumor proliferation. Finally, specific proteases can function to activate other latent enzymes, bind to cell adhesion receptors such as integrins, and thereby regulate cellular adhesion and migration *(24,27–29)*.

A final group of metastasis regulators include ECM components such as collagen, laminin, and fibronectin. Again, similar to the molecules discussed previously, ECM components can modulate tumor metastasis by a variety of mechanisms including cellular adhesion, migration, differentiation, apoptosis, signal transduction, and gene expression *(30–32)*. Thus, tumor metastasis is a highly complex cascade of events that is regulated by molecules that have distinct as well as overlapping regulatory functions.

1.4. Metastasis Models

A major complication in understanding tumor metastasis arises from the multitude of cellular, biochemical, and molecular events that contribute to this process. To this end, many investigators have developed unique in vitro models of tumor invasion including Boyden chamber (refer to Chapter 5 by Brown and Bicknell) /Matrigel invasion assays (refer to Chapters 7 and 8 by Hall and Brooks and by Hendrix et al.), three-dimensional collagen invasion assays (refer to Chapter 9 by Bracke et al.), and skin reconstruct invasion assays *(33–35)*. However, these in vitro models do not necessarily duplicate the physiological events that facilitate dissemination of tumors cells in vivo. Therefore, many in vivo assays described in other chapters in this volume have been developed including a number of murine models *(36,37)*. These animal models are not discussed in detail here, but instead this discussion is focused on the chick embryo metastasis model **(Fig. 2)**. The chick embryo has a long history as a useful and efficient in vivo model to study such complex physiological processes as embryonic development, angiogenesis, and tumor metastasis *(38–46)*. As a result of many elegant studies using the chick embryo, a wealth of physiological and biochemical information has been generated on these complex biological phenomena. The chick embryo has numerous advantages as compared to animal models of metastasis. For example, fertilized chick eggs are considerably less expensive than mice or rats. In addition, the chick embryo provides a model to study either spontaneous or experimental metastasis in a considerably shorter time, 7–9 d as compared to 4–10 wk for most typical murine models. Furthermore, because the chick embryo is a closed system, the half-life of many experimental antagonists including small peptides tends to be much longer in the chick as compared to other animal models. Thus, the chick embryo allows experimental evaluation of potential antimetastatic compounds that are in limited supply. The chick embryo also has the advantage of ease of experimental manipulation as well as offering versatility in studying tumorgenicity, local invasion, and metastases to a variety of organs including the lungs, liver, and kidney *(10,43,47,48)*. Recently, the chick embryo has also been used to study metastasis by intravital microscopy *(3)*. Finally, quantification of metastasis can be conducted by a variety of efficient and reproducible methods including flow cytometry (refer to Chapter 1 by Derek Davies), polymerase chain reaction (PCR) (refer to Chapters 17 and 19 by Tennant et al. and Haack et al. in the

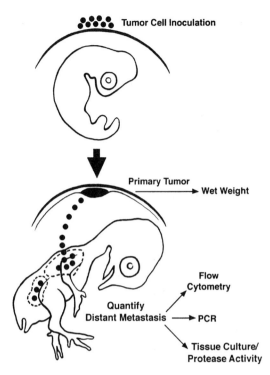

Fig. 2. The 9-d chick embryo metastasis assay. The chick embryo has been used to study numerous biological phenomena including tumor cell metastasis. The chick embryo metastasis assay involves the application of a single cell suspension of tumor cells to the chorioallantoic membrane of a 9-d-old chick embryo. The embryo is allowed to incubate for a total of 9 d to allow the tumor cells to metastasize to various organs. At the end of the 9-d incubation period, the primary tumor can be removed to quantify tumorgenicity, and specific embryonic organs such as the lungs can be assayed for metastatic tumor foci. Metastasis can be quantified by at least three independent methods including flow cytometry, PCR, or protease activity/tissue culture methods.

companion volume), and enzymatic and/or morphological culture methods *(10,44,49)*. In this chapter we describe in detail the chick embryo metastasis assay utilizing flow cytometry for quantification.

2. Materials

1. Egg incubator (Lyon Electric Co. Inc., Chula Vista, CA).
2. Egg candler (Lyon Electric Co. Inc., Chula Vista, CA).
3. Nine-day-old chick embryos (AA Labs, Irvine, CA).
4. Styrofoam egg holder.
5. Cordless rotary tool (Sears, Los Angeles, CA).
6. Small drill bit and cutting wheel (Sears, Los Angeles, CA).
7. Mineral oil (Sigma, St. Louis, MO).

8. 30 1/2-Gauge needles (Becton Dickinson, Lincoln Park, NJ).
9. 1-mL syringes (Becton Dickinson, Lincoln Park, NJ).
10. 70% Ethanol (VWR, Plainfield, NJ).
11. Curved forceps (VWR, Plainfield, NJ).
12. Transparent adhesive tape (VWR, Plainfield, NJ).
13. Vacuum pump (VWR, Plainfield, NJ).
14. Large dissecting scissors (VWR, Plainfield, NJ).
15. Small dissecting scissors (VWR, Plainfield, NJ).
16. 35-mm Petri dishes (Becton Dickinson, Lincoln Park, NJ).
17. Bacterial collagenase (Worthington Biochemical Co., Freehold, NJ).
18. Sterile phosphate-buffered saline (PBS).
19. 2.5% w/v bovine serum albumin (BSA)/PBS.
20. 15-mL tubes (VWR, Plainfield, NJ).
21. Fluorescence-activated cell sorter (FACS) tubes (VWR, Plainfield, NJ).
22. Aluminum foil (PCA, Northbrook, IL).

3. Methods

3.1. Preparation and Candling of the Eggs

The 9-d-old fertilized chick eggs should be immediately placed in a humidified incubator maintained at a constant temperature of 99.5°F and 51% relative humidity (*see* **Note 1**). During all procedures, the eggs should not be left out of the incubators for more than 30 min at any one time.

1. The shell of the eggs can be cleaned with 70% ethanol to remove any debris that may be associated with the outer shell surface. The process of candling the eggs is done to determine the viability of the embryos, to locate the optimal position for the addition of tumor cells, and to identify potential blood vessels for intravenous injections (**Fig. 3**).
2. To begin, remove only the number of eggs from the incubator that correspond to the investigators' speed, since it is critical that the embryos are not left outside the incubators for an extended period of time. With the egg candler, determine the position of the air sac (broad end of egg). Mark the middle zone of the air sac with a soft lead pencil. Next, rotate the egg close to the candle light to determine the position of prominent blood vessels on the lateral sides of the egg that are well anchored and close to the surface. The vessel selected for injection should branch in a direction opposite from the air sac (**Fig. 3**) to ensure proper direction of blood flow. The selected vessel should be of medium to small diameter to reduce the amount of bleeding after removal of the needle. Once the blood vessel is identified, draw a square around the selected vessel (5 mm × 10 mm) to mark the injection window (**Fig. 3**).
3. Within the marked area, draw a thin line to indicate the position of the blood vessel to be injected. The injection window should be held in a position horizontal to the egg holder. Next, mark a point on the top side of the egg (tumor cell window) which will serve as the site for tumor cell application. This point designates the area of the chorioallantoic membrane (CAM) that will be dropped and the position at which the tumor cells will be applied.

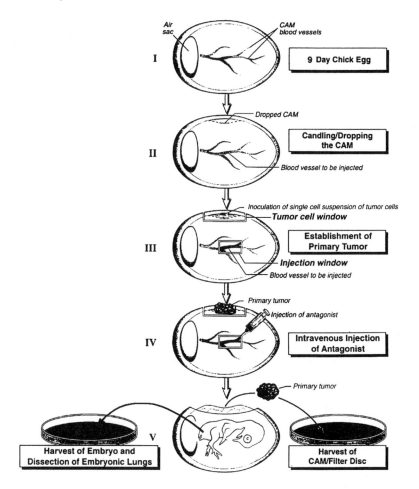

Fig. 3. The chick metastasis assay protocol, which can be divided into five general stages. Stage I involves obtaining and incubating the chick embryos. Stage II includes candling the chick eggs for the identification of blood vessels, establishment of tumor cell and injection windows, and dropping the CAM. Stage III involves application of the tumor cells to establish a primary tumor. Stage IV includes intravenous administration of potential antimetastatic compounds. Finally, stage V involves harvesting of the primary tumors and dissection of the embryonic organs for quantification of metastasis.

3.2. Dropping the CAM

Dropping the CAM involves separating the CAM from the egg shell membrane. This is accomplished by displacing the air from the air sac at the broad end of the egg to the top side where the CAM is pulled away from the shell membrane, creating a false air sac (**Fig. 3**).

1. Swab the egg shell (original air sac and tumor cell window) with 70% ethanol. Carefully drill a small hole through the egg shell at the broad end of the egg (original air sac). In a similar manner, drill a small hole on the top side of the egg at the position marked to indicate the tumor cell window. When drilling the hole at the tumor cell window (top side), extreme care should be taken to penetrate only the shell and not the shell membrane (*see* **Note 2**).

2. Place the egg next to the candler so that the air sac is illuminated (*see* **Note 3**). With forceps presoaked in 70% ethanol, gently place the forceps through the small hole and apply a downward pressure on the exposed shell membrane. This step will assist in detachment of the egg shell membrane from the CAM. Complete the process by applying a slight negative pressure at the hole at the air sac with a small vacuum hose. This should reduce the air in the air sac and facilitate separation of the CAM from the egg shell membrane (dropping CAM). Following this procedure, care must be taken to maintain the tumor cell window in the upright position to avoid contamination of the newly dropped CAM. Discard any eggs in which the CAM is broken or the air was displaced internally under the CAM.

3. Draw a small square window (tumor cell window) on the top side of the egg such that the newly created false air sac (dropped CAM) is centered within the window. Using the small grinding wheel, cut along the margins of the marked tumor cell window, being careful to cut only through the egg shell but not the shell membrane. Leave the corners of the tumor cell window intact and do not remove the shell. Gently remove any egg shell debris from the intact window before removing the cut shell. This procedure helps to limit contamination of the CAM tissue with shell fragments. Carefully place the embryos back in the incubator, making sure that the newly cut tumor cell window is facing up.

3.3. Preparation of the Tumor Cells

Selection of the tumor cell model to be used is dependent on the investigator's interests. It is important to note that the selection of the tumor cells used must be made empirically, as some tumor cells do not grow well on the chick CAM. In this report, we describe the use of the human epidermoid carcinoma cell line Hep-3, which has be used extensively in the chick embryo model *(43,47–49)*.

1. Subconfluent Hep-3 cells are removed from culture by standard trypsinization or EDTA treatment and washed 3× with serum-free media. Tumor cells are resuspend in serum-free Dulbecco's minimum essential medium (DMEM) (*see* **Note 4**). The number of tumor cells to be inoculated depends on the specific tumor type and should be determined by the investigator.

2. For Hep-3 cells, the washed tumor cells should be resuspended in DMEM (*see* **Note 4**) at a concentration of $6.25 \times 10^6/mL$ and 40 μL should be applied to each CAM (2.5×10^5). It is important that the cell density be adjusted for each tumor type to establish a tumor size that is not lethal to the embryo.

3.4. Application of the Tumor Cells to the CAMs

When preparing to apply the tumor cells, it is important to deliver the single cell suspension to the embryo within 30–45 min of dropping the CAM (*see* **Note 5**). Longer delays may lead to poor tumor take and thus poor metastasis. To prepare the eggs for inoculation, the eggs should remain in the incubator and care should be taken to avoid any unnecessary movements.

1. Next, remove the lid from the incubator and carefully remove the egg shell window by gently pushing a pair of sterile forceps through the cut shell, following the outline of the window.
2. Slowly pipet 40 µL of the cell suspension in three equal amounts, all at the same point directly on the exposed CAM (*see* **Note 5**).
3. Following the inoculation of the cells, the tumor cell window is sealed with clear adhesive tape, being careful not to move the embryo, as even small movements can cause the tumor cell suspension to spread out, resulting in poor tumor take (*see* **Note 6**). The embryos are left undisturbed for 24 h to allow the tumor cells to adhere to the CAM tissue.

3.5. Intravenous Administration of Potential Anti-Metastatic Compounds

To evaluate specific compounds for antimetastatic activity, various reagents can be administered intravenously. The concentrations of the antagonist are determined experimentally; however the antagonists should be injected in no more than 100 µL total volume. Although multiple injections are possible, it is not recommended because the number of accessible blood vessels is limited and further movement and trauma may significantly reduce embryo viability.

1. To prepare the injection window, the egg is carefully positioned in the egg holder and the candle is oriented such that the light is focused down through the tumor cell window on the top side of the egg. Make sure that the blood vessel that was previously selected is still positioned within marked border of the injection window, as the position of the vessel may change when the CAM is dropped.
2. Carefully cut along the margins of the previously marked window enclosing the blood vessel. Using extreme care, gently cut through the egg shell, being careful not to penetrate the shell membrane as the blood vessels are in close proximity to the shell at this point.
3. Place a drop of mineral oil along the upper margins of the cut shell and allow it to spread down between the shell and shell membrane. This procedure helps to loosen the shell from its underlying membranes, thus facilitating its removal. Gently remove the cut shell to expose the blood vessel.
4. Place a second drop of mineral oil on the exposed shell membrane, which will result in the membrane becoming translucent, thus facilitating visualization of the vessel.

5. Holding the 30-gauge needle beveled side up, inject no more than 100 μL of antagonists (*see* **Note 7**). Carefully watch the vessel as you are injecting, as you should be able to see the blood clearing from the vessel. Following the injection, wait 3–5 s before withdrawing the needle to ensure the return of blood flow (*see* **Note 8**). A small amount of bleeding is normal. If excess bleeding occurs, gently apply pressure to the area with a Kimwipe for approx 30 s.
6. The injection window should be sealed with adhesive tape and the eggs returned to the incubator. The embryos are allowed to incubate for a total of 9 d.

3.6. Resection of Primary Tumor and Dissection of Embryonic Lungs

Following the incubation period, the primary tumors will form on the surface of the CAM.

1. The eggs are next removed from the incubator and place on ice for 5–10 min.
2. Using large dissecting scissors, cut through the tumor cell window (top side) and remove the surrounding egg shell that covers the CAM and tumor. Sacrificing the embryos should be performed in accordance with any institutional and NIH guidelines for use of experimental animals.
3. Resect the primary tumor and place it in a 35-mm Petri dish containing 1 mL of PBS. The tumors should be trimmed free of surrounding CAM tissue and wet weights determined.
4. With large forceps grab the chick embryo and quickly decapitate it with large dissecting scissors. Place the carcass in a 100-mm Petri dish ventral side up and wash with PBS. Beginning posteriorly, make a continuous cut up the midline of the body. Carefully open the body cavity and remove the intestines, liver, and heart to expose the lungs. The lobes of the lungs lie in recessed cavities on either side of the body wall.
5. Again, wash the area with PBS and gently remove the lungs and place them in a 35-mm Petri dish for processing. Additional organs may also be harvested for further analysis.

3.7. Preparation of a Single Cell Suspension of Lung Tissue

1. Wash the lungs extensively with PBS. For each individual embryo, thoroughly mince the lung tissue with the small dissecting scissors and resuspend the lung mince in 1 mL of 0.25% crude bacterial collagenase and transfer the suspension to a 2-mL Eppendorf tube.
2. Incubate the lung suspension at 37°C for 2 h with vortex-mixing every 30 min. Vigorously pipet the lung suspension up and down to resuspend any clumps of tissue and let stand for stand for 1 min to allow any residual tissue clumps to settle to the bottom.
3. Being careful to avoid any tissue clumps, transfer the upper portion of the single-cell suspension to a 15-mL conical tube that contains 1.0 mL of 2.5% BSA–PBS. The cell suspension is next centrifuged at 2000 rpm for 5 min followed by four additional washes with 1.0 mL of 2.5% BSA–PBS.

4. The lung cell suspension is then resuspended in 500 μL of 1% paraformaldehyde and incubated for 15 min.
5. The fixed lung cell suspension is then washed 3× with 2.5% BSA–PBS. At this stage, the lung cell suspensions can be stored at 4°C in 1.0 mL of 2.5% BSA–PBS plus 0.02% sodium azide prior to the immunostaining. The samples should not be stored for more than 3 d before analysis.

3.8. Detection of Tumor Cells in Single-Cell Lung Suspensions

The tumor cells utilized in this model are of human origin and therefore can be detected within the background of the avian lung cells by indirect immunofluoresence staining with a human-specific monoclonal antibody that does not react with chick tissue. In a similar manner, murine tumor cells could be detected with murine-specific antibody reagents.

1. To stain the samples, a fraction of the lung cell suspension (250 μL) is washed 3× as described in **Subheading 3.7., step 5** to remove azide and incubated with a human-specific antibody (e.g., anti-MHC-1 Mab W6/32) for 2 h at room temperature. The concentration of the antibody is dependent on the antibody used, and must be determined by the individual investigator.
2. The cell suspensions are next washed 4× as described in **Subheading 3.7., step 5** and incubated with goat antimouse fluorescein isothiocyanate (FITC) conjugated IgG for 1 h a room temperature.
3. Finally, the cell suspensions are washed 5× as before and resuspended in 0.5% w/v BSA in PBS and covered with aluminum foil to prevent the fluorescence from fading. Lung suspensions prepared from chick embryos in the absence of tumor cells should also be immunostained as described previously. Cell fluorescence can be measured by a FACScan flow cytometer (Becton Dickinson) and side scatter and forward scatter can are measured simultaneously and data collected with FACScan research software (Becton Dickinson). All samples from each experimental condition (10 individuals per condition) should be analyzed by flow cytometry.

3.9. Quantification of Tumor Cell Metastasis

Flow cytometry setup parameters as well as negative control gates for fluorescence intensity are set corresponding to the fluorescence obtained from control lung suspensions stained in the presence of FITC-conjugated secondary antibody only. The percentage of cells within each sample staining positive (above background) are compared between experimental samples and control samples derived from embryos in the absence of a tumor cell inoculum. It should be noted that the percentage of human tumor cells detected is not an absolute number of tumor cells per lung but rather a relative percentage.

4. Notes

1. To increase consistency from experiment to experiment use the same vendor as CAM development, vascularization, and embryo viability can vary from different vendors.

2. To increase the efficiency of dropping the CAMs, begin dropping the CAMs within a few minutes after drilling the appropriate holes. Leaving embryos for longer than 30 min after drilling the holes results in drying and increased adherence of the CAM to the shell making it difficult to drop.
3. Minimize the time that the candle light is in close contact with the embryo, as the intense light can cause excessive heating of the embryo and may reduce viability.
4. Tumor cells should always be resuspended and applied to the CAM in serum-free media and not PBS, as PBS has been observed to cause reduced tumor growth in this model.
5. Application of the single cell suspension of tumor cells to the CAM should be completed within 30–45 min after dropping the CAM to ensure tumor take. In addition, gently touching the CAM itself with the end of the pipet tip during application of the cells helps in the establishment of a localized tumor. However, caution must be used to avoid damaging the CAM blood vessels and inadvertantly inoculating tumor cells directly into damaged vessels.
6. Always apply the tumor cells to the CAM with the eggs sitting in the incubator and do not move the eggs during inoculation of the cells. Small movements of the egg can cause the tumor cell suspension to spread out, reducing focal tumor growth.
7. When preparing antagonists for intravenous administration, be sure that the pH of the solution is between 7.0 and 7.5, as the embryos are sensitive to large pH changes. Moreover, do not inject more than 100 µL total volume of any antagonists, as this may significantly reduce embryo viability.
8. When withdrawing the needle following injection, wait 3–5 s for the blood to return to the vessel. In addition, be sure to remove the needle slowly and as straight as possible, as this will help minimize bleeding.

Acknowledgment

P. C. Brooks was supported in part by grants from the NCI (1R29CA74132-01) and the Stop Cancer Foundation of Los Angeles. E. Petitclerc was supported in part by postdoctoral fellowships from the Medical Research Council of Canada and The Fonds de la Recherche en Santé du Québec.

References

1. Varner, J. A., Brooks, P. C., and Cheresh, D.A. (1995) The integrin $\alpha v \beta 3$: angiogenesis and Apoptosis. *Cell Adhes. Commun.* **3,** 367–374.
2. Meyers, T. and Hart, I. R. (1997) Mechanisms of tumor metastasis. *Eur. J. Cancer.* **34,** 214–221.
3. Chambers, A. F., MacDonald, I. C., Schmidt, E. E., Koop, S., Morris, V. L., Khokha, R., and Groom, A. C. (1995) Steps in tumor metastasis: new concepts from intravital videomicroscopy. *Cancer Metast. Rev.* **14,** 279–301.
4. Quigley, J. P. and Armstrong, P. B. (1998) Tumor cell intravasation Alu-cidated: the chick embryo opens the window. *Cell* **94,** 281–284.
5. Jiang, W. G., Puntis, M. C. A., and Hallett, M. B. (1994) Molecular and cellular basis of cancer invasion and metastasis: implications for treatment. *Br. J. Surg.* **81,** 1576–1590.

6. Liotta, L. A., Steeg, P. S., and Stetler-Stevenson, W. G. (1991) Cancer metastasis and angiogenesis: an imbalance of positive and negative regulation. *Cell* **64,** 327–336.
7. Blood, C. H. and Zetter, B. R. (1990) Tumor interactions with the vasculature: angiogenesis and tumor metastasis. *Biochim. Biophysica. Acta* **1032,** 89–118.
8. Herlyn, M. and Malkowicz, S. B. (1991) Regulatory pathways in tumor growth and invasion. *Lab. Invest.* **65,** 262–267.
9. Rodeck, U. and Herlyn, M. (1991) Growth factors in melanoma. *Cancer Metast. Rev.* **10,** 89–101.
10. Brooks, P. C., Klemke, R. L., Schon, S., Lewis, J. M., Schwartz, M. A., and Cheresh, D. A. (1997) Insulin-like growth factor receptor cooperates with integrin $\alpha v \beta 5$ to promote tumor cell dissemination in vivo. *J. Clin. Invest.* **99,** 1390–1398.
11. Claffey, K. P., Brown, L. F., del Aguila, L. F., Tognazzi, K., Yeo, K., Manseau, E. J., and Dvorak, H. F. (1996) Expression of vascular permeability factor/vascular endothelial growth factor by melanoma cells increases tumor growth, angiogenesis and experimental metastasis. *Cancer Res.* **56,** 172–181.
12. Pedersen, P-H., Ness, G. O., Engebraaten, O., Bjerkvig, R., Lillehaug, J. R., and Laerum, O. D. (1994) Heterogenous response to the growth factors [EGF, PGDF (bb), TGF-α, bFGF, IL-2] on glioma spheroid growth, migration and invasion. *Int. J. Cancer* **56,** 255–261.
13. Plopper, G. E., McNamee, H. P., Dike, L. E., Bojanowski, K., and Ingber, D. E. (1995) Convergence of integrin and growth factor receptor signaling pathways within the focal adhesion complex. *Mol. Biol. Cell* **6,** 1349–1365.
14. Albelda, S. M. (1993) Role of integrins and other cell adhesion molecules in tumor progression and metastasis. *Lab. Invest.* **68,** 4–14.
15. Oka, H., Shiozaki, H., Kobayashi, K., Inoue, M., Tahara, H., Kobayashi, T., et al. (1993) Expression of E-cadherin cell adhesion molecules in human breast cancer tissues and its relationship to metastasis. *Cancer Res.* **53,** 1696–1701.
16. Hangan, D., Morris, V. L., Boeters, L., von Ballestrem, C., Uniyal, S., and Chan, B. M. C. (1997) An epitope on VLA-6 ($\alpha 6 \beta 1$) integrin involved migration but not adhesion is required for extravasation of murine melanoma b16F1 cells in liver. *Cancer Res.* **57,** 3812–3817.
17. Swada, R., Tsuboi, S., and Fukuda, M. (1994) Differential E-selectin-dependent adhesion effeciency in sublimes of a human colon cancer exhibiting distinct metastatic potentials. *J. Biol. Chem.* **269,** 1425–1431.
18. Quain, F., Vaux, D. L., and Weissman, I. L. (1994) Expression of the integrin $\alpha 4 \beta 1$ on melanoma cells can inhibit the invasive stage of metastasis formation. *Cell* **77,** 335–347.
19. Chan, B. M. C., Nariaki, M., Takada, Y., Zetter, B. R., and Hemler, M. E. (1991) In vitro and in vivo consequences of VLA-2 expression on rhabdomyosarcoma cells. *Science* **251,** 1600–1602.
20. Yun, Z., Menter, D. G., and Nicolson, G. L. (1996) Involvement of integrin $\alpha v \beta 3$ in cell adhesion, motility and liver metastasis of murine RAW117 large cell lymphoma. *Cancer Res.* **56,** 3103–3111.
21. Dedhar, S. (1995) Integrin mediated signal transduction in oncogenesis: an overview. *Cancer Metast. Rev.* **14,** 165–172.

22. Heino, J. (1996) Biology of tumor cell invasion: interplay of cell adhesion and matrix degradation. *Int. J. Cancer* **65,** 717–722.

23. Ruoslahti, E. and Obrink, B. (1996) Common principles in cell adhesion. *Exp. Cell Res.* **227,** 1–11.

24. Magnatti, P. and Rifkin, D. B. (1993) Biology and biochemistry of proteases in tumor invasion. *Physiol. Rev.* **73,** 161–185.

25. Chambers, A. F. and Matrisian, L. M. (1997) Changing views of matrix metalloproteinases in metastasis. *J. Natl. Cancer. Inst.* **89,** 1260–1270.

26. Johnson, M. D., Torri, J. A., Lippman, M. E., and Dickson, R. B. (1993) The role of cathepsin D in the invasiveness of human breast cancer cells. *Cancer Res.* **53,** 873–877.

27. Brooks, P. C., Stromblad, S., Sanders, L. C., von Schalscha, T. L., Aimes, R. T., Stetler-Stevenson, W. G., et al. (1996) Localization of matrix metalloproteinase MMP-2 to the surface of invasive cells by interaction with integrin $\alpha v\beta 3$. *Cell* **85,** 683–693.

28. Brooks, P. C., Silletti, S., von Schalscha, T. L., Friedlander, M., and Cheresh, D. A. (1998) Disruption of angiogenesis by PEX, a noncatalytic metalloproteinase fragment with integrin binding activity. *Cell* **92,** 391–400.

29. Byzova, T. V. and Plow, E. F. (1998). Activation of $\alpha v\beta 3$ on vascular cells controls recognition of prothrombin. J. *Cell. Biol.* **143,** 2081–2092.

30. Lester, R. B. and McCarthy, J. B. (1992) Tumor cell adhesion to the extracellular matrix and signal transduction mechanisms implicated in tumor cell motility, invasion and metastasis. *Cancer Metast. Rev.* **11,** 31–44.

31. Pasqualini, R., Bourine, S., Koivunen, E., Woods, V. L., and Ruoslahiti, E. (1996) A polymeric form of fibronectin has anti-metastatic effects against multiple tumor types. *Nature Med.* **2,** 1197–1203.

32. Adams, J. C. and Watt, F. M. (1993) Regulation of development and differentiation by the extracellular matrix. *Development* **117,** 1183–1198.

33. Jia, T., Liu, Y. E., and Shi, Y. E. (1999) Stimulation of breast cancer invasion and metastasis by synuclein. *Cancer Res.* **59,** 742–747.

34. Crescimanno, C., Foidart, J-M., Noel, A., Polette, M., Maquoi, E., Birembaut, P., et al. (1996) Cloning of choriocarcinoma cells show that invasion correlates with expression and activation of gelatinase A. *Exp. Cell Res.* **227,** 240–251.

35. Hsu, M-Y., Shih, D-T., Meier, F. E., Belle, P. V., Hsu, J-Y., Elder, D. E., et al. (1998) Adenoviral gene transfer of $\beta 3$ integrin subunit induces conversion from radial to vertical growth phase in primary human melanoma. *Am. J. Pathol.* **153,** 1435–1442.

36. Isoai, A., Goto-Tsukamoto, H., Yamori, T., Oh-hara, T., Tsuruo, T., Silletti, S., et al. (1994) Inhibitory effects of tumor invasion-inhibitory factor 2 and its conjugate on disseminating tumor cells. *Cancer Res.* **54,** 1264–1270.

37. Bagheri-Yarmand, R., Kourbali, Y., Rath, A. M., Vassy, R., Martin, A., Jozefonvicz, J., et al. (1999) Carboxymethyl benzylamide dextran blocks angiogenesis of MDA-MB435 breast carcinoma xenografted in fat pad and its lung metastases in nude mice. *Cancer Res.* **59,** 507–510.

38. Asprunk, D. H., Knight, D. R., and Folkman, J. (1975) Vascularization of normal and neoplastic tissues grafted to the chick chorioallantois. *Am. J. Pathol.* **79,** 597–618.

39. Flamme, I. (1989) Is extraembryonic angiogenesis in the chick embryo controlled by the endoderm. *Anat. Embryol.* **180,** 259–272.
40. Iruela-Arispe, M. L., Lane, T. F., Redmond, D., Reilly, M., Bolender, R. P., Kavanagh, T. J., and Sage, E. H. (1995) Expression of SPARC during development of the chicken chorioallantoic membrane: evidence for regulated proteolysis in vivo. *Mol. Biol. Cell.* **6,** 327–343.
41. Ganote, C. E., Beaver, D. L., and Moses, H. L. (1964) Ultrastructure of the chick chorioallantoic membrane and its reaction to inoculation trauma. *Lab. Invest.* **13,** 1575–1589.
42. Leeson, T. S. and Lesson, C. R. (1963) The chorio-allantois of the chick. light and electronmicrospic observations at various times of incubation. *J. Anat. (Lond.)* **97,** 585–595.
43. Gorden, J. R. and Quigley, J. P. (1986) Early spontaneous metastasis in the human epidermoid carcinoma Hep3/chick embryo model: contribution of incidental colonization. *Int. J. Cancer* **38,** 437–444.
44. Scher, C. D. (1976) The chick chorioallantoic membrane as a model system for the study of tissue invasion by viral transformed cells. *Cell* **8,** 373–382.
45. Rizzo, V. and DeFouw, D. O. (1993) Macromolecular selectivity of the chick chorioallantoic membrane microvessels during normal angiogenesis and endothelial differentiation. *Tissue Cell* **6,** 847–856.
46. Nguyen, M., Shing, Y., and Folkman, J. (1994) Quantitation of angiogenesis and anti-angiogenesis in the chick embryo chorioallantoic membrane. *Microvasc. Res.* **47,** 31–40.
47. Brooks, P. C., Lin, J-M., French, D. L., and Quigley, J. P. (1993) Subtractive immunization yields antibodies that specifically inhibit metastasis. *J. Cell Biol.* **122,** 1351–1359.
48. Ossowski, L. and Reich, E. (1980) Experimental model for quantitative study of metastasis. *Cancer Res.* **40,** 2300–2309.
49. Kim, J., Yu, W., and Ossowski, L. (1998) Requirement for specific proteases in cancer cell intravasation as revealed by a novel semiquantitative PCR-based assay. *Cell* **94,** 353–362.

17

Gene Transfection for Metastasis Research Using Animal Models

Ruth J. Muschel and Jin Hua

1. Introduction

One means of testing a candidate gene for involvement in the metastatic process is to alter the expression of that gene in a tumor cell and then to test the metastatic potential of the altered cells. In designing such experiments, it is crucial to take into account the factor of tumor heterogeneity *(1)*. Some cell lines or cultures contain highly heterogeneous populations in regard to metastasis. Upon cloning these cells, some clones will be highly metastatic, but others will not. Thus, selection of a clone itself might skew the results if only a few clones are evaluated. Furthermore, the use of pooled populations after transfection must be considered with caution because the population may contain cells with a variety of metastatic potentials. To avoid these problems, it is necessary to do a preliminary experiment in which the chosen parental cell is subcloned and the subclones are tested for metastatic behavior. If the subclones have a similar metastatic potential to the parental line, then it should be a suitable recipient for metastasis studies. If, however, there is considerable variability in the subclones, either the subclones can be tested for stability or another more stable cell line should be sought.

A stable recipient cell line will be transfected with expression vectors designed to alter the expression of the gene of interest. The alteration might also be affected via knockout by homologous recombination *(2)*. Transfection controls should include vectors coding for other proteins or in the case of antisense vectors or ribozymes, for other alternative RNAs that will lead to pairing with the similar secondary structure, but target other gene products. This is especially important because double stranded RNAs generated by

From: *Methods in Molecular Medicine, vol. 58:*
Metastasis Research Protocols, Vol. 2: Cell Behavior In Vitro and In Vivo
Edited by: S. A. Brooks and U. Schumacher © Humana Press Inc., Totowa, NJ

antisense are known to have biological effects and overexpression of proteins can also in itself cause alterations in cellular signaling, for example activation of the NFκB pathway *(3)*. If the recipient is a non- or poorly metastatic cell line, then the goal of the experiment will be to induce or enhance metastasis through transfection. Transiently transfected cells can then be used in the injection into mice. After selection, the pooled population can be tested or in addition individual clones could be isolated and tested in vivo. If the goal is to take a metastatic population and diminish metastasis, then it is unlikely that any form of transient transfection will affect enough (at least 50%) of the cells so that any alteration in metastatic potential would not be detected. Thus, individual clones must be isolated and tested individually in this case. The tests for metastasis can include the lung colonization assay in which cells are injected into the tail vein of mice and the number of lung colonies counted, the spontaneous metastasis assay in which cells are allowed to form tumors and at later times the necropsied animals are evaluated and other assays detailed in this volume. These strategies have been used to demonstrate the involvement of CD44, NM23, VLA, MMP-9, met, E-cadherin, and Tiam among others in metastasis *(4–13)*. Detailed methodology for metastasis models using nude mice are described in Chapter 19 by Price.

The construct of interest can be introduced into cells in different ways, and indeed different cells are more susceptible to some methods than others. In the following subheadings, we will detail the use of transfection of DNA precipitated with calcium phosphate, but sometimes electroporation or use of lipid micelles must be used. A preliminary assay using a vector encoding green fluorescent protein (methodology is specifically covered in Chapter 25 by Hoffman) can easily allow one to determine the transfection efficiency.

To follow are the methods that we have used to test the involvement of metastasis by members of the matrix metalloproteinase family. Chapter 3 by McWilliams and Collins also gives detailed protocols for the genetic modification of cell lines to enhance their metastatic capability, and the reader is directed to consult this chapter also.

2. Materials

All buffers and solutions are made up in deionized/distilled water.

2.1. Transfection and Selection

1. Cell culture media.
2. Selecting reagent: Antibiotics such as geneticin, hygromycin, etc.
3. Trypsin–EDTA: 0.05% trypsin, 0.53 mM EDTA in PBS (*see* **ref. 7**).
4. 0.1X TE: 1 mM Tris-HCl, 0.1 mM EDTA, pH 8.0; sterilize by autoclaving.
5. 2 M CaCl$_2$, filter to sterilize, aliquot and store at –20°C (*see* **Note 1**).

6. 2X HEPES-buffered saline (100 mL): Mix 1.6 g of NaCl, 0.074 g of KCl, 0.027 g of $Na_2HPO_4 \cdot 2H_2O$, 0.2 g of Dextrose and 1 g of HEPES (acid). Adjust pH to exactly 7.05 (*see* **Note 2**) with 0.5 N NaOH, bring to 100 mL, and filter. Then aliquot and store at –20°C.

7. 1X PBS: 8 g of NaCl, 0.2 g of KCl, 1.15 g of $Na_2HPO_4 \cdot 7H_2O$, 0.2 g of KH_2PO_4, adjust pH to 7.3 with NaOH, bring to 1 L with water, and autoclave.

8. Cloning cylinders: Put cloning cylinders vertically in a glass dish layered with vacuum grease and sterilize by autoclaving.

2.2. Metastasis and Tumorigenicity Assays

1. 1X PBS: 8 g of NaCl, 20.2 g of KCl, 1.15 g of $Na_2HPO_4 \cdot 7H_2O$, 0.2 g of KH_2PO_4, adjust pH to 7.3 with 10 N NaOH, bring to 1 L with water, and autoclave.
2. Cell culture media.
3. Trypsin–EDTA.
4. Sterile 30-gauge needles and syringes.
5. Mouse holder.
6. Light bulb.
7. 75% Ethanol.

3. Methods

3.1. Calcium Phosphate Transfection and Selection of Clones (see Note 3)

1. On d 1, seed 2×10^5 cells /10-cm tissue culture dish in 10 mL of media.
2. On d 2, replace media 3 h before transfection. Precipitate 30 µg of DNA (expression vector) in ethanol and resuspend in 438 µL of 0.1× TE and 62 µL of 2 M $CaCl_2$. Add dropwise to 500 µL of 2X HEPES-buffered saline (*see* **Note 2**) in a 50-mL tube while bubbling air, then vortex-mix for 2 s. Allow to stand for 30 min. Distribute to a 10-cm dish evenly and agitate gently to mix.
3. On d 3, wash with media twice and replace with media overnight.
4. On d 4, replace with selection media 24 h after the wash.
5. Replace with selection media every 2 d later on and grow for 10–14 d until individual clones are formed.
6. When selecting, wash clones with 1X PBS, remove all media carefully, and firmly place a cloning cylinder right on a clone using autoclaved forceps. Touch the rim of the cloning cylinder to autoclaved vacuum grease to allow a water tight seal to be formed. Add one drop of trypsin into cloning cylinder. Observe the clone under the dissecting microscope to demonstrate that it has been detected. Transfer trypsinized clones into a 6-well plate to grow.

3.2. Metastasis and Tumorigenicity Assays

All manipulations on mice should be done under aseptic conditions.

1. Obtain and house aseptically 4–6-wk-old female *nu/nu* mice.

2. Grow cells to subconfluence. Wash cells once with 1X PBS, trypsinize, and harvest by centrifugation. Then resuspend cells in serum-free media. Examine the cell suspensions microscopically to ensure that cells are single-cell suspensions. Transfer cells into a 1.5-mL tube and put on ice before using.

3. For metastasis assays, place a mouse in a mouse holder and warm the tail using light bulb until the tail veins are clearly seen and clean tail with 75% ethanol.

4. Utilize a 32-gauge needle to withdraw cells and inject into the lateral vein with 5×10^4 single cells/0.1 mL (*see* **Note 4**). No more than 0.2 mL should be used, as increased amounts can compromise the animal. Maintain the animals for several weeks, checking them at least twice per week. Metastases will usually develop between 2 and 8 wk.

5. Labored breathing or cachexia may be a sign of metastasis. Mice are killed when they exhibit labored breathing. Perform a necropsy and remove any organs with suspected tumors and fix in 10% w/v formalin.

6. Use a dissecting microscope to count the tumors for evidence of metastasis. Sections can also be taken to confirm the presence of metastasis histologically. The use of lung weight while a guide to metastasis formation is more correctly a measure of tumor growth rate in the lung and is a less direct measure than the colony number.

7. For tumorigenicity assays, inject mice subcutaneously in the flank with 5×10^5 cells/0.1 mL.

8. Measure the tumor size with calipers every 2 d.

4. Notes

1. Do not repeatedly freeze and thaw 2 M CaCl$_2$.
2. The pH of 2X HEPES-buffered saline is critical for transfection efficiency.
3. Alternatively, Lipofectamine reagent (Gibco-BRL, Gaithersburg, MA) may be used as a method of transfection; however, the transfection conditions should be optimized.
4. Single-cell suspensions are important for metastasis assays. Cell clumps will lead to tumors and even pulmonary infarction. It is critical to use only the lateral tail veins, not the dorsal or ventral arteries. These injections are difficult to perform. If the fluid flows in easily, it is likely to have been good. If force was applied, it is likely that the vein was missed.

References

1. Heppner, G. H. and Miller, F. R. (1998) The cellular basis of tumor progression. *Int. Rev. Cytol.* **177,** 1–56.
2. Stroeken, P. J., van Rijthoven, E. A., van der Valk, M. A., and Roos, E. (1998) Targeted disruption of the beta1 integrin gene in a lymphoma cell line greatly reduces metastatic capacity. *Cancer Res.* **58,** 1569–1577.
3. Pahl, H. L. and Baeuerle, P. A. (1997) The ER-overload response: activation of NF-kappa B. *Trends Biochem. Sci.* **22,** 63–67.
4. Vleminckx, K., Vakaet, L. Jr., Mareel, M. Fiers, W., and van Roy, F. (1991) Genetic manipulation of E-cadherin expression by epithelial tumor cells reveals an invasion suppressor role. *Cell* **66,** 107–119.

5. Chan, B. M., Matsuura, N., Takada, Y., Zetter, B. R., and Hemler, M. E. (1991) In vitro and in vivo consequences of VLA-2 expression on rhabdomyosarcoma cells. *Science* **251,** 1600–1602.

6. Leone, A., Flatow, U., VanHoutte, K., and Steeg, P. S. (1993) Transfection of human nm23-H1 into the human MDA-MB-435 breast carcinoma cell line: effects on tumor metastatic potential, colonization and enzymatic activity. *Oncogene* **8,** 2325–2333.

7. Bernhard, E. J., Gruber, S. B., and Muschel, R. J. (1994) Direct evidence linking expression of matrix metalloproteinase 9 (92-kDa gelatinase/collagenase) to the metastatic phenotype in transformed rat embryo cells. *PNAS* **91,** 4293–4297.

8. Habets, G. G., Scholtes, E. H., Zuydgeest, D., van der Kammen, R. A., Stam, J. C., Berns, A., and Collard, J. G. (1994) Identification of an invasion-inducing gene, Tiam-1, that encodes a protein with homology to GDP-GTP exchangers for Rho-like proteins. *Cell* **77,** 537–549.

9. Michiels, F., Habets, G. G., Stam, J. C., van der Kammen, R. A., and Collard, J. G. (1995) A role for Rac in Tiam1-induced membrane ruffling and invasion. *Nature* **375,** 338–340.

10. Hua, J. and Muschel, R. J. (1996) Inhibition of matrix metalloprotinase 9 expression by a ribozyme blocks metastasis in a rat sarcoma model system. *Cancer Res.* **56,** 5279–5284.

11. Gunthert, U., Hofmann, M., Rudy, W., Reber, S., Zoller, M., Haussmann, I., et al. (1991) A new variant of glycoprotein CD44 confers metastatic potential to rat carcinoma cells. *Cell* **65,** 13–24.

12. Giordano, S., Bardelli, A., Zhen, Z., Menhard, S., Ponzetto, C., And Comoglio, P. M. (1997) A point mutation in the MET oncogene abrogates metastasis without affecting transformation. *PNAS* **94,** 13868–13872.

13. Sehgal, G., Hua, J., Bernhard, E. J., Sehgal, I., Thompson, T. C., and Muschel, R. J. (1998) Requirement for matrix metalloproteinase-9 (gelatinase B) expression in metastasis by murine prostate carcinoma. *Am. J. Pathol.* **152,** 591–596.

18

Theoretical Considerations in Using Animal Models of Metastasis and Brief Methodology for In Vivo Colorectal Cancer Models in SCID and Nude Mice

Sue A. Watson and Teresa M. Morris

1. Introduction

1.1. In Vivo Colorectal Cancer Models

Metastatic spread is generally responsible for the mortality of colorectal cancer patients. There are no adequate treatments for advanced colorectal cancer, and novel therapeutic modalities are urgently required. To this end, valid metastatic models, which accurately mimic the disease process, are needed. When deciding upon a metastasis model, the goals of the investigation will dictate the complexity of the model chosen. If biological mechanisms are being investigated, only a small number of experimental animals may be required, and a more complex, surgically intensive model may be used. If a therapeutic agent is being evaluated, owing to group sizes required to generate statistically significant effects, a less complex, less surgically intensive model may be preferable. The latter, however, may encompass only a particular phase of metastasis rather than reflecting all aspects of the metastatic cascade.

In colorectal cancer models, the site of implantation is dictated by the common sites of metastasis in humans, mainly the liver, with the lungs being involved in a minimal way, often as tertiary spread. To achieve growth within the liver, the main sites of implantation are the spleen, the peritoneal cavity, and orthotopically into the colon or cecal wall. The former two models mimic only the last phase of metastasis, that is, extravasation from the bloodstream into the liver parenchyma, and are thus experimental. The latter model encompasses all aspects of true spontaneous metastasis. Other sites of implantation

From: *Methods in Molecular Medicine, vol. 58:*
Metastasis Research Protocols, Vol. 2: Cell Behavior In Vitro and In Vivo
Edited by: S. A. Brooks and U. Schumacher © Humana Press Inc., Totowa, NJ

exist that model metastasis to lung. A simple method of initiating experimental metastasis in the lung involves injection of cells intravenously, generally into the tail vein. This results in multiple lesions within the lung, is generally aggressive, and simply involves an extravasation step. A spontaneous lung metastasis model involves implantation of cells into the muscle layer of the abdominal wall. This results in the development of a well-vascularized primary tumor and spontaneous spread to the lungs.

1.2. Syngeneic vs Xenogeneic Models

In selecting an animal model in the field of cancer research, several factors should be taken into consideration before a study begins. Most of these will be concerned with the scientific aspects of the study. Do the investigations elucidate mechanisms of metastatic spread? Is a therapeutic agent to be investigated, and if so what is its mode of action? What body system will be principally affected? Is the basis of the work to repeat existing studies? What comparisons to existing data, clinical and preclinical, will be made? What statistical evaluation will be performed? However, some considerations must reflect more mundane, but important, questions. What facilities and resources are available? How much will the study cost? Paramount to all these considerations (in the UK) is that the necessary authorization, in the form of a project license, must be in place.

Subsequently, a choice must be made between a xenogeneic system, that is, human tissue grown in an immunodeficient animal or a syngeneic system where a spontaneous tumor, which has previously formed in a particular strain of mice or rats, is subsequently passaged into animals of the same strain. These animals will generally be immunocompetent. The main advantage of xenograft models is that, by the use of human tumor cell lines, they allow direct investigation of human tissue. It may be that the target of a therapeutic drug varies between humans and rodents, making it imperative to use such a model. In addition, the xenograft models may be established with well-characterized cell lines, many passages away from the patient from whom they were derived or from tissue recently derived from a clinical sample. The latter may be a more heterogeneous cell population, with a lower level of characterization, but any therapeutic response may be more reflective of that likely to be achieved in a clinical study. The disadvantages of xenogeneic models relate to the necessity to grow human tumors in immunodeficient animals. Such animals are expensive to purchase and require sterile isolator containment, as they are prone to infections. In addition, the use of human tissue necessitates animals to be maintained in Advisory Committee for Dangerous Pathogens (ACDP) Containment Level 2. Immunodeficient mice lack a fully functional immune system; nude mice (1) have no functional T cells (spontaneous and experimental xenograft metastasis models in nude mice are described in Chapter 19 by Janet Price) and severe combined immuno-deficient (SCID) *(2)* mice no functional B or T cells (an experimental colon and breast cancer metastasis model in the SCID mouse is described in Chapter 20 by Schumacher and Brooks). Therefore, if a particular therapeutic agent works by modulation of the immune response to a tumor, a xenograft model would be inappropriate. Similarly, if tumor–stroma interactions are important, for example, in the area of matrix metalloproteinase (MMP) research, xenograft models may be disadvantageous. MMP expression and activation involve complex interactions between tumor and stroma that may be compromised if the two tissue components are from different species.

A wide range of human colorectal tumor cell lines is available. These can be purchased from the American Type Tissue Collection (ATCC) *(3)* and the European Cell Culture Collection (ECACC) *(4)* held at Porton Down in the UK. In addition, detailed protocols are in place showing the derivation of tumors from surgically resected human tumor tissue *(5)*.

Syngeneic models use immunocompetent animals bearing spontaneous tumors, which originated in the same strain. Thus a fully functional immune system is generally in place that will allow immunomodulation to be investigated. The experimental animals can be kept under conventional conditions that are likely to be in place in a standard animal facility. However, if a therapeutic agent is human-specific then a syngeneic model will be of no use. In addition, the tumors tend to be aggressive and give a short time frame both for detailed observations and studies on established tumors to be performed. A syngeneic murine model of B16 melanoma is described in Chapter 21 by Giavazzi and Garofalo.

Examples of syngeneic colorectal models are as follows:

Mouse

MC26 in Balb/C mice	When injected intravenously into the tail vein form lung metastases.
KLN205 in DBA/2 mice	Form lung metastases from intervenous implantation.
CMT93 and CMT9369 in C57/Bl mice	" " " " " "

Rats

WB2054M in Brown Norway × Wistar Furth F_1 rats	Form spontaneous lung metastases following implantation into muscle layer of abdominal wall.
DHDK12 in BDIX rats	Form spontaneous lung metastases following implantation into muscle layer of abdominal wall.

1.3. Spontaneous vs Experimental Metastasis

Spontaneous metastasis is defined as the full cascade of tumor spread. This should involve invasion of a primary tumor through the extracellular matrix and basement membrane and intravasation of cells into the bloodstream. Cells then travel in the bloodstream to a particular organ, where they will extravasate, invade into the tissue, and subsequently grow. In the same way, cells may travel within the lymphatic system following entry into a draining lymph node. Derivation of in vivo models, which reflect this complex process, has been an area of active interest for well over a decade. A major breakthrough has been in the use of orthotopic transplantation *(6)* which, in the field of colorectal cancer metastasis models, principally involves injection of tumor cells into the lymphoid follicle of the cecum *(7)*. Clinically accurate orthotopic mouse models of cancer are described in Chapter 23 by Hoffman. In initial studies, injection of India ink or fluorescent particles into the follicle demonstrated distribution within the draining lymphatics. Following injection of tumor cells and partial resection of the cecum, tumor developed within the lymph nodes, and subsequently spread to the liver. Orthotopic xenografting has also been carried out, small pieces of tumor tissue being sutured onto the colon wall. Problems with such models include:

1. The surgically intensive nature of their initiation, limiting the number of mice that can be set up at any time point.
2. Potentially low take rate in the secondary organ of interest which would limit the use of this model in therapeutic terms.
3. The need to initiate large numbers of animals for therapeutic experiments to obtain statistically valid results.
4. Either technique may result in leakage or shearing of cells into the peritoneal cavity, leading to peritoneal tumor deposits, necessitating early termination of mice.
5. Cells may invade the liver directly and bypass phases of the metastatic cascade.
6. Cells have to be prepared in acutely small volumes which may leach out of the injection site leading to inaccuracies in cell inocula.

A simpler model of establishing spontaneous metastasis of a human colorectal tumor has recently been described by our research group *(8)*. In this model the human colorectal line, AP5LV, which was previously selected from an experimental lung tumor (*see* **Subheading 3.2.**) is implanted into the muscle layer of the abdominal wall of SCID mice. After a 35–40 d time period, during which the primary tumor is left *in situ*, there is metastatic spread to the lungs in 30–40% of the mice. Again due to the ease of initiation, this model also lends itself to large-scale therapy determinations as well as evaluation of the biological/mechanical characteristics of invasion.

Experimental metastasis is a process that models a single aspect of the metastatic cascade. It can be invasion and intravasation from the primary site or extravasation and growth within the secondary site. This usually involves transplantation of cells directly into an organ, or into a site that allows easy access to the organ of interest. For example, injection into the spleen *(9)* or portal vein allows access to the liver. The former may ask more of the cells in terms of passage through one organ and into another whereas the latter is purely associated with lodging of cells in the capillary bed and invasive growth.

A further experimental metastasis model involves intraperitoneal injection of the human colorectal tumor cell line, C170HM2 *(10)*. Cells have been selected to invade and grow specifically on the liver by in vivo and in vitro selection, which will be outlined below theoretically and practically. This models the end stage of metastasis but relies on the cells homing to the liver, adhering to the surface, invading the liver capsule and growing within the liver parenchyma. This process also involves the overexpression of both adhesive cell-surface antigens and invasive enzymes *(10–12)*. Such a model, owing to the simplistic method of initiation, lends itself to large-scale therapy experiments with novel anti-metastatic agents, as have been recently described *(13)*.

1.4. Derivation of Cell Lines with Specific Invasive Characteristics

There are two main ways of deriving cell lines with invasive characteristics

1. By selection either in vitro or in vivo of clones with enhanced metastatic properties.
2. By genetic modification.

Detailed methodology for the latter is given in Chapters 3 and 17 by McWilliams and Collins and by Muschel and Hua.

Cell lines with specific metastatic characteristics in vivo can either arise spontaneously or be induced by manipulating the injection route or organ environment. The heterogeneous nature of the cell population within the tumor may give rise, by selection or mutational events, to clones of cells having increased metastatic capabilities. Should these then become the dominant population within the tumor, the metastatic potential of that tumor will be increased. Therefore, any tumors exhibiting changes in phenotype, for example, invasion into the body cavity, or specific organ invasion, which may have resulted from the outgrowth of such clones, could potentially become new metastatic models. These can be isolated and serially passaged either in vivo or in vitro.

To stimulate the development of specific clones that may be present within the cell population, the same cell line may also be administered via different routes in order to develop sublines with differing metastatic potential *(14)*.

The two cell lines described in the following, C170HM2 and AP5LV, were both developed in our Unit using a combination of in vivo and in vitro techniques. In both cases a clone of cells exhibiting particular characteristics in vivo were established in vitro, reinitiated in vivo, reestablished in vitro, etc. until a stable phenotype was achieved. Other models have also been established in our Unit in the same way, notably a gastric ascites model in SCID mice.

Confirmation of the human origin of newly derived metastatic cell lines can be carried out, for example, using isozyme analysis (Authentikit; Corning

Medical). This would appear to have greater importance as recent publications have suggested that spontaneous mouse tumors can be stimulated by implantation of human tumor xenografts *(15)*.

2. Materials

1. Animal strain: MF1 nude mice (Harlan Olac) 4–6 wk old. Originally both male and female used, now cells grow more reproducibly in male mice giving approx an 80% take rate. In females, take rate can fall to 50%.
2. Animal strain: SCID mice (Cancer Studies Unit, University of Nottingham) 4–6 wk old, both male and female used.
3. Husbandry: Animals are maintained in sterile Pathoflex isolator units (Elwyn Roberts Isolators, UK). Food and bedding are purchased irradiated (2.5 Mrad) from commercial sources (food—Special Diet Services R/M 3 [E] type, bedding—Datesand, UK) Water is autoclaved. Cages, water bottles, and all materials entering the isolators are autoclaved. Virkon disinfecting solution is used to spray the outer surface of all items entering the isolator. Nude mice are maintained at slightly higher than normal temperatures, 26–28°C, with 12-h light and 12-h dark cycles.
4. C170HM2 cells are maintained in vitro in RPMI 1640 culture medium (GIBRO, Paisley, UK) containing 10% v/v heat-inactivated fetal bovine serum (FBS) (Sigma, Poole, UK) at 37°C in 5% CO_2 and humidified conditions. Cells from semiconfluent monolayers are harvested with 0.025% EDTA, washed twice in the culture medium described in the preceeding, and resuspended at 1.5×10^6/mL in sterile phosphate-buffered saline, pH 7.4 (PBS).
5. AP5LV cells were maintained in vitro in RPMI 1640 culture medium (GIBRO, Paisley, UK) containing 10% v/v heat inactivated FBS (Sigma, Poole, UK) at 37°C in 5% CO_2 and humidified conditions. Cells from semiconfluent monolayers were harvested with 0.025% EDTA, washed twice in the culture medium described in the preceeding, and resuspended at 1×10^6 in 50 µL in sterile PBS, pH 7.4.

3. Methods
3.1. Establishment of C170HM2 Liver-Invasive Tumors

The parental cell line, the human colorectal carcinoma C170, was injected subcutaneously into female nude mice. The subsequent tumor was resected, dissagregated enzymatically, and 2×10^6 cells, resuspended in 1 mL of medium, were injected intraperitoneally into 10 female MF1 nude mice (Harlan Olac). Fifty-nine days later 4/10 mice had developed very large liver tumors (replacing between 40% and 90% of normal liver tissue). These tumors were again dissagregated and 4×10^6 cells were injected into 3 female nude mice, the subsequent liver tumors being again dissagregated and reinjected. The process was repeated 4 times in vivo. Following this, cells were established in vitro in RPMI tissue culture medium containing 10% heat-inactivated fetal calf serum (FCS) on irradiated mouse 3T3 fibroblast feeder layers. The cells were reintroduced, via the peritoneal cavity, and selected 10 times in the same manner. After this, the tumor line was shown to selectively invade the liver in 70–80% of mice and have extremely limited growth elsewhere in the peritoneal cavity *(10)* (*see* **Notes 1–8**). Owing to the latter, tumor growth may continue for 40–50 d before termination, allowing a large window for therapeutic studies. Thus, the effects of drugs, in both advanced and adjuvant settings, can be compared. The metastatic clone may be compared to the parental line for specific metastasis-associated characteristics. This has previously been carried out for C170HM2 and the parental line, C170 *(12)*. The liver-invasive clone was shown to express elevated levels of MMP1 and MMP-9 by competitive reverse transcriptase-polymerase chain reaction (RT-PCR). Such studies confirm that a more highly invasive clone has been derived and expresses the characteristics expected of such a clone in that it correlates with the MMP expression of metastatic human colorectal tumors *(16)*. Interestingly, C170HM2 grows with greater reliability within the liver of male nude mice. In female mice the take rate drops to approx 50%. This emphasises the sex differences that may be encountered which always must be taken into account when planning such studies.

3.2. Establishment of AP5LV Lung-Invasive Tumors

The parental cell line, the human colorectal tumor AP5, was injected intravenously into 8–10-wk-old male SCID mice, at a dose of 10^5 cells in a 100 μL volume. Within 21–30 d, experimental lung tumors had formed in the mice. These were dissected free and mechanically disaggregated into tissue culture medium (RPMI + 10% heat-inactivated FCS). Cells were then refed on a daily basis until all the lung debris was removed and small colonies of tumor cells were allowed to establish over a 2–3-wk period. The cells were harvested and 5×10^6 cells in 50 μL were injected into the peritoneal muscle wall of 10 SCID mice. Using a sterile procedure, the mice were anaesthetized with Hypnorm (Janssen)/ Hypnovel(Roche), shaved on their right flanks, and a small incision made. The skin was undercut and the muscle wall overlying the peritoneal cavity, exposed. The cells were injected into the muscle wall so that a bleb appeared, indicating a successful injection has occurred. The skin was closed using michelle clips. At termination, one mouse was found to have developed lung nodules in addition to the primary tumor in the peritoneal muscle wall. The lung tumors were removed and again mechanically dissaggregated and established in vitro. The cell line was then renamed AP5LV (lung variant). A group of mice was then established with intra-abdominal wall injection of AP5LV cells (*see* **Notes 9–16**). The metastatic potential of the cell line, when reintroduced into the muscle layer of the abdominal wall, increased, with 60–70% of the mice developing lung nodules. The metastasis rate is higher in female when compared to male mice, again emphasizing the importance of correcting for sex differences *(8)*. Also, it is important that all metastatic variants are chromosome typed to confirm they are of human origin.

4. Notes

Any adverse effects should be listed in the 19b section of a project license. They are limited by careful observation and monitoring, restriction of the study length, and humane killing where necessary.

1. Once a stable phenotype is established, initiation of the model is by simple intraperitoneal injection. In order that a good distribution within the peritoneal cavity is achieved, the cell innoculum is injected in a volume of 1 mL. Smaller volumes have been found to result in solid tumors at the injection site. Anesthesia/analgesia are therefore unnecessary. In fact, to maintain the normal "flow" of fluid within the peritoneal cavity it is preferable for the animal to be mobile.
2. At induction, care should be taken with the intraperitoneal injection. We prefer not to inject straight into the abdomen (using a "stabbing" method), which may result in injection of the cells into part of the gut. Holding the mouse in the left hand we insert a 24-gauge needle, held at right angles to the line of the body, between the last two nipples, so that the needle can be seen clearly entering the peritoneal cavity. The needle is then gently pushed along inside the cavity toward the mid-line. The cell inoculum is gently expressed.
3. Occasionally the liver tumors may develop in such a way that liver function is disrupted. In this case animals may develop an obvious jaundice and their clinical condition will rapidly deteriorate. These animals should be terminated as soon as this becomes apparent.
4. The cells have been found to adhere to the plastic of the syringe and it is preferable therefore to either load one at a time or ask an assistant to load the syringes.
5. The duration of the model is normally approx 40 d. At this time 1–4 liver tumors will be present (these may have replaced up to 80% of normal liver tissue, however they should remain within the 10% of initial body weight recommended by the UKCCCR guidelines).
6. Monitoring throughout the study is by measurement of body weight. Visual signs of tumor burden or loss of muscle mass, especially visible behind the head of nude mice when the bone structure can clearly be seen. An abdominal mass may also be visible or palpable. With an advanced tumor, movement may become restricted due to abdominal tumor load.
7. Any tumors developing either at the injection site or in the peritoneal cavity will necessitate early termination of the mice as the tumor burden will become too great.
8. Quantification at termination. Because the tumor tissue is more solid than the normal liver parenchyma, it is relatively easy to dissect free the liver tumors. These can be measured using callipers, and weighed.
9. For initiation of AP5LV peritoneal wall tumors, injected anaesthetic is used. Hypnorm (Roche) Hypnovel (Jannsen) are combined with water in 1:1:5 combination. 100–150 µL is injected intraperitoneally.
10. It has been found that it is easier to gently hold the anaesthetized animal in the left hand during the procedure, enabling gentle tension to be exerted on the muscle layer of the abdominal cavity.

11. No special postoperative care is required, the procedure being comparable to a subcutaneous graft.
12. The AP5LV primary tumor develops by invading along and through the peritoneal muscle wall. It is therefore difficult to accurately assess tumor size, which tends to be masked by the "iceberg effect," that is, a greater proportion of the tumor grows inwards. It is therefore important to adhere to the predetermined time scale of the study or the tumor size may exceed UKCCCR guidelines and cachexia may develop.
13. Normally the tumor growing into the peritoneal cavity will be encapsulated. Occasionally, however, the capsule breaks down and cells may slough off into the cavity. This results in extensive diffuse peritoneal tumor developing, often accompanied by ascites. This will result in weight loss, loss of clinical condition, and rapid deterioration. Any animals exhibiting this should be humanely killed.
14. Monitoring throughout the study is by measurement of body weight. The nature of the peritoneal wall tumor will not allow calliper measurements to be made, although gentle palpation is possible to determine the approximate size.
15. The duration of the model is normally approx 40 d. At this time the primary peritoneal wall tumors should remain within the 10% of initial body weight (recommended by the UKCCCR guidelines).
16. Quantification at termination. The primary tumor can be dissected free, measured and weighed as for a subcutaneous tumor. The lungs are removed and fixed in formal saline.

References

1. Flanagan, S. P. (1966) Nude, a new hairless gene with pleiotropic effects in the mouse. C*ancer Res. Camb.* **8,** 295–309.
2. Bosma, G. C., Custer, P. R., and Bosma, M. J. (1983) A severe combined immunodeficiency mutation in the mouse. *Nature* **301,** 527–530.
3. American Type Culture Collection, 12301 Parklawn Drive, Rockville, MD 20852.
4. ECACC, Dept. of Cell Resources, Centre for Applied Microbiology and Research, Porton Down, Salisbury, Wiltshire SP4 0JG, UK.
5. Moyer, M. P., Armstrong, A., Bradley-Aust, J., Levine, B. A., and Sirinek, K. R. (1986) Effects of gastrin, glutamine and somatostatin on the *in vitro* growth of normal and malignant human gastric mucosal cells. *Arch. Surg.* **121,** 285–288.
6. Manzotti, C., Audisio, R. A., and Pratesi, G. (1993) Importance of orthotopic implantation for human tumors as model systems: relevance to metastasis and invasion. *Clin. Exp. Metast.* **11,** 5–14.
7. Schackert, H. K. and Fidler, I. J. (1989) Development of an animal model to study the biology of recurrent colorectal cancer originating from mesenteric lymph system metastases. *Int. J. Cancer* **44,** 177–181.
8. Watson, S. A., Michaeli, D., Morris, T. M., Clarke, P., Varro, A., Griffin, N., et al. (1999) Antibodies raised by Gastrimmune inhibit the spontaneous metastasis of a human colorectal tumor, AP5LV. *Eur. J. Cancer* **35(8),** 1286–1291.

9. Giavazzi, R., Jessup, J. M., Campbell, D. E., Walker, S. M., and Fidler, I. J. (1986) Experimental nude mouse model of human colorectal cancer liver metastases. *J. Natl. Cancer Inst.* **77,** 1303–1307.

10. Watson, S. A., Clifford, T., Robinson, E., and Steele, R. J. C. (1995) Gastrin sensitivity of primary human colorectal cancer: the effect of gastrin receptor antagonism. *Eur. J. Cancer* **31A,** 2086–2092.

11. Watson, S. A., Morris, T. M., Robinson, G., Crimmin, A., and Brown, P. D. (1995) Inhibition of organ invasion by metalloproteinase inhibitor, BB-94 in 2 human colon metastasis models. *Cancer Res.* **55,** 3629–3633.

12. Collins, H. M., Tierney, G. M., and Watson, S. A. (1997) Expression of matrix metalloproteinases (MMPs) and TIMPs in colorectal cancer cell lines using RT-PCR. *Gut* **41,** p. A254.

13. Watson, S. A., Skelton, L., Jackman, A., Morris, T. M., Page, M., and Rholff, C. (1999) A novel, orally administered nucleoside analog, OGT-719 inhibits the liver invasive growth of a human colorectal tumor, C170HM2. *Cancer Res.* in press.

14. Morikawa, K., Walker, S. M., Jessup, M. J., and Fidler, I. J. (1988) In vivo selection of highly metastatic cells from surgical specimens of different primary human colon carcinomas implanted into nude mice. *Cancer Res.* **48,** 1943–1948.

15. Pathak, S., Nemeth, M. A., and Multani, A. S. (1998) Human tumour xenografts in nude mice are not always of human origin. *Cancer* **78,** No. S1, p. P63.

16. Kelly, S. R., Gough, A. C., and Primrose, J. N. (1998) Downregulation of tissue inhibitors of metalloproteinases (TIMPs) in hepatic tissue surrounding colorectal carcinoma metastases *Br. J. Cancer* **78,** No. S1, p. P63.

19

Xenograft Models in Immunodeficient Animals

I. Nude Mice: Spontaneous and Experimental Metastasis Models

Janet E. Price

1. Introduction

The growth of metastases is the end result of a multistep process in which cancer cells invade through basement membranes, extravasate into bloodstream or lymphatic vessels, survive transit in the circulation, arrest, and then grow in the new site *(1)*. Tissue culture traits that reliably predict the metastatic ability of cancer cells are rare, possibly because any particular assay, for example, invasion through extracellular matrix *(2)*, or growth in semisolid agarose *(3)* can evaluate only a tumor cell's ability to perform one step in the multistep process. Thus, animal models using transplantable tumors that produce a predictable number of metastases in suitable recipients are the standard test systems for analyzing the metastatic phenotype, and for evaluating the efficacy of antimetastatic agents. The discovery that tumor tissue could be xenografted into the mutant athymic "nude" mouse strain opened a new area for experimental studies with human tumor cells, including the analysis of their metastatic properties *(1,4)*. Additional immunodeficient mouse strains are also available for human tumor experimentation. The combination of the nude and beige mutations produced athymic mice with reduced NK cell activity. The triple deficient beige *(bg)*/nude *(nu)*/xid mouse is functionally depleted of T and B cells and lack precursors of lymphokine activated killer (LAK) cells. Severe combined immune-deficient (SCID) mice, homozygous for the mutant gene *scid*, are severely deficient in both T and B cells (SCID mouse xenograft models of metastasis are described in Chapter 20 by Schumacher and Brooks). In comparisons of tumor take and metastasis of several human tumor cell lines in different immunodeficient mice, some differences were seen. Some cell lines produced a higher incidence of

From: *Methods in Molecular Medicine, vol. 58:*
Metastasis Research Protocols, Vol. 2: Cell Behavior In Vitro and In Vivo
Edited by: S. A. Brooks and U. Schumacher © Humana Press Inc., Totowa, NJ

metastasis in the SCID vs nude mice *(5,6)*. However, in another example, the incidence of metastasis of a human breast cancer cell line was lower in the triple deficient *bg/nu/xid* mice than in nude mice *(4)*, suggesting that using a mouse with a more profound immunodeficiency does not guarantee that the implanted tumor cells will grow more aggressively. Ultimately, the choice of the strain will be dictated by the design of the experiment, as well as availability and expense. The procedures described in this chapter can be applied to any of the different immuno-deficient animals.

There are two types of experimental design for metastasis models. The spontaneous metastasis models assess the ability of cells to spread from a tumor implanted into a local site, commonly from subcutaneous (s.c.) or intramuscular (i.m.) injections, or injections into tissues reflecting the origin of the tumor cell line (orthotopic injections). Depending on the site of injection, the growth of the local tumor can be monitored as part of the experiment. The use of orthotopic models has arisen from the observation that implanting tumor cells or fragments into the equivalent mouse tissue or organ can promote local tumor growth and subsequent metastasis. Hence, growth of human prostate cancer cells can be assessed in the prostate gland, colon cancer in the cecum, breast cancer in the mammary fatpad, etc. *(7–9)* and clinically accurate orthotopic mouse models of cancer are described in Chapter 23 by Hoffman. While the exact mechanisms of how the tissues can influence the tumor cell phenotype have not been fully defined, the role of stromal cell derived factors that influence angiogenesis and proteolytic enzyme release by the tumor cells has been implicated in some studies *(10,11)*. This chapter describes a subcutaneous model, suitable for human melanoma cells *(12)*, and a model for breast cancer cells injected into the mammary fatpad of mice *(9)*. Experimental metastasis models assess the ability of tumor cells to arrest, extravasate, and grow in a particular organ following intra-vascular injection. Intravenous (i.v.) injection into the lateral tail vein is the most commonly used model, generally resulting in lung metastases. Injection of cells into the spleen is commonly used to determine the ability of colon cancer cells to form liver metastases; within 10 min of injection of radiolabeled cells into the spleen, 90% of the cells arrest in the liver *(13)*. This procedure and tail vein injections are described in this chapter.

2. Materials

1. Human tumor cell line, free of *Mycoplasma* and murine pathogenic viruses (reovirus type 3, pneumonia virus, K virus, Theiler's encephalitis virus, Sendai virus, minute virus, mouse adenovirus, mouse hepatitis virus, lymphocytic choriomeningitis virus, ectromelia virus, lactate dehydrogenase virus). Checking the cell lines for these viruses will reduce the risk of introducing pathogens into the animal facility.
2. Nude mice age (6 wk old at start of experiment) and sex-matched.

3. Culture medium with serum.
4. Phosphate-buffered saline (PBS) without Ca^{2+} and Mg^{2+}.
5. Trypsin–EDTA: 0.25% w/v trypsin and 0.02% w/v EDTA in PBS without Ca^{2+} and Mg^{2+}. Prepare a fresh trypsin solution before harvesting cell cultures.
6. Sterile instruments for necropsy and surgery (forceps, scissors, and 12-mm wound clips and wound clip applier if performing survival surgery).
7. Sterile gauze squares, 2-in. and 4-in. sterile cotton swabs (used for surgical procedures).
8. Mouse restraint device (for tail vein injections) and warming lamp. The restraint should secure the mouse with the tail extended outside.
9. Sterile 1-mL tuberculin syringes and 27-gauge (G) ¥ 1/2-in. (13 mm) needles; 0.5-mL insulin syringes with 28 G –1/2-in. needles for spleen injections.
10. Metofane (methoxyflurane) for anesthesia. Moisten a piece of sterile gauze with the Metofane, place it in a small glass dressing jar, and cover with a wire mesh to prevent contact between the Metofane and the mouse.
11. Alcohol wipes and Betadine scrub (or equivalent antiseptic scrub solution).
12. 10% Neutral buffered formalin.

Two critical elements for working with immunodeficient mice are the facility in which they are housed and the areas used for experimental manipulations. Ideally, the animals should be housed in a Specific Pathogen Free (SPF) Barrier Facility, in microisolator cages. All manipulations should be performed in laminar airflow workstations, or an area that is designated solely for work with immunodeficient animals. Depending on the facility, working with the immunodeficient mice may require changing into surgical scrubs, sterile coveralls, caps, masks, shoe covers, and gloves. Work patterns should be organized such that working with and monitoring immunodeficient animals precedes any work with immunocompetent mice in the same day. Use of the anesthetic Metofane requires a fume hood to reduce exposure to this potential carcinogen.

3. Methods
3.1. Preparation of Cells for Injection

1. Aspirate culture medium from cultures of tumor cells that are between 75% and 90% confluent (plate cells, or add fresh medium the previous day to obtain actively growing cultures) (*see* **Note 1**). Wash with 10 mL of PBS per 75-cm^2 flask; add 1–2 mL of the trypsin–EDTA solution. Incubate for 30 s–1 min, then agitate, shake, or tap the flask in the palm of one hand to detach the cells.
2. Resuspend the cells in 10 mL of culture medium and transfer to a centrifuge tube. Centrifuge at 200g for 10 min, and resuspend the pellet in PBS.
3. Determine cell number, and adjust the concentration for the appropriate inoculum volume, by centrifugation and resuspension in a smaller volume of PBS.
4. Place the suspension in ice and proceed immediately to inject the cells.

3.2. Experimental Metastasis Assays

3.2.1. Tail Vein Injections

1. Place mice in a clean cage under a warming lamp, ensuring that they do not get overheated or burnt. This is to dilate the tail veins.
2. Vortex-mix the cell suspension briefly, then draw an aliquot into a 1-mL syringe without a needle, or using a 18-gauge needle. Passing the suspension through a small gauge needle may damage the cells. Place a 27-gauge needle on the syringe, and dispel any air bubbles. Adjust the needle so that the bevel is facing up, and the gradations on the syringe barrel are visible. For tail vein injection, use a volume of 0.1–0.2 mL. For the A375 human melanoma cell line, inject 5×10^5 cells per mouse.
3. Place a mouse in the restraint device, with a firm grip on the tail extending out of the device.
4. Wipe the tail with an alcohol wipe. Insert the needle into one of the lateral veins in the tail, choosing the side of the tail where a vein is clearly visible. Track the needle along the tail before inserting into the vein, and hold the tail and needle steady. Gradually inject the required volume. If resistance is felt, the needle is not in the vein. Withdraw, and try again in another part of the same vein, or the vein on the opposite side of the tail. First attempts should be made in the middle, or more distal in the tail so that if the first attempt is unsuccessful, the next injection can be made nearer the base of the tail, and the inoculum will not leak from the first hole.
5. After successfully injecting the full inoculum, withdraw the needle and return the mouse to the cage. Clearly mark the cage label with the details of the experiment (cell line, route of injection, date).
6. Monitor the mice daily, for signs of developing tumor burden such as weight loss, reduced mobility, hunched posture, and ruffled fur in SCID mice (*see* **Note 2**). For metastatic A375 human melanoma cells injected into nude mice, a typical experiment ends 6 wk after the injection (*see* **Note 3**).
7. Euthanize the mice with CO_2 or anesthetic overdose followed by cervical dislocation.
8. Secure the mouse to a dissection board, and necropsy. The principal organ where experimental metastases will be found following intravenous injection is the lungs, although the abdomen should also be examined. Examine the lungs, under a dissecting microscope if available, and count visible surface lesions (*see* **Note 4**).
9. Remove lungs, rinse in water to remove blood, and fix in formalin, if histology is required, or counting and measuring of metastases will be performed at a later time.

3.2.2. Intrasplenic Injection

1. Anesthetize a mouse, until its breathing is slow and regular and there is no toe-pinch reflex.
2. Place the mouse on its right side on the work area, and clean the skin on the left of the body.
3. Make a 5–10 mm incision through the skin and peritoneum to expose the spleen. Gently grasp connective tissue at the distal end of the spleen and pull the organ out of the abdominal cavity. Lay the spleen on a sterile gauze sponge. Do not allow the spleen to dry; if there is a delay in injecting the cells, moisten the spleen with sterile saline solution.

4. Continue to hold the spleen firmly with forceps. Using a low-dose syringe fitted with a 28-gauge needle, inject 0.05 mL of inoculum under the capsule of the spleen. For the HT-29 human colon cancer cell line, use an inoculum of 1×10^6 cells. Compress the injection site with a sterile cotton swab and withdraw the needle.

5. Replace the spleen in the abdominal cavity, grasp the peritoneum and skin with forceps, and close the wound with surgical clips or sutures.

6. Monitor the mouse for uneventful recovery from surgery, then return it to the cage.

7. Observe mice daily for signs of tumor burden, including hunched posture, bloated abdomen, and loss of mobility. Euthanize before the mice become moribund. The end of a typical experiment of HT-29 cells injected into the spleen is 6–8 wk after injection *(13)*. Dissect out the spleen and liver, and record the presence and amount of tumor. Spleen tumors can be dissected out and weighed. Count the numbers of liver colonies visible at the surface of the organ. Fix tissues in formalin if required.

3.3. Spontaneous Metastasis Models
3.3.1. Subcutaneous Injection

1. Vortex-mix the cell suspension, draw up into a 1-mL syringe. Place a 27-gauge needle on the syringe, and dispel any air bubbles.

2. Grasp a mouse firmly in one hand. Hold the scruff of the neck between thumb and forefinger with the tail between the third and fourth fingers and the palm of the hand. Alternatively, have an assistant hold the mouse securely. Wipe the skin of the flank with an alcohol swab.

3. Insert the needle through the loose skin of the flank, not deep enough to puncture the peritoneum or muscle. Inject 0.1 mL of inoculum (5×10^5 cells is sufficient for 100% tumor take of A375 human melanoma cells in nude mice).

4. Monitor mice daily for overall condition, and measure tumor growth once or twice weekly (depending on the rate of growth). Holding the mouse as described previously, use calipers to measure two diameters of the tumor. Calculate the mean diameter to graph out tumor growth over time. The diameter measurements can also be used to estimate tumor volume, using the formula:

$$\text{Tumor volume} = \frac{x^2 y}{2}$$

where x is the smaller diameter of the tumor and y is the larger.

5. Kill the mice when the maximum tumor size is reached (1.5-cm diameter). Alternatively, perform survival surgery to remove the local tumor and allow established micrometastases to grow to a more readily detectable size. Anesthetize mouse and clean the skin around tumor with Betadine and 70% ethanol. Remove the tumor and close the incision with wound clips. Monitor closely to ensure uneventful recovery from the surgery and anesthetic. Remove the wound clips 10–14 d after surgery.

6. At euthanasia (when tumors are 1.5 cm, or 6 wk after tumor removal), necropsy and examine lungs and abdominal organs for metastases. Fix organs in formalin for histology as required.

3.3.2. Mammary Fatpad Injections of Human Breast Cancer Cells

1. Anesthetize a female mouse, lay it on one side, and clean the skin of the opposite side in preparation for surgery. Make a 5-mm incision in the skin over the lower lateral thorax. Open a pocket under the skin in a cranial direction with the blades of the scissors, so that the mammary fatpad can be seen.
2. Vortex-mix the cell suspension and draw it up into a 1-mL syringe. Place a 27-gauge needle on the syringe and expel any air bubbles.
3. Insert the needle into the fatty tissue of the mammary fatpad, and inject 0.1 mL with 2×10^6 cells for the MDA-MB-435 breast cancer cell line (*see* **Note 5**). The inoculum should form a bubble inside the fatpad, and not leak into the subcutaneous space. Close the incision with wound clips, and monitor the mouse until recovered from the anesthesia. Return the mouse to a clean cage.
4. Monitor the mice daily, and measure tumor growth weekly, using caliper measurements as described above.
5. When the tumor reaches a maximum size of 1.5 cm, either kill the mouse or remove the tumor (as described above for subcutaneous tumors). The MDA-MB-435 cell line can form tumors of this size in 10–12 wk. If the tumors are removed, kill mice 4–6 wk later.
6. Euthanize mice and examine for metastases, principally in lungs and lymph nodes, but examine the abdomen also. Fix the lungs in formalin and prepare sections for histology if required. If a mouse had been showing abnormal balance or movements, remove the brain for histology.

4. Notes

1. Preparation of cell suspensions: Some of the variability in repeat experiments with a particular cell line, or from published results from other laboratories, may arise from inconsistencies in techniques or poor quality preparation of the cells for injections. To optimize the results and consistency between experiments, thaw a vial from frozen stocks of the cell line and expand the cells in tissue culture to obtain the required cell number. The cells should be in subconfluent, actively growing cultures. The cells from confluent cultures are more likely to form cell clumps or aggregates, depending on the cell type. In addition, the degree of confluence in vitro has been reported to regulate gene expression, which might impact on the in vivo behavior *(14)*. The important point is to be consistent in using good cell preparation techniques. High viability is essential. The method described generally yields cell suspensions with high viability (98–100%, by trypan blue dye exclusion). If a suspension has < 90% viability, or if the cells are in clumps, it would be best to discard these cells and start with a fresh culture. For experimental metastasis assays (primarily the intravenous route) injecting clumps of cells, or dead cells mixed with live tumor cells can artificially increase the number of lung colonies formed *(15)*. Using the Ca^{2+} and Mg^{2+}-free buffer will retard formation of clumps, and gentle vortex-mixing may help to break up loose clusters, but if cells come off the plastic in clumps, it is best to start with fresh, less confluent cultures. Too vigorous pipetting or mixing is more likely to

damage the cells than break up the clumps. As stated previously, once the suspension has been prepared, proceed to inject as soon as possible. Keeping the suspension on ice will reduce the formation of cell aggregates.

2. All of the animal procedures (housing conditions, experimentation, surgical procedures, euthanasia and anesthesia, etc.) will probably be regulated by an institutional body such as an Institutional Animal Care and Use Committee. In the United States, this committee is charged with ensuring compliance with guidelines and requirements established by the Public Health Service (PHS) *Policy on Humane Care and Use of Laboratory Animals*, the US Department of Health and Human Services *Guide for the Care and Use of Laboratory Animals*, and the Animal Welfare Act of 1966 as amended. Experimental design should take into account the well being of the mouse and use appropriate procedures to reduce pain and suffering. In the context of this chapter this means careful monitoring of mice for development of tumor burden, appropriate animal handling and surgical procedures, and the humane use of euthanasia. Using a moribund endpoint rather than a death endpoint for a study is more practical if the point of the study is to assess the extent of tumor spread. Autolysis of mouse tissues starts rapidly, and it is easier to monitor, measure, and recover metastases from freshly killed mice than from those dead for more than an hour or two. Furthermore, if tissues are needed for analyses such as nucleic acid extraction or immunohistochemistry, these should be harvested immediately after killing the mouse. If a veterinary medicine department is administering the animal facility, this is a source for advice on small animal surgery and anesthesia. Inhalation of Metofane is a rapid and easy means of anesthesia, and is ideal for short procedures such as those described, as the mice will recover rapidly. Metofane is a hazardous agent, and should therefore only be used in a suitable fume hood or with appropriate ventilation. (Note added in proofs: Metofane is no longer generally available. Use of an alternate inhaled anesthetic, e.g., Isoflurane, may require gas scavenging apparatus and approval by occupational safety and animal care and use committees.) Injectable anesthetics such as Nembutal (sodium pentobarbital, 50 mg/kg injected i.p.) or Ketamine-HCl have longer induction and recovery times. When using anesthesia on nude mice take precautions to prevent hypothermia, and do not be too liberal with ethanol and surgical scrub fluids. Use a warming pad or lamp during the recovery phase, but do not let the mouse overheat either.

3. The dose of tumor cells required, and the length of time before metastases develop may differ from what has been published for a particular cell line. In addition, the distribution of metastases in different organs may vary from previous publications. In the first experiment with a cell line monitor the mice closely and, if necessary, wait longer than expected for the mice to show signs of metastatic tumor burden. Killing mice at different timepoints can also be done to monitor and establish the time course of growth of metastases (assessed macroscopically or in histological sections). No or fewer metastases than expected could be the result of a number of factors, including the health and housing conditions of the mice, and the cell preparation techniques. Variants of some human tumor cell lines have arisen, possibly resulting from different tissue culture techniques, that

vary considerably in their tumorigenic and metastatic phenotypes. To save time and resources, it may be prudent to obtain a particular cell line from an investigator who is currently using the cells for in vivo studies.

4. Counting the metastases: The simplest method is to count the numbers of metastases visible on the surface of the target organs. An alternative to aid detection of metastases is to fix the organs in Bouin's fixative. The metastases will be white lesions (or black with some melanoma cell lines) against the yellow stained normal tissue. Counting surface lesions does not include microscopic disease, which can be detected in histological sections, although quantitation of the metastases in multiple organ sections is labor intensive and not highly practical. Depending on the model used and site of metastasis, the weights or volumes of organs may be used to estimate the tumor burden (discussed in **ref. *15***). How the metastatic burden is measured will dictate the choice of test used for statistical analysis. For comparisons of numbers of metastases estimated by surface counting, use a nonparametric test such as the Mann–Whitney rank sum test. One aspect of in vivo experiments, especially with immunodeficient mice, is variability within experimental groups. To try and overcome this, if possible use at least 10 animals per group. Loss of one or two mice (from early morbidity, or reasons unrelated to the experiment) will still leave enough data points for valid statistical analyses.

5. Breast cancer models: The method described uses an estrogen-receptor (ER) negative breast cancer cell line. Cell lines that express ER may not grow unless the nude mice are supplemented with estrogen. One commonly used method is the implantation of slow release pellets of 17β-estradiol (from Innovative Research of America, Sarasota, Florida). A 60-day release 0.72-mg pellet will support the growth of the ER-positive MCF-7 breast cancer cell line (from injection of 5×10^6 cells into the mammary fatpad).

References

1. Fidler, I. J. (1990) Critical factors in the biology of human cancer metastasis: twenty-eighth G. H. A. Clowes Memorial Award Lecture. *Cancer Res.* **50,** 6130–6138.
2. Xie, H., Turner, T., Wang, M. H., Singh, R. K., Siegal, G. P., and Wells, A. (1995) In vitro invasiveness of DU-145 human prostate carcinoma cells is modulated by EGF receptor-mediated signals. *Clin. Exp. Metast.* **13,** 407–419.
3. Li, L., Price, J. E., Fan, D., Zhang, R. D., Bucana, C. D., and Fidler, I. J. (1989) Correlation of growth capacity of human tumor cells in hard agarose with their in vivo proliferative capacity at specific metastatic sites. *J. Natl. Cancer Inst.* **81,** 1406–1412.
4. Price, J. E. (1996) Metastasis from human breast cancer cell lines. *Breast Cancer Res. Treat.* **39,** 93–102.
5. Garafalo, A., Chirivi, R. G. S., Scanziani, E., Mayo, J. G., Vecchi, A., and Giavazzi, R. (1993) Comparative study on the metastatic behavior of human tumors in nude, beige/nude/Xid and severe combined immunodeficient mice. *Invas. Metast.* **13,** 82–91.
6. Xie, X., Brunner, N., Jensen, G., Albrectsen, J., Gotthardsen, B., and Rygaard, J. (1992) Comparative studies between nude and scid mice on the growth and metastatic behavior of xenografted human tumors. *Clin. Exp. Metast.* **10,** 201–210.

7. Morikawa, K., Walker, S. M., Nakajima, M., Pathak, S., Jessup, J. M., and Fidler, I. J. (1988) Influence of organ environment on the growth, selection, and metastasis of human colon carcinoma cells in nude mice. *Cancer Res.* **48,** 6863–6871.

8. Stephenson, R. A., Killion, J. J., Dinney, C. P. N., Gohji, K., Ordonez, N. G., and Fidler, I. J. (1992) Metastatic model for human prostate cancer using orthotopic implantation in nude mice. *J. Natl. Cancer Inst.* **84,** 951–957.

9. Price, J. E., Polyzos, A., Zhang, R. D., and Daniels, L. M. (1990) Tumorigenicity and metastasis of human breast carcinoma cell lines in nude mice. *Cancer Res.* **50,** 717–721.

10. Singh, R. K., Bucana, C. D., Gutman, M., Fan, D., Wilson, M., and Fidler, I. J. (1994) Organ-site dependent expression of basic fibroblast growth factor in human renal cell carcinoma cells. *Am. J. Pathol.* **145,** 365–374.

11. Fabra, A., Nakajima, M., Bucana, C. D., and Fidler, I. J. (1992) Modulation of the invasive phenotype of human colon carcinoma cells by organ specific fibroblasts of nude mice. *Differentiation* **52,** 101–110.

12. van Golen, K. L., Risin, S., Staroselsky, A., Berger, D., Tainsky, M. A., Pathak, S., and Price, J. E. (1996) Predominance of the metastatic phenotype in hybrids formed by fusion of mouse and human melanoma clones. *Clin. Exp. Metast.* **14,** 95–106.

13. Price, J. E., Daniels, L. M., Campbell, D. E., and Giavazzi, R. (1989) Organ distribution of experimental metastases of a human colorectal carcinoma injected in nude mice. *Clin. Exp. Metast.* **7,** 55–68.

14. Koura, A. N., Liu, W., Kitadai, Y., Singh, R. K., Radinsky, R., and Ellis, L. M. (1996) Regulation of vascular endothelial growth factor expression in human colon carcinoma cells by cell density. *Cancer Res.* **56,** 3891–3894.

15. Welch, D. R. (1997) Technical considerations for studying cancer metastasis *in vivo. Clin. Exp. Metast.* **15,** 272–306.

Further Reading

Other experimental metastasis models can be used to target tumor cells to different organs. Injection of cells into the left ventricle of the heart can result in metastases in the bone and bone marrow, adrenal glands and the brain. Direct injection of cells into the carotid artery will produce metastases in the brain. Both of these techniques have been used for studying human tumor metastases in immunodeficient mice, and are well described in the cited references.

Arguello, F., Baggs, R. B., and Frantz, C. N. (1988) A murine model of experimental metastases to bone and bone marrow. *Cancer Res.* **48,** 6879–6881.

Verschraegen, C. F., Giovanella, B. C., Mendoza, J. T., Kozielski, A. J., and Stehlin, J. S., Jr. (1991) Specific organ metastases of human melanoma cells injected into the arterial circulation of nude mice. *AntiCancer Res.* **11,** 529–536.

Schackert, G., Price, J. E., Bucana, C. D., and Fidler, I. J. (1989) Unique patterns of brain metastasis produced by different human carcinomas in athymic nude mice. *Int. J. Cancer* **44,** 892–897.

20

Xenograft Models in Immunodeficient Animals

II. The Use of SCID Mice in Metastasis Research:
Breast and Colon Cancer Models of Metastasis

Udo Schumacher and Susan A. Brooks

1. Introduction
1.1. Background and Advantages of the SCID Mouse Model

Metastasis is a multistep phenomenon, and all steps have to be successfully and consecutively followed through until a clinically manifest metastasis occurs. Although all of these steps have been defined and individual steps can be mimicked in vitro, the rate-limiting step of metastases formation is unknown. Hence the significance of a particular in vitro test to the overall process of metastases formation is undefined. For example, a particular cell line may prove to have excellent capabilities to degrade the extracellular matrix, which would be one prerequisite to enter the circulation but be highly vulnerable to pro-apoptotic factors within the circulation. Although matrix degrading in vitro assays would indicate high metastatic potential, this cell line would be very unlikely to form metastasis in an in vivo (clinical) situation because of the subsequent cell death within the circulation. This is why whole organism animal models, which cover the entire process of the formation of metastases, are still needed to place defined in vitro assays into a broader perspective.

Several animal models of metastasis have been proposed and evaluated over the past few decades. However, the main problem of these models is their relevance to the clinical situation. Murine breast cancer, for example, is caused by the mammary tumor virus and is not hormone dependent. In contrast, a considerable proportion of human breast cancer is estrogen-dependent and no viral causes of human breast cancers have been shown. Therefore murine breast cancer is of limited use as a model for human breast cancer (1).

From: *Methods in Molecular Medicine, vol. 58:*
Metastasis Research Protocols, Vol. 2: Cell Behavior In Vitro and In Vivo
Edited by: S. A. Brooks and U. Schumacher © Humana Press Inc., Totowa, NJ

Not only do the different biological behaviors of animal cancers compared to human ones make it difficult to assess the clinical relevance of the animal models but also differences in antigen expression have to be taken into account and pose a problem. Most of the monoclonal antibodies that react with human epitopes do not crossreact with other species, making it impossible to evaluate the usefulness of a particular monoclonal antibody in cancer diagnosis and treatment using animal derived tissues.

To overcome these problems, human cancers have been transplanted into immunodeficient animals, mainly mice. The first widespread model of an immunodeficient animal was the nude mouse *(2)*. Detailed methodologies for spontaneous and experimental metastasis models in nude mice are given in Chapter 19 by Price. Besides lacking hair, this mouse is characterized by the absence of a functional thymus, hence mature and functionally active T lymphocytes are lacking. However, a T-cell-independent B-cell response is still present in this mouse. The T-cell-independent B-cell immune response is mainly active against polysaccharides such as those occurring in bacterial capsules. Many thousand studies in which human tumors were xenografted into nude mice have been published, but metastases of human tumors is rarely observed; hence, the nude mouse is disappointing as a model for metastases *(2)*. In recent years a number of reports on the successful metastatic spread of human tumors transplanted orthotopically in the nude mouse model have been published *(3–6)*; the methodology for this approach is given in Chapter 23 by Hoffman.

An alternative model in metastasis research is the severe combined immunodeficient (SCID) mouse. This mouse strain lacks the enzyme recombinase, which links the specific with the nonspecific parts of the immunoglobulins and the T-cell receptor, respectively. The original SCID mouse was derived from the Balb/c mouse and looks phenotypically normal but lacks both immunoglobulins and functional T cells, but macrophages and natural killer (NK) cells are still present *(7)*. Because of this extended immunodeficiency the SCID mouse has attracted our attention as a tool for metastasis research *(8)*.

1.2. Choice of Appropriate Cell Lines

A complete model of metastasis formation does not only require an appropriate animal (the "soil") but also requires the choice of the right cell line (the "seed"). A general assumption often made is that tumor cells derived from metastatic sites, for example, from pleural effusions or from lymph node metastases, are metastatic while those derived from an apparently localized primary tumor are nonmetastatic. However, there is no experimental proof that this assumption is correct. Therefore it is helpful to assess the metastatic potential of human tumor cell lines before they are transplanted into the animals to obtain a correlation with the clinical situation.

Such an analysis of metastatic capabilities for breast and colon cancer has been performed by us and others using the lectin *Helix pomatia* agglutinin (HPA; refer to Chapter 4 by Brooks and Hall in the companion volume). This lectin-labeled primary tumor cells in clinical material from patients who had a poor prognosis and hence suffered from a metastatic tumor *(9)*. It does not work as a prognostic marker in all types of tumors *(10)* but seems to be of particular value in adenocarcinomas (for review, *see* **ref. 9**). According to the expected clinical behavior, human HPA positive breast and colon cancer cell lines metastasise in scid mice, whereas HPA-negative ones generally do not do so *(8)*. Tumors other than adenocarcinomas (squamous cell carcinoma, small cell carcinoma of the lung) do not metastasize in SCID mice (the author's unpublished observations). The reason for this is failure to metastasize is unclear. This may be due to the selection of the cell lines or to the general nonsuitability of the SCID mouse as a host for these types of tumors. It may well be that adenocarcinomas in general, or at least of certain types, provide the appropriate seed and soil mechanisms for homing of metastasis and that other tumor types use different recognition systems that are not represented in SCID mice, and hence are unsuitable as a host to mimic metastatic spread.

Any other prognostic marker besides HPA can be applied for this kind of study. The only thing in common is the correlation between the expression of the marker of metastasis in clinical studies and in human tumor cells grown in the SCID mouse to give the model some clinical relevance.

1.3. Scope of this Chapter

The handling of SCID mice, the treatment of the human tumor cell lines, and their processing are described in the following sections.

2. Materials
2.1. Maintenance of the SCID Mouse Colony

The SCID mouse can be obtained from any of the large animal breeding farms (e.g., Jackson Laboratory).

2.2. Treatment of the Cells for Injection into SCID Mouse

1. 250-mL Flasks of cells cultured according to standard laboratory protocols.
2. Standard cell culture medium appropriate for cell lines to be used (*see* **Note 1**).
3. Sterile phosphate-buffered saline (PBS, pH 7.1): Dissolve 8.5 g of sodium chloride, 1.07 g of disodium hydrogen phosphate (anhyd.; Na_2HPO_4), 0. 39 g of sodium dihydrogen phosphate ($NaH_2PO_4 \cdot 2 H_2O$) dissolved in 850 mL of distilled water (*see* **Note 2**). Adjust to pH 7.1 with 0.1 *M* HCl or NaOH. Make up to 1 L in a measuring cylinder and filter under a sterile hood with 2-µm filter (*see* **Note 2**).
4. Trypsin–EDTA solution is supplied by GIBCO-BRL (cat. no. 45300-019).
5. Standard cell culture medium appropriate for the cell lines used, containing 10% v/v fetal calf serum.

6. Cell counting chamber, for example, Neubauer.
7. 1-mL Sterile syringes fitted with small-gauge needles (e.g., Becton Dickinson Microlance 2, 27G 3/4).
8. Saturated picric acid solution in distilled water.

2.3. Harvesting the Metastases for Microscopic Examination and Analysis

1. 70% v/v Ethanol in distilled water.
2. Neutral buffered formalin, pH 7.1: 100 mL of formalin (40% formaldehyde in water) is added to 900 mL of PBS (*see* **Note 3**).
3. 4% w/v Difco Agar Noble.

3. Methods
3.1. Maintenance of SCID Mouse Colony

1. SCID mice are, despite their immunodeficiency, relatively easy to handle. Most pathogens that challenge the mice are bacteria, and because they are combated by granulocytes that are functional in SCID mice, these mice can resist infection. However, special care needs to be taken.
2. It is advisable to house SCID mice in a separate room within the animal house facility. Animal technicians should always take care of the SCID mouse colony first in the morning before they deal with other animal colonies to avoid cross-contamination. A barrier room to change clothes is advisable. Use disposable face masks, hoods, and sterilized gowns such as used in operating theaters before entering the SCID mouse colony. Use fresh clothes every time you enter the colony. The cages have to be filter top cages to minimize infection, and food, water bedding, and cages have to be sterilized. The sterilization procedure can take place within the normal sterilizing procedure already in use for routine purposes in the animal facility. The changing of the cages has to be done under sterile conditions in a laminar flow hood. Change cages once a week. These conditions have allowed us to maintain the scid mouse colony without special incubator facilities ("bubble"). The mice should weigh approx 18–20 g when the experiments are started.

3.2. Treatment of the Cells for Injection into SCID Mice

1. Grow the cell lines (for choice of cell line *see* **Note 4**) in their usual culture medium in the large culture flask (250 cm^2). When confluent, remove the culture medium with a suction pipet. Rinse the cells with 15–20 mL of sterile PBS solution and aspirate the PBS.
2. Add 5 mL of trypsin–EDTA solution to the flask. Incubate the flask for 5 min at 37°C. Tilt the flasks occasionally. The cells should come off by this time. The cells form white layers in the solution, which lift off from the bottom from the flask (*see* **Note 5**).
3. Add 5 mL of culture medium with 10% foetal calf serum (FCS) added (*see* **Note 6**). Aspirate the solution with a 10-mL pipet several times to help loosen the cells from each other. Empty this suspension into a sterile 15-mL centrifuge tube.

4. Rinse the bottom of the cell culture flask with an additional 5 mL of medium and centrifuge this plus the initial solution at 1000*g* for 10 min.
5. Aspirate the supernatant, pool the cells and resuspend in 5 mL of culture medium. Count the cell number using a cell counting chamber (e.g., Neubauer). Adjust the cell number to 1×10^6 cells in a total volume of 200 µL. Use 1-mL syringes for injection and a small-gauge needle (*see* **Note 7**).
6. Before injection of the cells, the mice should be weighed, individually labeled, and a record book should be initiated. Use saturated picric acid in water (itself a sterile solution) and apply the solution with cotton wool to the fur of the animal (*see* **Note 8**). Inject 200 µL of the cell solution between the scapulae of scid mice (*see* **Note 9**).

3.3. Harvesting Metastases for Microscopic Examination and Analysis

1. The mice should be killed when the tumor reaches 20% of the body weight at the beginning of the experiments, or when the tumors start to ulcerate (*see* **Note 10**). Consult your local animal care guidelines.
2. The mice should be killed by a schedule 2 method. To harvest the primary tumors, moisturize the skin over the tumor with 70% ethanol solution to ease cutting and incise the skin over the tumor with a pair of scissors. Using forceps, hold one of the two sides of the skin flap open and dissect the tumors out of their bed. Fix the tumors in neutral buffered formalin for 2 d or stored frozen in sealed containers in liquid nitrogen (*see* **Note 11**).
3. Turn the mouse round, moisturise the fur over the rib cage and open it using a pair of scissors. Remove the lung *en bloc* by cutting it out beginning at the trachea. Fix the lung *en bloc* in neutral buffered formalin for 2 d (*see* **Note 12**).
4. Now the abdominal cavity is fully opened and the internal organs are removed and placed into neutral buffered formalin for 2 d (*see* **Note 13**). Alternatively, they can be stored in liquid nitrogen.
5. After the 2 d, the lungs are sliced using a stereomicroscope. Cover graph paper with a glass plate and put this in the viewing field of the microscope. Section the lungs with a razor blade in 2-mm thick slices. Place all the slices on a histological glass slide and cover the slices in 4% agar (*see* **Note 14**).
6. When the agar has solidified, trim the edges of the agar block without any tissue slices away and routinely process to paraffin wax in the same way as a piece of solid tissue (*see* **Note 15**). Cut 7-µm-thick sections on a microtome and prepare routine hematoxylin and eosin slides for microscopy (*see* Chapter 4 by Brooks and Hall in the companion volume). Use ×100 magnification to search for metastases (*see* **Note 16**).

4. Notes

1. Different cell lines often require different cell culture media and this makes the culture of a bank of cell lines expensive and difficult to maintain. By careful adjustment, many cell lines can be brought to grow in one of the better (and more expensive) media such as RPMI 1640. The ease of handling only one medium more than compensates for the extra costs of RPMI 1640.

2. Use fresh distilled water, which can vary considerably in pH. For cell culture purposes, it is advisable to use water supplied in 1-L bottles for clinical use. This is pyrogen free and tested. Instead of filtering, this solution can be autoclaved, which is cheaper. If some of the water has evaporated after autoclaving it has to be adjusted to 1 L again using sterile water.

3. During storage formaldehyde decays to formic acid and hence the pH drops. Buffering is therefore necessary. For optimal results, it should neutral or slightly alkaline. Check solution before use. Prepare enough solution for optimal fixation results, 9 vol of buffered formalin should be added to 1 vol of tissue.

4. The particular value of this system is the correlation between the behavior of the tumor cells in the clinical studies and the behavior of the human tumor cell lines grown in SCID mice. HPA-positive cell lines were: breast: T47D, MCF-7; colon: HT29. HPA-negative cell lines were: breast: BT20, HS578T, HBL 100; colon: COLO 320DM, SW 480; SW 620 (*see* **ref. 9**). This type of analysis can be performed with any other marker under consideration. It should be borne in mind that antigen and glycotope expression can vary considerably between in vitro grown cells and tumor cells grown in vivo in SCID mice (*see* **ref. 12**). Therefore the analysis of tumor cells from both sources is recommended.

5. Trypsin inhibitors in the serum block its activity.

6. If the cells do not come off, incubate them for 1 min longer in the trypsin–EDTA solution. Depending on the cell junctions, different cell lines need different incubation times, which have to be established for every cell line. If the cell line is embedded in agar to compare antigen expression of cells grown in vitro as compared to grown in situ in SCID mice no trypsin should be used as this may digest the antigen under study. The use of agar-embedded cells will allow the processing of the cells according to the same protocol as blocks of tissue. Under those circumstances, cells should be harvested with a rubber policeman, fixed in buffered formalin and embedded in agar for further processing.

7. Epithelia tend to self aggregate. Take the cell suspension in a sterile centrifuge tube to the mouse colony. Shake the cells gently before injection because some cell lines can aggregate while in the centrifuge tube or even in the syringe.

8. Devise a labeling scheme (mark on left foreleg = 1, right foreleg = 2, left hindleg = 3, right hindleg = 4, no label = 5, etc). House up to five animals in a small cage or up to 10 animals in a large cage.

9. For normal subcutaneous injection, the mice do not need to be anesthetised. One person should hold the mouse while another person injects the cells. The cells should be injected in a skin flap and should not be injected too deeply (subcutaneous!).

10. At least in the HT29 model, the size (and weight) of the primary tumor has a considerable influence on the number of metastases detected in the lungs. Primary tumors weighing below 1 g rarely show metastatic spread to the lungs, while primary tumors weighing > 1.6 g lead to hundreds of metastases in both lungs.

11. Primary tumors and lungs can be removed aseptically at this stage if further in vitro culture experiments are envisaged.

12. For most monoclonal antibodies, cryostat sections are necessary. Pretreatment of the sections with microwave or digestion with trypsin will allow the use of

paraffin sections (*see* Chapter 2 by Brooks in the companion volume). These give a superior morphology and are easier to handle for serial sections than frozen sections. If these pretreatment methods for antigen retrieval fail, one lung should be embedded in wax, serially sectioned, and the number of metastases counted. The other lung can be stored frozen and if the individual animal has sufficient numbers of metastases, this lung can be used for immunocytochemistry.

13. We generally only use liver, spleen, and sternum for histological examination. However, so far only spontaneous metastases have been found in the lungs, so that not so much emphasis is placed on the examination of these organs. Only sample sections are cut, no serial sections are prepared. It is, however, not unexpected that metastases are absent from these sites. In the HT29 colon cancer model, metastases occur after about 21 d when the primary tumor is already large. In the clinical situation, the primary tumor is often removed before gross anatomically visible metastases occur. To mimic this situation, the primary tumor should be removed at an earlier stage and the metastases should be allowed to grow independently (*see* **ref. *11***). Under these experimental conditions the brain might additionally be investigated for the presence of metastases.

14. To prepare the agar solution, heat 100 mL of distilled water in a 200-mL beaker in a larger beaker used as a waterbath on a hot plate stirrer. Adjust the magnetic stirrer to a slow to medium rotation. Add 4 g of agar. Stir until the agar is dissolved, boiled, and turned into a yellowish solution. Use preheated glass pipets to add the liquid agar onto the lung slices. This will enable you to cut the whole lung in one block which is only about 2 mm thick. This will largely reduce the workload for histological examination.

15. Process primary tumor, lungs, and internal organs except for the sternum, which has to be decalcified, in parallel. If differences in the results of immuno- or lectin histochemistry between the primary tumor and its metastases are detected, different processing procedures as the reason for the results can be discounted.

16. Human tumor cells are in general larger than the surrounding normal cells of the mouse lung. It is often helpful to compare the morphology of the tumor cells in the primary tumor with those in the lungs when in doubt. Particularly the structure of the often heterochromatin-rich large nucleus and the basophilic cytoplasm of the tumor cells are of help in assessing the presence of a metastatic cell. If in doubt, immunohistochemistry for human- or tumor-specific antigens will help. SCID mice do not have immunoglobulins so that all mouse-derived monoclonal antibodies directed against human antigens can be used without background staining.

References

1. Van de Vijver, M. J. and Nusse, R. (1991) The molecular biology of breast cancer. *Biochim. Biophys. Acta* **1072,** 33–50.
2. Giovanella, B. C. and Fogh, J. (1985) The nude mouse in cancer research. *Adv. Cancer Res.* **44,** 69–120.
3. Fu, X., Guadagni, F., and Hoffman, R. M. (1992) A metastatic nude-mouse model of human pancreatic cancer constructed orthotopically with histologically intact patient specimens. *Proc. Natl. Acad. Sci. USA* **89,** 5645–5649.

4. Kubota, T. (1994) Metastatic models of human xenografted in the nude mouse: the importance of orthotopic transplantation. *J. Cell. Biochem.* **56,** 4–8.
5. Furukawa, T., Kubota, T., Watanabe, M., Kitajima, M., and Hoffman, R. (1993) A novel "patient-like" treatment model of human pancreatic cancer constructed using orthotopic transplantation of histologically intact human tumor tissue in nude mice. *Cancer Res.* **53,** 3070–3072.
6. Furukawa, T., Kubota, T., Watanabe, M., Kitajima, M., and Hoffman, R. M. (1993) Orthotopic transplantation of histologically intact clinical specimens of stomach cancer to nude mice: correlation with metastatic sites in mouse and individual patient donors. *Int. J. Cancer* **53,** 608–612.
7. Bosma, C. G., Custer, R. P., and Bosma, M. J. (1983) A severe combined immunodeficiency in the mouse. *Nature* **301,** 527–530.
8. Schumacher, U. and Adam, E. (1997) Lectin histochemical HPA-binding pattern of human breast and colon cancers is associated with metastases formation in severe combined immunodeficient mice. *Histochem. J.* **29,** 677–684.
9. Mitchell, B. S. and Schumacher, U. (1999) The use of the lectin *Helix pomatia* agglutinin (HPA) as a prognostic indicator and as a tool in cancer research. *Histol. Histopathol.* **14,** 217–226.
10. Schumacher, D. U., Randall, C. J., Ramsay, A. D., and Schumacher, U. (1996) Is the binding of the lectin *Helix pomatia* agglutinin (HPA) of prognostic relevance in tumors of the upper aerodigestive tract? *Eur. J. Surg. Oncol.* **22,** 618–620.
11. Mitchell, B. S., Horny, H.-P., and Schumacher, U. (1997) Immunophenotyping of human HT29 colon cancer cell primary tumors and their metastases in severe combined immunodeficient mice. *Histochem. J.* **29,** 393–399.
12. Schumacher, U., Mohamed, M., and Mitchell, B. S. (1996) Differential expression of carbohydrate residues in human breast and colon cancer cell lines grown *in vitro* and *in vivo* in SCID mice. *Cancer J.* **9,** 247–254.

21

Syngeneic Murine Metastasis Models
B16 Melanoma

Raffaella Giavazzi and Angela Garofalo

1. Introduction

Animal studies are costly, time consuming, and subject to several restrictive regulations. However, the metastatic process is one of the research areas in which the in vivo studies remain most relevant *(1)*. In fact, the in vitro studies are not fully predictive of the metastatic behavior of a tumor cell, probably because in vitro, it is difficult to reproduce the complexity of the metastatic process in itself and the interaction with the host.

Several tumor models of murine and of human origin have been described as being metastatic in syngeneic or immunodeficient mice *(2,3)*. Perhaps one of the most used to study the mechanisms associated with the metastastatic process is the murine B16 melanoma. The B16 melanoma is a transplantable tumor, which originated spontaneously in a C57/BL6 mouse in 1954, and then was established in vitro after passages in syngeneic recipients.

After its original selection as a metastatic tumor line to the lung *(4)*, a variety of cell lines have been derived, in vitro or in vivo, having different metastatic behavior. In this chapter, for simplicity, we refer to the bahavior of the main metastatic cell variants described by Fidler and colleagues: the B16-F1 an unselected tumor cell line that metastasizes poorly; the B16-F10 selected in vivo for its ability to colonize the lung after intravenous administration; the B16-BL6 cell line that, selected in vitro for its invasiveness throughout the wall of the mouse bladder, produces a high incidence of spontaneous metastases after trasplantation in the foot pad *(5,6)*. While all the three variants are used to study artificial metastases (*see* **Subheading 2.2.**), spontaneous metastases are mainly studied with the B16-BL-6. Conventionally, with spontaneous metastasis, we mean the formation of a tumor at the site of

From: *Methods in Molecular Medicine, vol. 58:*
Metastasis Research Protocols, Vol. 2: Cell Behavior In Vitro and In Vivo
Edited by: S. A. Brooks and U. Schumacher © Humana Press Inc., Totowa, NJ

transplantation (primary tumor) followed by distant metastases, whereas with experimental or artificial metastases, often simply called tumor colonies, one means tumor cells directly injected in the circulation (mainly intravenously) *(2,7)*. The respective relevance of the two different assays in studying the metastatic process is discussed elsewhere, in Chapter 1 by Davies, Chapter 2 by Clarke and Davies, and Chapter 7 by Hall and Brooks. For the reader it is, however, useful to know that tumor cells into the circulation can be obtained also via arterial or cardiac injection followed by diffuse tumor colonies in different organs; the injection in the spleen, followed by tumor colonies in the liver is also considered an artificial metastatic models *(2)*. Details on these methodologies are not part of this chapter's objective and therefore will not be covered here. Here we describe the methods to obtain artificial metastases to the lung by intravenous injection of the B16 melanoma cells and spontaneous metastases following its growth in the foot pad *(5,6,8)*. We will mainly refer to lung metastases; however, extrapulmonary metastases to lymph nodes and to visceral organs such as liver or to the brain have been often found in the B16 melanoma animal model. The reader will realize that several conditions, described in the Notes, are critical to consider when planning and executing metastatic studies. These aspects, originally described by Fidler in detail *(9)*, have been recently revised *(10)*.

2. Materials
2.1. Mice

1. Specific-pathogen free C57BL/6N 4–6 wk-old mice (*see* **Note 1**). A minimum of 10 mice per group is required to accommodate statistical analysis with inherent variability of the assays.

2.2. Tumor Lines (see Note 2)

1. Lung colonization: B16-F1 (low); B16-F10 (high); B16-BL6 (low–high) *(5)*.
2. Spontaneous metastasis: B16-BL6 (high) *(6)*.

2.3. Media and Solutions

1. Culture medium (CMEM) for B16 melanoma cell lines: Eagle's minimum essential medium supplemented with 2 nM L-glutamine, 1 nM sodium pyruvate, and 10% fetal calf serum (FCS).
2. Washing medium (HBSS): Ca^{2+}, Mg^{2+}-free Hank's Balanced Salt Solution.
3. Trypsin–EDTA solution: 0.25% Trypsin + 0.02% EDTA in Ca^{2+}, Mg^{2+}-free phosphate-buffered saline (PBS).
4. Trypan blue solution (0.4%).
5. Bouin's fixative solution (picroformol acetic acid).

2.4. Lung Colonization Assay

1. A 1-cc tuberculin syringe with a 27G × 1/2-in. needle.

2. A mouse vise (animal holder) for intravenous injection.
3. 150-watt Infrared lamp.
4. Bouin's fixative solution (*see* **Subheading 2.3., item 5**).

2.5. Spontaneous Metastasis Assay

1. A 1-cc tuberculin syringe with a a $25G \times 5/8$-in. needle.
2. Surgery table at 37°C.
3. Sterile surgery instruments: scalpel, scissors, and forceps.
4. Surgery thread (nylon, 45-cm, FS-2 needle) and metal wound clips (9 mm).
5. Caliper.
6. Injectable anesthetic.
7. Bouin's fixative solution (*see* **Subheading 2.3., item 5**).

3. Methods
3.1. Preparation of Tumor Cell Suspension

1. Culture B16 tumor cells as usual (*see* **Note 2**).
2. At 4–5 d prior to the experiment, split cells (1:10–1:20) and plate them in 75-cm^2 flasks so that they do not grow over semiconfluency. Calculate to obtain approx 6–8×10^6 cells in each flask (*see* **Note 3**).
3. 24 h before harvesting for injection, refeed them with culture medium.
4. Control condition of cells before detaching, then empty medium and wash monolayer with HBSS once.
5. Empty medium from the flask and overline with trypsin–EDTA and pour off (leave a thin layer) (*see* **Note 4**).
6. One minute later, tap the flask until cells come off.
7. Add 10 mL of CMEM (need FCS), pipet up and down to obtain a single cell suspension, and then transfer to a 50-mL polypropylene conical tube (*see* **Note 4**).
8. Wash them by centrifugation (1200 rpm × 10 min) and then twice again with HBSS.
9. Count cells by trypan blue esclusion and adjust cells at the concentration of 2.5×10^5/mL or 8×10^6/mL for intravenous injection (*see* **Subheading 3.2.**) or foot pad injection (*see* **Subheading 3.3.**), respectively (*see* **Note 4**).

3.2. Lung Colonization Assay

1. Place mice in a cage under a heat lamp for a few minutes, until tail vein dilates (*see* **Note 5**).
2. Place one mouse in a mouse vise (animal holder) one at a time for intravenous injection.
3. While holding the tail, inject cell suspension into the lateral tail vein (two lateral veins can be clearly seen) by gently inserting the needle just below the skin with the bevel facing upward. The cells are injected using a tuberculin syringe with a 27G 1/2-in. at an inoculum dose of 5×10^4 cells in 0.2 mL (*see* **Note 6**). Perform a slow steady rate injection. Successful inoculation is evident by the lack of resistance during the process; if any resistance is felt, the process should be

redone. It is best to begin injections at the most distal part of the tail; if the injection is missed or needs to be repeated, one can proceed cranially.

4. Withdraw the needle slowly to minimize leakage and backwash and then replace the mouse in the cage (transfer injected mice to a separate cage).
5. Kill mice after 3–4 wk and collect the lung. Try to avoid touching the lung surface with forceps, as this could cause some damage to the lung parenchyma. Wash the lung briefly in a beaker with cold water to eliminate excess blood (*see* **Note 7**).
6. Count metastases (visible lung nodule) or fix the lung in Bouin's solution to preserve them for future count. With this treatment tumor nodules are seen as raised black/opaque foci against a yellow background.
7. Count lung nodules (number and size of metastatic foci) (*see* **Note 8**) with the aid of a dissection microscope.

3.3. Spontaneous Metastasis Assay

1. Hold the junction of the hind leg and the foot of the mouse and inject the cell suspension into the foot pad. Tumor cells are injected at a dose of 4×10^5 in 0.05 mL of HBSS (*see* **Note 9**).
2. Withdraw the needle slowly, avoiding backwash, and replace the mouse in the cage.
3. Monitor the growth of the tumor in the pad and measure size with the aid of a caliper until approx 250 mg (range 140–320 mg) is reached, or 0.8×0.8 cm in diameter.
4. Place an anesthetized mouse onto the surgery table warmed at 37°C. Work in aseptic/sterile conditions.
5. Open the skin with a small incision, and close the femoral artery proximal to the surgical cut with a small suture. Amputate the leg bearing tumor proximal at the popliteal lymph nodes (at mid-femur). Close the skin with metal wound clips (*see* **Note 10**).
6. Kill mice 3 wk post-excision of the primary tumor. Collect lung and wash it briefly in a beaker with cold water to eliminate excess blood (*see* **Note 7**).
7. Count metastases immediately (visible lung nodule) or fix the lungs in Bouin's solution to preserve them for a future count (*see* **Note 8**).

4. Notes

1. Syngeneic mice should be used, as they reproduce most accurately the history of tumor development and progression. We prefer to use female mice because they are easier to handle and have fewer tendencies to fight than males. As a general rule, it is recommended that mice as young as possible, especially for artificial metastases, be used; however, opposite findings have been reported (*11*). Specific pathogen-free mice should be used. Bacterial, viral, and parasitic infections can profoundly impact the outcome of metastasis. This is likely due to alterations in the host's immune response. Hyperchlorinated water from one side and hepatitis virus (MHV) from the other are two typical examples of the conditions that have been shown to impair metastasis from B16 melanoma (*10*). Subclinical infections are perhaps the most insidious because they are often overlooked. Although the use of imbred animals together with the routine test of the breeding stocks should prevent genetic drift,

changes in metastatic behavior with the same stock of tumor deriving from one laboratory to another have been observed, especially because the same strains of mice but, purchased from different vendors, were used. In conclusion, to obtain reproducible results, our suggestion is to standardize the animal source and characteristics as well as monitor husbandry conditions and animal health carefully. For guidelines for laboratory animal care and use *see also* **refs.** *12* and *13*.

2. The B16 cell lines should be grown and their stocks frozen down in liquid nitrogen. Stocks should be checked and they should be free of mycoplasma, as it is known that infected cells vary in their metastatic behavior. Cell lines should not be maintained in culture for long periods to avoid the drift of their metastatic behavior; once every 2–3 mo (approx 15–20 passages) of being continuously in in vitro culture, a new batch from the stock needs to be recovered to guarantee the phenotypic stability of the cell line.

3. Culture confluence affects the metastatic bahavior. It is important that cell culture is in the growth phase. Cells maintained in culture for too long without passage are difficult to detach from the plastic (*see* use of trypsin in **Note 4**), have difficulty producing cell suspensions and ultimately lose viability.

4. The length of trypsinization does affect the metastatic potential of the cell, therefore make sure you do not overtrypsinize *(14)*. Cells need to be evenly dispersed. Use only suspensions containing single cells of >90% viability. Dead cells do not form metastases; however, they influence the behavior of viable cells. The number of metastases is also influenced by tumor cells present as emboli *(15)*. The preparation of a single-cell suspension is influenced by the way in which the cells are prepared. Most small clumps can be eliminated by gentle pipetting. Try to avoid the use of small-pore pipets or syringes, as too small a diameter can result in cell killing. Cells can easily be maintained in cell suspension by suspending them in ice-cold Ca^{2+}, Mg^{2+}-free medium or saline (it is mandatory that there be no serum). We routinely inject 5×10^4 cells, ranging between 10^4 and 10^5, to produce lung tumor colonies by B16 melanoma but note that there is not always a linear correlation between cell number injected and the number of metastases.

   All the proceeding notes are fundamental for the injection of cells intravenously (artificial metastases), but not necessarily for spontaneous metastases that require the growth of a primary tumor, although in this case the tumor take and growth rate can be affected. Taken together, these observations (*see* **Notes 2–4**) show that cell culture conditions can significantly influence the metastatic bahavior. Conditions for culturing and preparing cells for injection must be carefully reported and repeated consistently.

5. Intravenous injections can be done without dilating the tail, but this procedure facilitates the process. This can be done by dipping the tails in hot water, swabbing with irritants such as xylene, or warming them under a heat lamp. We use an infrared lamp, but this requires close monitoring to avoid the animals becoming overheated.

6. When loading the syringe, it is important that the needle is not in place, to avoid cell killing; once fluid is drawn into the syringe, the needle should be placed onto the syringe for injection. Gently suspend tumor cells every time you load a syringe. It is

important that a filled syringe with cell suspension not be allowed to stand for extended periods prior to injection to limit variability. For intravenous injection in a mouse a volume of no more than 0.2 mL is recommended, to avoid that plasma blood volume does not exceed the normal range which influences the cell distribution.

7. To kill the mice, use the method of euthanasia approved by the Institutional Animal Care Committee, but consider that carbon dioxide causes a number of petechia in the lung, generating confusion in distinguishing tumor foci; cervical dislocation can cause clots in the lung. Perhaps the best way to obtain a clean lung is the use of an overdose of anesthetic.

8. Identification of macroscopic metastasis is easy for B16 melanoma which colorates differently from the parenchyma. The majority are melanotic (black or semiblack) metastases; a few amelanotic metastases can be observed. In general, they are 1–3 mm in size; those ≥5 mm are rare. We use Bouin's fixative to fix the lung for future count; however, alternative methods such as injecting India ink in neutral formalin in the trachea have been used. The limitation of the Bouin's fixation is that it makes the preparation of the tissue for histological analysis difficult in case one needs further confirmation. We suggest the lung be fixed in buffered formalin if histological analysis is anticipated. Most investigators evaluate the number of mice with metastases and count the number of metastases. However, the evaluation of tumor burden should also include the size of the colonies; as metastases from B16 are for the most part spherical, we extrapolate the tumor volume in milligrams from their size *(8)*. With B16 melanoma, the principal site for metastasis is the lung; however, extrapulmonary metastases are frequent. We suggest that a careful autopsy of the viscera, lymph nodes, and brain always be performed.

9. Always hold the extremity of the mouse hind leg with some pressure during injection and direct the injection toward the foot extremity; this helps to prevent tumor spread.

10. When the tumor reaches a large size and it is not removed, it ulcerates quickly causing toxicity. Since, the Institutional Animal Care Committee might not allow the amputation of the leg in the experimental protocol, an alternative to amputation would be to kill the mice with approx 1 cm tumor size, collect the lungs, and then fix them in buffered formalin. Microscopic metastases can now be detected by histopathological analysis (*see also* **Note 8**).

References

1. Poste, G. and Fidler, I. J. (1980) The pathogenesis of cancer metastasis. *Nature* **283,** 139–145.
2. Giavazzi, R. (1991) Metastatic models, in *The Nude Mouse in Oncology Research* (Boven, E. and Winograd, B., eds.), CRC Press, Boca Raton, FL, pp. 117–132.
3. Rygaard, J. (1994) Animal models in cancer research, in *Handbook of Laboratory Animal Science* (Svendsen P. and Hau, J., eds.), CRC Press, Boca Raton, FL, pp. 199–208.
4. Fidler, I. J. (1973) Selection of sucessive tumor lines for metastasis. *Nature New Biol.* **242,** 148–149.

5. Talmadge, J. E. and Fidler, I. J. (1982) Cancer metastasis is selective or random depending on the parent tumour population. *Nature* **297,** 593–594.

6. Hart, I. R. (1979) Selection and characterization of an invasive variant of the B16 melanoma. *Am. J. Pathol.* **97,** 587–600.

7. Stackpole, C. W. (1981) Distinct lung-colonizing and lung-metastasizing cell populations in B16 mouse melanoma. *Nature* **289,** 798–800.

8. Chirivi, R. G. S., Garofalo, A., Crimmin, M. J., Bawden, L. J., Stoppacciaro, A., Brown, P., and Giavazzi, R. (1994) Inhibition of the metastatic spread and growth of B16-BL6 murine melanoma by synthetic matrix metalloproteinase inhibitor. *Int. J. Cancer* **58,** 460–464.

9. Fidler, I. J. (1978) General considerations for studies of experimental cancer metastasis, in *Methods in Cancer Research,* Vol. XV, Busch, H. (ed.), Academic Press, New York, pp. 399–439.

10. Welch, D. R. (1997) Technical considerations for studying cancer metastasis *in vivo. Clin. Exp. Metastast.* **15,** 272–306.

11. Hirayama, R., Hirokawa K., and Makinodan, T. (1985) Change in the metastatic mode of B16 malignant melanoma in C57BL/6 mice with ageing and sex. IARC Scientific Publications, **58,** 85–96.

12. Institute for Laboratory Animal Research (1996) *Guide for the Care and Use of Laboratory Animals.* National Academy Press, Washington, DC.

13. UKCCCR Committee. (1998) United Kingdom Coordinating Committee on Cancer Research (UKCCCR) Guidelines for the Welfare of Animals in Experimental Neoplasia (Second Edition). *Br. J. Cancer* **77,** 1–10.

14. Hagmar, B. and Norrby K. (1973) Influence of cultivation, trypsinization and aggregation on the transplantability of melanoma B16 cells. *Int. J. Cancer* **11,** 663–675.

15. Fidler, I. J. (1973) The relationship of embolic heterogeneity, number size and viability to the incidence of experimental metastasis. *Eur. J. Cancer* **9,** 223–227.

22

Transgenic Animal Models

Chantale T. Guy and Gizela Cardoso

1. Introduction

Cancer is a prevalent and poorly understood disease in human populations. It is generally viewed as a complex, genetic, multistep process involving a series of independent events, each of which creates an incremental phenotypic aberration. For example, the capabilities for extended proliferation, invasion of adjacent tissue, and distant metastasis might each be acquired independently by a cancer cell *(1–4)*. The molecular basis underlying the ability of tumor cells to metastasize from the primary site of growth to other tissues is a major challenge in understanding oncogenesis.

Although most in vitro experiments have provided a significant amount of information regarding the role of oncogenes and tumor suppressor genes in oncogenesis, they do not view malignant progression in its natural in vivo context. For example, tissue culture experiments do not take into account the effects of epigenetic factors such as hormonal conditions, surrounding tissue, extracellular matrix, and humoral factors on tumor development and progression. Thus, directly correlating in vitro observations to in vivo consequences can be misleading. To overcome the intrinsic limitations of these studies, a number of laboratories have turned to the transgenic mouse as an experimental animal model system to assess the genetic requirements of this disease.

A number of techniques are available for making transgenic mice. They include (1) retroviral integration into an early-developing embryo, (2) injection of DNA into the pronucleus of a newly fertilized egg, and (3) genetic manipulation of embryonic stem cells. All three methods have been employed to generate transgenic mice. However, microinjection of DNA into the pronucleus of a zygotic embryo is the most efficient and reliable method *(5)*. This method involves injecting several hundred copies of the DNA into a newly

From: *Methods in Molecular Medicine, vol. 58:*
Metastasis Research Protocols, Vol. 2: Cell Behavior In Vitro and In Vivo
Edited by: S. A. Brooks and U. Schumacher © Humana Press Inc., Totowa, NJ

fertilized egg or zygote and then allowing the embryo to develop in a pseudopregnant mother. Of the animals born, 10–30% should contain exogenous DNA stably integrated into their genome. The DNA typically integrates randomly into the host chromosome, usually at one locus as a multicopy head-to-tail concatomer *(6)*. The transgenic animal that is born is called a founder, and when crossed with a normal animal, the exogenous DNA is transmitted to subsequent generations in normal Mendelian fashion.

The expression of the transgene is regulated by promoter/regulatory sequences present at the 5' end of the gene. Trangenic animals prepared with gene constructs in which promoter/regulatory sequences from one gene are fused with coding sequences of another gene express protein in the tissues specific for the promoter function. Thus, promoters with very high cell type specificity can be employed to direct expression of oncogenes, growth factors, receptors, and others to a variety of target cells in transgenic animals. Consequently, analysis of transgenic mice that express oncogenes in different tissues has revealed that both cell type and oncogene type influence the tumor phenotype *(7–9)*.

The generation of transgenic animal models that spontaneously develop pathology similar to what is seen in humans has allowed us to gain insight into the role and function of various genes in tumor progression.Therefore, the transgenic mouse provides one of the best systems to study the role of genes in tumor progression and metastasis.

1.1. Transgenic Mouse Model of Metastasis

Over the last 20 years, a plethora of transgenic mouse lines have been generated that express activated oncogenes in a variety of tissue types. Although many of these strains develop heritable malignancies, both phenotypes and kinetics vary greatly. The induction of tumors in most of these transgenic models is a multistep process in which transgene expression, although required, is not sufficient for conversion of a normal cell to a transformed phenotype. Their expression induces hyperplastic lesions that may eventually progress to neoplasia with the cooperation of additional genes and the participation of other tumor progression factors that are involved in processes such as apoptosis, angiogenesis, and cell adhesion *(10–13)*. However, in a few exceptional transgenic strains, tumor progression can occur very rapidly, suggesting that, if additional genetic events are required, they occur very quickly *(14,15)*. Because no intermediate lesion has been found in these models, it is believed that malignancies may emerge immediately from normal cells in a one-step progression once the oncogene is expressed or oncogene expression exceeds a given threshold.

It is notable that metastasis is infrequent in most transgenic mouse models of cancer. **Table 1** summarizes the most relevant transgenic models of metastasis *(16–36)*. As tabulated, fewer than 30% of these models demonstrated a

Table 1
Summary of Transgenic Mouse Models of Metastasis

Strain	Promoter/Gene	Onset of tumor formation	Tumor type	Percent metastatic tumors	Ref.
FVB	MMTV/PyV MT	100% by 37 d	Mammary adenocarcinomas	~100% Pulmonary	15
FVB	MMTV/erb 2 (protooncogenic form)	100% by 270 d	Mammary adenocarcinomas	72% Pulmonary	16
C57BL/6 × SJL F1	Wap/Ha-ras	50% by 365 d	Mammary and salivary adenocarcinomas	18% Pulmonary	17
FVB	MMTV/int-1	80% by 219 d	Mammary and salivary adenocarcinomas	Rare pulmonary	18
FVB	MMTV/int-3	100% by 210 d	Mammary adenocarcinomas	High frequency, pulmonary	19
FVB	Wap/int-3	50% by 150 d	Mammary adenocarcinomas	~100% Pulmonary	20
FVB	Wap/c-myc	Mean of 210 d	Mammary adenocarcinomas	21% Pulmonary	21
FVB	Wap/TGFa × Wap/c-myc	100% by 120 d	Mammary adenocarcinomas	28% Pulmonary	22
C57BL/6 × SJL F1	MMTV/FGF8	85% by 365 d	Mammary and salivary adenocarcinomas	40% Pulmonary	23
FVB	MMTV/mts-1 × GRS/A (MMTV provirus)	70% by ~150 d	Mammary adenocarcinomas	40% Pulmonary	24
BDF1	Drosophila heat shock protein 70/SV40 Tag	100% by 217 d	Various smooth muscle tumors and osteosarcomas	50% Brain, 33% liver, 16% lung from osteosarcoma	25
C57BL/6	Rat probassin/SV40 Tag: TRAMP model	80% by 90 d	Autochonous prostate carcinomas	100% Lymphatic, 67% Pulmonary	26
C57BL/6 × CBA	Fetal Gγ-globin/SV40 Tag	100% by 140 d	Prostate adenocarcinomas	100% Lymphatic, some in various sites	27
FVB	Mouse cryptdin-2/SV40 Tag	100% by 180 d	Prostate adenocarcinomas	40% at various sites	28
FVB	Uroplakin-2/SV40 Tag	100% by 150 d	Bladder traditional cell carcinomas	~100% Pelvic lymph nodes and liver	29
FVB	Metallothionein (MT-1)/hepatocyte growth factor	22% by 480 d	Amelanotic melanomas of skin and subcutaneum	21% at various sites	30

Table 1 (cont.)
Summary of Transgenic Mouse Models of Metastasis

Strain	Promoter/Gene	Onset of tumor formation	Tumor type	Percent metastatic tumors	Ref.
CD-1	HPV 16 LCR/*HPV16*	86% by 365 d	Carcinomas in various organ, T-cell lymphomas	70% at various sites	*31*
CB6	Tyrosinase related protein-1/*SV40 Tag*	100% by 120 d	Adenocarcinomas of the retinal pigmented epithelium	100% Lymph node and 30% in spleen	*32*
C57BL/6	Rat Insulin/*SV40 Tag* (*Rip1 Tag 2*) × NCAM null	80% by 112 d	Pancreatic β-cell tumors	16% at various sites	*33*
C57BL/6	Rat Insulin/*SV40 Tag* (*Rip1 Tag 2*)× E cadherin null	~100% by 84 d	Pancreatic β-cell tumors	3.5% Lymphatic	*34*
C57BL/6	*Rip1 Tag 2*× rat insulin/polyoma small *Tag* (Rip2PyST1)	100% by 98 d	Pancreatic β-cell tumors, intestinal tumors	High frequency in lymph node and liver	*35*
FVB	MMTV/*erbB-2* (oncogenic form)× S100A4 (*mts-1*, genomic clone)	67% by 420 d	Mammary adenocarcinomas	37% Pulmonary	*36*

100% penetrance of the metastatic phenotype *(15,20,21,26,27,29,32)*. Although it is clear that all these models have acquired an invasive phenotype, the degree of penetrance and time of onset implies that invasiveness is not the only requirement for metastasis and that additional components of the metastatic phenotype exist. A variety of cellular changes have been implicated in invasion and metastasis *(37)*. These include changes in expression of various proteases that are thought to play important roles in the turnover of basement membrane components such as collagen, glycoproteins, and proteoglycans. Evidence from a number of studies has also suggested that the balance between expression of proteolytic enzymes and their inhibitors plays an important role in tumor invasion *(38)*. Furthermore, metastasis may also involve alterations of cell surface determinants such as CD44, growth and motility factors, oncogenes, or the function of cell type specific adhesion molecules, and finally loss of tumor or metastatic suppressor genes *(39–41)*. The paucity of metastatic disease in cancer models is possibly due to the fact that oncogene expression selectively promotes proliferative steps in tumor progression. Tumors in transgenic mice expressing oncogenes often progress from benign hyperplasia to development of vascular tumors, while both invasiveness and metastasis occur as late-stage events. It appears that the time at which invasiveness is turned on may dramatically influence the subsequent characteristics of the cancer.

On the other hand, evidence for genetic control or modulation of metastasis is growing. A recent study from Hunter et al. has identified strain-dependent modifiers of metastasis using transgenic mice expressing the polyoma virus middle T antigen under the control of the MMTV promoter *(15,42)*. These mice develop mammary tumors and extensive pulmonary metastases in a heritable and highly penetrant manner, making it an excellent model to perform genetic screens for metastasis modifier/suppressor genes. The transgenic animal was bred to 27 different inbred strains of mice and the rate of pulmonary metastasis was monitored. Thirteen different genetic backgrounds had a reduction in their metastatic index whereas the AKR/J strain showed a higher rate of metastasis. The further development of these model systems will likely provide great tools for the identification of metastatic modifiers *(42)*.

In the course of this chapter, we intend to provide a basic procedure for generating such a transgenic model. The purpose is not to illustrate the only way to proceed, but rather help to establish a basis and simplify some of the decisions that need to be made when a laboratory begins to do research with transgenic mice.

2. Materials

2.1. Animals

1. Ten immature 4–6-wk-old FVB/N females. These mice serve as egg donors for microinjection *(see* **Note 1**).

2. Ten mature 2 to 12-mo-old FVB/N stud males. These mice are required for mating with the immature female to generate fertilized zygotes (*see* **Note 2**).
3. Five to eight mature (>8 wk) pseudopregnant CD-1 females. These mice are generated by breeding with vasectomized males. All plugged animals are used as egg transfer recipients (*see* **Note 3**).
4. Vasectomized males (*see* **Note 4**).

2.2. Solutions and Media

1. TBE electrophoresis buffer: 2 mM EDTA, 89 mM Tris, and 89 mM boric acid, pH 8.0.
2. Sample buffer: 10 mM EDTA, 0.25% w/v bromophenol blue, and 50% v/v glycerol.
3. Tris-buffered phenol–chloroform: Melt the phenol in a water bath at 56°C and add 0.1 M Tris-HCl, pH 7.4, until the mixture pH reaches 7.4. Allow solution to separate. Mix an equal volume of buffered phenol (lower phase) and chloroform.
4. Chloroform isoamyl alcohol: Add 24 vol of chloroform to 1 vol of isoamyl alcohol.
5. Injection buffer: 10 mM Tris-HCl, pH 7.4, and 0.1 mM EDTA in MilliQ water. Filter through a 0.2 μm membrane (Ultra-MC, Millipore, cat. no. UFC3 OGC 00).
6. Pregnant mare serum (PMS): Resuspend lyophilized PMS powder (Sigma cat. no. G 4527) at 50 IU/mL in sterile 0.9% saline. Aliquot and store at –20°C.
7. Human chorionic gonadotropin (hCG): Resuspend lyophilized hCG powder (Sigma cat. no. C 8554) at 50 IU/mL in sterile 0.9% saline. Aliquot and store at –20°C.
8. Hyaluronidase: Prepare a stock solution of 10 mg/mL in M2 medium using type IV-S from bovine testes (Sigma cat. no. H 3884). Aliquot and keep at –20°C.
9. M2 medium: A modified Krebs–Ringer solution with HEPES buffer. Purchase from Sigma (cat. no. M 5910).
10. M16 medium: Similar to Whitten's bicarbonate medium. Purchase from Sigma (cat. no. M 1285).
11. Avertin: A stock of 100% is made by mixing 10 g of 2,2,2-tribromoethyl alcohol (Aldrich cat. no. T4, 840-2) with 10 mL of tertiary amyl alcohol (Aldrich cat. no. 24, 048-6). Dilute stock to a 2.5% working solution in water. Use approx 0.015 mL/g body wt. Store at 4°C, protected from light.
12. Light paraffin oil (Fluka cat. no. 76235).
13. Fluorinert electronic fluid FC77 (Sigma cat. no. F 4758).

2.3. Tools

Glass capillaries from most suppliers do not require any cleaning or sterilization but particular attention should be given to contamination from dust particles and grease. Capillaries should not be handles with powdered gloves. Pipets should be pulled the same day they are to be used. Unused capillaries should be kept in sealed packages. Avoid touching ends of pipets with fingers. Nucleases can be transfered this way and destroy your stock of DNA. We also find that it is not necessary to bevel or siliconize the pipet.

2.3.1.Transfer Pipets

Transfer pipets are used to pick up eggs from the hyaluronidase solution and move them through different washes and into microdrop cultures. Pasteur pipets or hard glass capillaries can both be used to make this tool.

1. Hold a 9-in. Pasteur pipet at both ends and soften the glass by rotating it over a small blue flame of a Bunsen burner. The flame should be placed underneath the glass, where the thin portion of the pipet begins to widen.
2. Withdraw the pipet from heat as soon as the glass melts and quickly pull from both ends to yield a thin-walled shaft of glass of about 6–10 cm long.
3. Hold the drawn tube to allow the glass to cool and harden (approx 5 s).
4. Continue to pull the glass so as to snap the glass at its thinnest point. The break should be clean and straight with no sharp edges. Bending it can also snap pipets.
5. Check for size and shape under a stereomicroscope. The outer diameter should be approx 0.2 mm, the inner shaft about 120 µm, and the drawn-out piece no more than 3 cm long. The ideal pipet is one that is slightly larger then a the diameter of an egg.
6. Polish the opening of the transfer pipet by passing the tip through the blue flame.
7. Check the degree of polishing under the stereoscope.
8. Repeat **steps 1–7** four to five times before proceeding.
9. Fit the transfer pipet to the end of a plastic mouthpiece that is held between the teeth and connected to a rubber tube.

2.3.2. Holding Pipets

These pipets are designed to hold eggs in place while injection is in progress **(Fig. 1)**.

1. Use thick-walled borosilicate capillaries 15 cm long with an outside diameter of 1 mm and an inside diameter of approx 0.5 mm (Leitz glass capillaries, Leitz cat. no. 520119).
2. Pull the pipet on a horizontal or vertical needle puller so that it has a suitable tip diameter of approx 50–100 µm. The pipet puller settings necessary to accomplish this will be different in each situation and will need to be assessed by the operator. Note settings for future use.
3. Move to a microforge.
4. Melt a small bead of glass on the filament of the microforge using a discarded capillary.
5. Clip the pulled pipet at an angle of 30° off the horizontal plane above the glass bead on the microforge filament.
6. Turn on the reostat until the bead just begins to glow (orange in color). The pipet is lowered to contact the bead. Turn off the heat as soon as contact is made. The capillary is now fused to the glass bead. As the filament contracts on cooling, the fused bead and pipet will break to form the tip of the pipet.
7. Pull back the pipet. This should create a clean, vertical break in the capillary.

Holding Pipet

Injection pipet

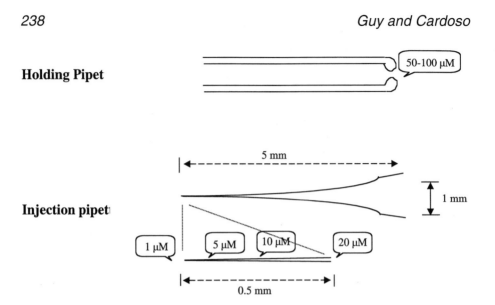

Fig. 1. Dimension and shape of holding and injection pipets.

8. Polish the end of the holding pipet by moving the pipet vertically over a hot filament until the open tip just begins to melt.
9. Monitor the internal diameter of the holding pipet. It should be no smaller than 15–20 µm.
10. Prepare several extra pipets before starting the experiment.

2.3.3. Injection Pipets

The injection pipet is used to physically introduce DNA into the pronucleus of a one-cell fertilized egg **(Fig. 1)**.

1. Use a thin-walled borosilicate glass capillary (15 cm long) containing an internal glass filament (World-Precision Instrument TW100F). This filament allows the pipet to be filled with DNA by its blunt end through the capillary.
2. Pull the capillary on a vertical or horizontal pipet puller. The settings necessary to pull the perfect pipet will be different for each situation and need to be assessed by the operator. Note settings for future use.
3. Verify that the inner opening of the pipet is no larger than 1 µm. The taper between the tip and the shoulder of the pipet should be approx 5 mm long.
4. Prepare several extra pipets before starting the experiment.

2.4. Major Equipment

1. A humidified tissue culture incubator set at 37°C and 5% CO_2 (v/v).
2. An inverted microscope equipped with a fixed stage, a 10× eyepiece, and a 40× objective lens is suitable. Nikon Diaphot-TMD with Nomarski differential interference contrast optics is widely used for microinjection.

3. Micromanipulators: A set of Nikon micromanipulator is used with the Nikon Diaphot-TMD microscope.
4. A set of micropipet holders to hold the injection and holding pipets in place.
5. A programmable Sutter micropipet puller (Model P-87/PC).
6. A microforge (Narishige model MF-83).
7. A Narishige Pico-Injector (PLI-188) that allows preprogrammed regulation of fluid delivery volume, time, and pressure.
8. A dissecting microscope.
9. An antivibration table (Kinetic Systems) that supports solid stainless steel surfaces on four nitrogen-driven pistons.
10. An oil-driven microsyringe assembly (Nikon) fitted with Tygon tubing (ID 1/8, OD 1/4, and wall 1/16 in.) to connect to the holding micropipet holder.

3. Methods

3.1. DNA Preparation

Because prokaryotic cloning vector sequences can interfere with transgene expression, we purify construct elements from plasmid sequences as much as possible prior to microinjection. Doubled cesium chloride purified DNA should be use as starting material. Transgenic mice can be generated with either a linear or supercoiled form of DNA. Generally, we favor linear DNA fragments because of their higher integration frequency compared to circular molecules (approx fivefold) (*see* **Note 5**).

1. Digest your plasmid containing transgene overnight with appropriate restriction enzymes to generate enough material to yield approx 50 µg of transgene fragments.
2. Add 1 vol of sample buffer to 4 vol of DNA preparation. Aim to obtain 1–5 µg/mL of DNA.
3. Load samples onto a submarine horizontal 0.5% agarose gel and electrophorese at 80 V/cm using 0.5% TBE running buffer containing 0.5 µg/mL of ethidium bromide.
4. Visualize on an UV transilluminator.
5. Cut the appropriate DNA–agarose band representing your transgene using a clean scalpel blade.
6. Electroelute the DNA from agarose in a small dialysis bag containing 500 µL of running buffer at high voltage (~200 V/cm) for 20 min.
7. Reverse the voltage for 2 min and pipet the DNA–buffer mixture to a clean tube.
8. Add 1 vol of a 1:1 mix of Tris-buffered phenol and chloroform.
9. Mix thoroughly by repeated inversion and centrifuge for 5 min at 13,000g in a benchtop centrifuge.
10. Remove the majority of the upper aqueous phase and place into a fresh clean Eppendorf tube. Avoid drawing up any of the organic phase.
11. Repeat **steps 8–10** five times.
12. Add 1 vol of a 24:1 mix of chloroform and isoamyl alcohol.
13. Mix thoroughly by repeated inversion and centrifuge for 5 min at 13,000g in a benchtop centrifuge.

14. Remove the majority of the upper aqueous phase and place into a fresh clean Eppendorf tube. Avoid drawing up any of the organic phase.
15. Repeat **steps 12–14** five times.
16. Add 2 vol of cold 100% ethanol.
17. Mix by repeated inversion and let sit on ice until DNA is precipitated (approx 60 min).
18. Pellet the DNA by centrifugation at 13,000g for 20 min at 4°C.
19. Resuspend the DNA in 300 µL of injection buffer and repeat **steps 16–18** two more times.
20. Dialyze the DNA solution against 2000 mL of the same injection buffer for 2 d at 4°C with two exchanges per day.
21. After dialysis, visualize 10 µL of the DNA on a 1% agarose gel to confirm adequate recovery and absence of degradation.
22. Dilute the DNA to a final concentration of approx 1–3 µg/mL, corresponding approx 200–500 copies/pL of a 5-kb DNA fragment
23. Filter the DNA sample through a 0.2-µm microfilter.
24. DNA used for microinjection is stored at 4°C and should be used within 2 wk. Prior to experiment, DNA is centrifuged at 13,000g for 15 min at 4°C and only the top 80% of the solution is transferred to a clean tube and used.

3.2. Superovulation of Female Donors

1. Set the light cycle for the animal room on a 14-h light–10-h dark program (lights on at 6 a.m. and off at 8 p.m.) at least 2 wk prior to any experiment.
2. Inject intraperitoneally ten 4–6-wk-old FVB females with 5 IU of PMS in a dose of 0.1 mL between 12 p.m. and 1 p.m.
3. At 46–48 h later inject the same set of animals as in **step 2** with 5 IU of hCG in a dose of 0.1 mL (*see* **Note 6**).
4. Place one superovulated FVB female in a cage with one stud FVB male immediately after hCG injection.
5. Collect all females the next morning and examine for the presence of copulation plugs in the vagina. The animals that are scored positive for plugs are ready for zygote collection.

3.3. Zygote Collection

1. Kill rapidly all plugged female donors using CO_2 inhalation or cervical dislocation.
2. Place the animal on its back and spray 70% ethanol on its abdomen to keep fur in place.
3. Grab the skin with a finger at the midline and pull the skin toward the head and tail until the abdomen is completely uncovered and free of fur.
4. Open the abdomen wall with forceps and scissors; push aside all organs; and locate the uterus, ovaries, and oviducts.
5. Remove the ovary, oviducts, and a small part of the uterine horn by first passing the blade of your scissors along the mesometrium while holding the tissues by the fat pad present on top of the ovary. Cut first in between the ovary and the fat pad, then a second time between the oviduct and the uterine horn.

6. Collect all tissues in a 30 mm tissue culture dish containing M2 medium at room temperature.
7. Transfer one oviduct at a time into a deep 3-well depression glass slide containing M2 medium supplemented with 300 mg/mL of hyaluronidase at room temperature and view the swollen striated ampulla through a stereomicroscope with transmitted light base at 20× magnification.
8. Tear open the ampulla with two fine forceps and observe the release of fertilized eggs and associated cumulus cells. If no eggs flow out, gently squeeze the oviduct to push them out.
9. Repeat **steps 7** and **8** until all oviducts have been emptied.
10. Wash all zygotes several times in fresh M2 medium to remove debris and traces of hyaluronidase solution by moving them to different wells using a sterile transfer pipet.
11. Prepare a microdrop culture by filling a depression slide with M16 medium and cover its surface with light mineral oil or Fluorinert.
12. Place the microdrop culture in a humidified incubator at 37°C, 5% CO_2 for equilibration to occur (approx 20 min).
13. Transfert zygotes from M2 medium to the prewarmed and CO_2 equilibrated M16 microdrop.
14. Return to the incubator until ready for microinjection.

3.4. Microinjection of Mouse Zygote

3.4.1. Setting up the Microinjection Chamber

1. A glass depression slide is used to prepare the injection chamber, as plastic is not compatible with Nomarski optics.
2. Place a large, flat drop of M2 medium in the center of the depression slide (approx 100 µL).
3. Cover the medium with a layer of light paraffin oil to prevent evaporation.
4. Divide your drop area in two using a marker so you have an upper and a lower area.
5. Transfer 20–30 fertilized eggs from the microdrop culture in the incubator to the top area of your drop using a transfer pipet and a mouthpiece.
6. Place the slide on the stage of an inverted microscope.

3.4.2. Setting up the Holding Pipet

1. Load a microsyringe with Fluorinert.
2. Connect the syringe to the holding pipet and holder via flexible Tygon tubings.
3. Fill the tubing, the micropipet holder, and the holding pipet by increasing the pressure on the syringe, allowing the liquid to come out of the opening of the pipet. All air bubbles should be purged out, as they will dampen the control. If no liquid comes out, the holding pipet is probably inadequate (overpolished or too small of an opening).
4. Adjust the pressure on the syringe to where no liquid comes out of the holding pipet but no air bubble is formed.
5. Lower the holding pipet into the center of the injection chamber.
6. Dial back the microsyringe to reduce the flow of Fluorinert and draw M2 medium into the holding pipet to about 1 cm.

3.4.3. Setting up the Injection Pipet

1. Connect the micropipet holder to the automatic injection system using Tygon tubing.
2. Fill the injection pipet with DNA by plunging its blunt end into DNA solution. The clear solution should fill the tip (approx 4 mm in distance).
3. Position the injection pipet to its holder.
4. Using the micromanipulator, lower the pipet to the center of the microinjection chamber. To avoid breaking the tip, ensure that the injection pipet does not contact the bottom of the injection chamber.
5. Bring the tip of the injection pipet into the same horizontal plane as the tip of the holding pipet. Verify that the injection pipet is sufficiently open by applying pressure using the regulator and look for a spray. If nothing happens, try chipping the very tip of the injection pipet on the holding pipet, creating a larger opening.

3.4.4. Microinjection of DNA

1. Focus the microscope so that all pipets tips and eggs are on the same horizontal plane.
2. Hold one egg from the top part of the microinjection chamber by sucking it on the holding pipet by decreasing the pressure on the syringe (**Fig. 2**).
3. Locate the largest pronucleus and position it as close as possible to the injecting pipet by increasing and releasing the pressure on the syringe filled with Fluorinert. This will cause the egg to rotate into a better position.
4. Place the tip of the injection pipet next to the egg and focus to bring both elements on a same horizontal plane. The tip of the pipet and the edge of the pronucleus should be clearly focused.
5. Push the injection pipet through the zona pellucida toward the pronucleus. Enter the pronucleus and inject the DNA by pressing the inject button of the Pico-injector. You should see a swelling of the pronucleus. Quickly remove the pipet from the egg so that it does not attach itself to nuclear components (*see* **Note 7**).
6. Move the holding pipet and the injected egg to the lower part of the chamber and release the egg by blowing the zygote away.
7. Repeat **steps 2–6** for all remaining eggs.
8. Transfer all injected eggs to a fresh M16 microdrop culture clearly labeled and keep in the incubator at 37°C until all eggs have been injected. In one session of injection, it is better to work only with as many eggs as you can inject in about 15 min, as their survival decreases with time.
9. Select all healthy looking injected eggs from the lysed ones and move them to a new M16 microdrop. A healthy zygote is bright and has a space between the egg and the zona pellucida whereas a lysed one has no space and appears gray (*see* **Note 8**).

3.5. Embryo Transfer

Following microinjection, the eggs must be transferred to the reproductive tract of pseudopregnant female mice to complete development of the embryos. Injected zygotes can either be implanted the same day into the oviduct of a

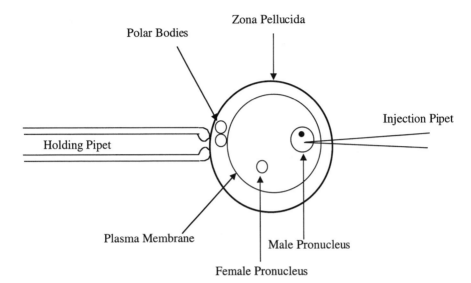

Fig. 2. DNA microinjection. Diagram of DNA microinjection into a pronuclear murine zygote. A large holding pipet holds a fertilized egg through suction. The injection pipet containing the DNA solution is inserted into the male pronucleus; the DNA is then slowly expelled into the pronucleus, which swells.

pseudopregnant female or cultured overnight and transferred at the two-cell stage embryo. In rare instances, the eggs can be cultured in vitro in M16 medium to the blastocyst stage and transfered into the uterus of a 2.5-d post-coitus pseudopregnant female mouse. We do not recommend using this strategy routinely; in our view, culture only reduces the likelihood of survival.

1. Generate five to eight pseudopregnant females (0.5-d post-coitus) by mating ten vasectomized males with ten 6–8-wk-old females in estrus.
2. Check for the presence of a copulation plug in the vagina of the females early the next morning (before 8 a.m., as the plug dissolves over time or falls off).
3. Pool all plugged females together. These mice are ready to receive the injected embryo.
4. Anesthetize one animal at a time using a dose of 0.015 mL of 2.5% avertin per gram of body weight. While the mouse goes under proceed to the next step.
5. Prepare a transfer pipet filled with M2 medium by loading it under the microscope with light mineral oil then with alternating regions of medium and air to create bubbles (*see* **Note 9**) (**Fig. 3**).
6. Take the injected eggs out of the incubator and load 30 injected eggs or 15 two-cell embryos into the prepared transfer pipet tip. Aspirate each egg as close as possible to the next one to minimize the overall amount of medium transferred. Once all eggs have been aspirated, one air bubble is created at the end of the tip to prevent leakage while you prepare the animal for surgery.

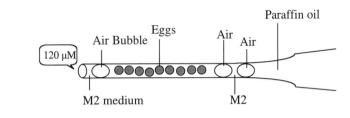

Fig. 3. Loading of eggs in the transfer pipet. Oil is first drawn into the tip of the pipet followed by M2 medium and two air bubbles. The addition of air bubble provides a greater precision in egg movement. Following injection of the air bubbles, the eggs are drawn side by side into the pipet. A last air bubble completes the loading.

7. Rest the loaded pipet aside, pay particular attention to the tip of the instrument by perching it on a monticule of Plasticine.
8. Place the mouse on its side with the head placed on your left. Spray ethanol on the flank and make a small incision in the skin about 1 cm from the spinal cord, behind the last rib.
9. Slide the incision around with forceps to locate the ovary or its fat pad. The ovary should be visible through the muscle wall. Cut the body wall just over the ovary and avoid blood vessels.
10. Grasp the fat pad with blunt forceps and gently pull the ovary, the oviduct, and part of the uterus out of the body cavity (**Fig. 4**). Lay the tissue toward the back of the animal such as to expose the bursa and oviduct better.
11. Attach a Dieffenbach clamp to the fat pad to prevent the tissue from sliding back into the body.
12. Place the animal under a dissecting stereomicroscope and locate the bursa, which is a thin clear membrane covering the oviduct and the ovary. Locate the infundibu-lum by gently probing the left side of the bursa in between the ovary and oviduct.
13. Rip the bursa while taking special care to avoid any large blood vessels and fold it around the ovary. Bleeding will obstruct your view and clog the pipet during transfer of the embryo.
14. Hold the mouthpiece attached to the prepared transfer pipet between you teeth and, with two fine forceps in hands, pick up an edge of the infundibulum using your left forceps. Switch the right forceps for the prepared pipet without losing sight of the infundibulum.
15. Insert the pipet into the opening of the oviduct until the tip reaches the first kink. Blow gently the eggs out of the pipet and observe the position of the bubbles. The transfer is successful when you can locate the leading bubble into the ampulla and one or two bubbles at the entrance of the oviduct.
16. Remove the mouse from under the microscope and unclip the Dieffenbach clamp. Push the ovary and oviduct back into the body cavity and sew up the body wall with two stitches. Close the skin with two wound staples.
17. Warm and observe the animal until recovery and return it to its cage.
18. Proceed with the next animal (*see* **Note 10**).

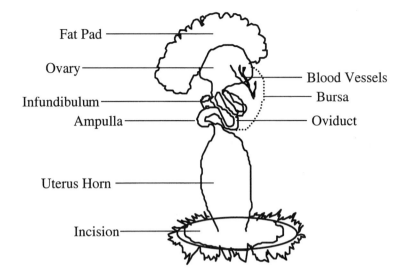

Fig. 4. Female reproductive tract. The fat pad is pulled outside of the body wall and reproductive organs are exposed. The fertilized eggs are located in the swollen ampulla. During egg transfer, the bursa is torn to expose the infundibulum. Embryos are blown through the opening into the ampulla.

4. Notes

1. In the production of fertilized eggs for DNA injection, we usually prefer inbred strains because of their stable and defined genetic backgrounds. Our laboratory routinely uses the inbred mouse strain FVB/N. This strain is widely used in transgenic experiments because of the large size of the pronucleus, their resistance to lysis, and its good reproductive characteristics. Many laboratories have also used hybrid F1 females to generate their fertilized eggs. From these hybrids, you may obtain a greater number of eggs but it is often preferable to study the effects of a transgene in a consistent genetic background. In general, if starting with 10 animals, 80–90% of the females will mate and yield an average of 100–200 eggs, of which about 80% will be fertilized zygotes ready for microinjection.

2. Fertile stud male mice: To produce an average of 100–200 fertilized eggs per day (approx 10 females) you will need to keep a stock of 30 fertile FVB/N stud males. They should be caged individually to avoid fighting and reduction in testosterone. Stud males can be used between the ages of 2 and 8 mo. A record of their performance (plugging efficiency) should be kept to eliminate any potential non-breeder. A rest of 24–48 h is recommended between mating, as the sperm count will usually decrease after mating.

3. Pseudopregnant females: Either outbred mice such as CD-1 which have very large ampulla or F1 hybrid females (B6 × CBA) are generally good mothers and can be used for mating. Females in estrus can be identified by the color, moistness, and

swelling of the vagina. It should be pink to red, moist, and swollen. One female is bred to one vasectomized male. Unplugged females can be reused 10–15 d later once they have completed their cycle.

4. Vasectomized males: Any outbred or F1 hybrid strain is good to use to generate sterile males. Vasectomized males may be purchased from a supplier or produced in house. Before using any vasectomized male, test for sterility by breeding the male for a week and scoring for pregnancy. A stock of 30 vasectomized male should be kept to produce five to eight pseudopregnant females a day. A rest of 24–48 h is recommended before using the same male a second time.

5. Microinjection DNA should be free of all contaminants. It should be dissolved in a Tris buffer containing no more then 0.2 mM EDTA as higher concentrations of EDTA or minute amounts of $MgCl_2$ are toxic to eggs. A high concentration of DNA also results in toxicity. A concentration of 1–5 µg/mL is optimal for a construct of 5 kb, as a lower concentration reduces the frequency of integration.

6. Hormones: PMS is used to mimic follicule-stimulating hormone (FSH), and hCG is used to mimic luteinizing hormone (LH). The age and weight of the female donor will affect the percentage of eggs that will be superovulated by the hormones. Prepubescent 4–6-wk-old mice are optimal for most mouse strains. They respond to PMS well and yield a peak amount of follicle release. In addition to age, weight is also critical. On average, mice between 12 and 14 g will produce the largest amount of viable fertilized eggs.

7. When injecting DNA, avoid touching the nucleolus as it will attach itself to the injection pipet and be drawn outside the egg, causing its death. A new pipet will also have to be used as it will clog it.

8. About 75% of the eggs should survive the injection. If this number is lower, verify your technique, sizes of pipets, and quality of medium.

9. Transfer pipet: The main purpose of the oil and bubbles is to slow the capillary action of the pipet and gain more control on the loading of the eggs in the pipet and the expulsion of the eggs in the oviduct. This is achieved by dipping the pipet in light mineral oil and forcefully aspirate the oil filling the tip. Move the pipet to M2 medium; dip in, then pull out, sucking on the mouthpiece to create an air bubble. The tip is dipped again in medium and the process is repeated two times. These pockets of air also serve as indicator once the eggs are transferred, as they are visible through the oviductal wall.

10. Reimplantation of injected eggs: This technique should be practiced using a dye on a cadaver before beginning into a real experiment. Test your ability by transferring uninjected eggs and scoring for pregnancy. Many investigators use both sides of the reproductive tract for implantation of embryos. Remember to turn the animal around 180° such that the head faces the left. The infundibulum will then be in the same position as for the first surgery.

References

1. Foulds, L. (1954) The experimental study of tumor progression: a review. *Cancer Res.* **14,** 327–339.

2. Fearon, E. R. and Vogelstein, B. (1990) A genetic model for colorectal tumorigenesis. *Cell* **61,** 759–767.

3. Vogelstein, B. and Kinzler, K. W. (1993) The multistep nature of cancer. *Trends Genet.* **9,** 138–141.

4. Kinzler, K. and Vogelstein, B. (1996) Lesson from hereditary colorectal cancer. *Cell* **87,** 159–170.

5. Gordon, J. W., Scangos, G. A., Plotkin, D. J., Barbosa, J. A., and Ruddle, F. H. (1980) Genetic transformation of mouse embryos by microinjection of purified DNA. *Proc. Natl. Acad. Sci. USA* **77,** 380–384.

6. Constantini, F. and Lacy, E. (1981) Introduction of a rabbit β-globin gene into the mouse germ line. *Nature* **294,** 92–94.

7. Corey, S. and Adams, J. M. (1988) Transgenic mice and oncogenesis. *Annu. Rev. Immunol.* **6,** 25–48.

8. Hanahan, D. (1988) Dissecting multistep tumorigenesis in transgenic mice. *Annu. Rev. Genet.* **22,** 479–519.

9. Adams, J. M. and Cory, S. (1991) Transgenic models of tumor development. *Science* **254,** 1161–1167.

10. Cardiff, R. D. and Muller, W. J. (1993) Transgenic mouse models of mammary tumorigenesis. *Cancer Surv.* **16,** 97–113.

11. Christofori, G. and Hanahan, D. (1994) Molecular dissection of multistage tumorigenesis in transgenic mice. *Semin. Cancer Biol.* **5,** 3–12.

12. Webster, M. A. and Muller, W. J. (1994) Mammary tumorigenesis and metastasis in transgenic mice. *Semin. Cancer Biol.* **5,** 69–76.

13. Macleod, K. F. and Jacks, T. (1999) Insights into cancer from transgenic mouse models. *J. Pathol.* **187,** 43–60.

14. Muller, W. J., Sinn, E., Pattengale, P. K., Wallace, R., and Leder, P. (1988) Single-step induction of mammary adenocarcinoma in transgenic mice bearing the activated c-neu oncogene. *Cell* **54,** 105–115.

15. Guy, C. T., Cardiff, R. D., and Muller, W. J. (1992) Induction of mammary tumors by expression of polyomavirus middle T oncogene: a transgenic mouse model for metastatic disease. *Mol. Cell Biol.* **12,** 954–961.

16. Guy, C. T., Webster, M. A., Schaller, M., Parsons, T. J., Cardiff, R. D., and Muller, W. J. (1992) Expression of the *neu* protooncogene in the mammary epithelium of transgenic mice induces metastatic disease. *Proc. Natl. Acad. Sci. USA* **89,** 10578–10582.

17. Andreas, A. C., Schonenberger, B., Groner, B., Henninghausen, L., Le Meur, M., and Gerlinger, P. (1987) Ha-*ras* oncogene expression directed by milk protein gene promoter; tissue specificity, hormonal regulation, and tumor induction in transgenic mice. *Proc. Natl. Acad. Sci. USA* **84,** 1299–1303.

18. Nielsen, L. L., Discafani, C. M. Gurnani, M., and Tyler, R. D. (1991) Histopathology of salivary gland and mammary gland tumors in transgenic mice expressing a human Ha-*ras* oncogene. *Cancer Res.* **51,** 3762–3767.

19. Tsukamoto, A. S., Grosschedl, R., Guzman, R. C., Parslow, T., and Varmus, H. E. (1988) Expression of the *int-1* gene in transgenic mice is associated with mammary gland hyperplasia and adenocarcinomas in male and female mice. *Cell* **55,** 619–625.

20. Jhappan, C., Gallahan, D., Stahle, C., Chu, E., Smith, G.H., Merlino, G., and Callahan, R. (1992) Expression of a Notch related *int-3* transgene interferes with cell differentiation and induces neoplastic transformation in mammary and salivary glands. *Genes Dev.* **6,** 345–355.

21. Gallahan, D., Jhappan, C., Robinson, G., Hennighausen, L., Sharp, R., Kordon, E., et al. (1996) Expression of a truncated Int3 gene in developing mammary epithelium specifically retards lobular differentiation resulting in tumorigenesis. *Cancer Res.* **56,** 1775–1785.

22. Sandgren, E. P., Schroeder, J. A., Qui, T. H., Palmiter, R. D., Brinster, R. L., and Lee D. C. (1995) Inhibition of mammary gland involution is associated with transforming growth factor α but not c-*myc*-induced tumorigenesis in transgenic mice. *Cancer Res.* **55,** 3915–3927.

23. Daphna-Iken, D., Shankar, D. B., Lawshe, A., Ornitz, D. M., Shackleford, G. M., and MacArthur, C. A. (1998) MMTV-Fgf8 transgenic mice develop mammary and salivary gland neoplasia and ovarian stromal hyperplasia. *Oncogene* **17,** 2711–2717.

24. Ambartsumian, N. S., Griogorian, M. S., Larsen, I. F., Karlstrom, O., Sidenius, N., Rygaard, J., et al. (1996) Metastasis of mammary carcinomas in GRS/A hybrid mice transgenic for the *mts*1 gene. *Oncogenes* **13,** 1621–1630.

25. Wilkie, T. M., Schmidt, R. A., Baetscher, M., and Messing, A. (1994) Smooth muscle and bone neoplasms in transgenic mice expressing SV40 T antigen. *Oncogenes* **9,** 2889–2895.

26. Gingrich, J. R., Barrios, R. J., Morton, R. A., Boyce, B. F., DeMayo, F. J., Finegold, M. J., et al. (1996) Metastatic prostate cancer in a transgenic mouse. *Cancer Res.* **56,** 4096–4102.

27. Perez-Stable, C., Altman, N. H., Mechta, P. P., Deftos, L. J., and Roos, B. A. (1997) Prostate cancer progression, metastasis, and gene expression in transgenic mice. *Cancer Res.* **57,** 900–906.

28. Garabedian, E. M., Humphrey, P. A., and Gordon, J. I. (1998) A transgenic mouse model of metastatic prostate cancer originating from neuroendocrine cells. *Proc. Natl. Acad. Sci. USA* **95,** 15382–15387.

29. Zhang, Z-T., Pak, J., Shapiro, E., Sun, T-T., and Wu, X-R. (1999) Urothelium-specific expression of an oncogene in transgenic mice induced the formation of carcinoma in situ and invasive transitional cell carcinoma. *Cancer Res.* **59,** 3512–3517.

30. Otsuka, T., Takayama, H., Sharp, R., Celli, G., LaRochelle, W. J., Bottaro, D. P., et al. (1998) c-Met autocrine activation induces development of malignant melanoma and acquisition of the metastatic phenotype. *Cancer Res.* **58,** 5157–5167.

31. Yang, J-T., Liu, C-Z., and Iannaccone, P. (1995) The HPV 16 genome induces carcinomas and T-cell lymphomas in transgenic mice. *Am. J. Pathol.* **147,** 68–78.

32. Penna, D., Schmidt, A., and Beermann, F. (1998) Tumors of the retinal pigment epithelium metastasize to inguinal lymph nodes and spleen in tyrosinase-related protein-1/ SV40 T antigen transgenic mice. *Oncogene* **17,** 2601–2607.

33. Perl, A. K., Wilgenbus, P., Dahl, D., Semb, H., and Christofori, G. (1998) A causal role of E-cadherin in the transition from adenoma to carcinoma. *Nature* **392,** 286–291.

34. Perl, A. K., Dahl, D., Wilgenbus, P., Semb, H., and Christofori, G. (1999) Reduced expression of neural cell adhesion molecule induces metastatic dissemination of pancreatic B tumor cells. *Nat. Med.* **5,** 286–290.
35. Grant, S. G. N., Seidman, I., Hanahan, D., and Bautch, V. L. (1991) Early invasiveness characterizes metastatic carcinoid tumors in transgenic mice. *Cancer Res.* **51,** 4917–4923.
36. Davies, M. P. A., Rudland, P. S., Robertson, L., Parry, E. W., Jolicoeur, P., and Barraclough, R. (1996) Expression of the calcium-binding protein S100A4 (p9Ka) in MMTV-neu transgenic mice induces metastasis of mammary tumours. *Cancer Res.* **13,** 1631–1637.
37. Nicolson, G. A. (1988) Cancer metastasis: tumor cell and host organ properties important in metastasis to specific secondary sites. *Biochem. Biophys. Acta* **948,** 175–224.
38. Liotta, L. A. (1986) Tumor invasion and metastases-role of the extracellular matrix. *Cancer Res.* **46,** 1–7.
39. Gunthert, U., Hofmann, M., Ruby, W., Reber, S., Zoller, M., Haubmann, I., et al. (1991) A new variant of glycoprotein CD44 confers metastatic potential to rat carcinoma cells. *Cell* **65,** 13–24.
40. Liotta, L. A., Steeg, P. S., and Stetler-Stevenson, W. G. (1991) Cancer, metastasis and angiogenesis: an imbalance of positive and negative regulation. *Cell* **64,** 327–336.
41. Marshall, C. J. (1991) Tumor suppressor genes. *Cell* **64,** 313–326.
42. Lifsted, T., Le Voyer, T., Williams, M., Muller, W., Klein-Szanto, A., Buetow, K. H., and Hunter, W. (1998) Identification of inbred mouse strains harboring genetic modifiers of mammary tumor age of onset and metastatic progression. *Int. J. Cancer* **77,** 640–644.

Further Reading

Hogan, B., Beddington, R., Constantini, F., and Lacy, E. (1994) *Manipulating the Mouse Embryo: A Laboratory Manual.* 2nd edition. Cold Spring Harbor Laboratory Press, Cold Spring Harbor, NY.
Gordon, J. W. (1993) Transgenic animals: pronuclear injection, in *Methods in Enzymology, Guide to Techniques in Mouse Development* (Wassarman, P. M. and DePamphilis, M. L., eds.), Academic Press, San Diego, CA, pp. 747–799.
Murphy, D. and Carter, D. A., eds. (1993) *Transgenesis Techniques: Principles and Protocols.* Humana Press, Totowa, NJ.

23

Clinically Accurate Orthotopic Mouse Models of Cancer

Robert M. Hoffman

1. Introduction

1.1. Background of Surgical Orthotopic Implantation Mouse Models of Human Cancer

In the past 10 years, we have developed a new approach to the development of a clinically accurate rodent model for human cancer based on our invention of surgical orthotopic implantation (SOI). The SOI models have been described in approx 70 publications *(2–72)* and in four patents.* SOI allows human tumors of all the major types of human cancer to reproduce clinical-like tumor growth and metastasis in the transplanted rodents *(2–72)*. The major features of the SOI models are reviewed here and also compared to transgenic mouse models of cancer.

1.2. Previous In Vivo Screening Systems

1.2.1. Early Screening Systems

Early screening in vivo systems for drug discovery included the L1210 mouse leukemia *(74)*. A more sensitive mouse leukemia, P388, was introduced somewhat later *(75)*. The possibility of more relevant screening was expanded when Rygaard utilized the newly isolated athymic nude mouse to transplant human tumors *(76)*. Screening with human xenografts started with the colon CX-1, lung LX-1, and breast MX-1 tumors *(77)*. The US National Cancer Institute *(84)* and the Central Institute of Experimental Animals of Japan *(83)* and the Cancer Research Campaign of the United Kingdom *(85)* have greatly expanded the number of human tumor cell lines that can grow in nude mice.

*US Patent Nos. 5,569,812 and 5,491,284; European Patent No. 0437488; Japanese Patent No. 2664261.

From: *Methods in Molecular Medicine, vol. 58:*
Metastasis Research Protocols, Vol. 2: Cell Behavior In Vitro and In Vivo
Edited by: S. A. Brooks and U. Schumacher © Humana Press Inc., Totowa, NJ

However, the early nude mouse models were quite distinct from clinical cancer. The human tumors were implanted subcutaneously, which is a very different microenvironment from the tissue of origin of the tumors. The subcutaneous environment usually precludes the tumors from metastasizing. Workers such as Sordat and Fidler *(1)* have partly addressed this point, by introducing orthotopic transplantation of suspensions of tumor cell lines in nude mice as detailed in the following subheading.

1.2.2. Orthotopic Injection of Suspensions of Established Cell Lines

Fidler *(1)* noted that the subcutaneous microenvironment for human visceral tumors is very different from their original milieu. He postulated that this difference may result in the lack of metastases and the altered drug responses seen in the subcutaneous models. Indeed radical differences have been noted by Fidler *(78)* and us *(21)* in the drug responses of tumors in the orthotopically transplanted site vs the tumor growing subcutaneously. Despite species difference, the corresponding nude mouse organ more closely resembles the original patient microenvironment than the subcutaneous milieu.

Injecting tumor cell suspensions into the analogous or orthotopic mouse sites occasionally allowed relevant metastases. For example, disaggregated human colon cancer cell lines injected into the cecum of nude mice produced tumors that eventually metastasized to the liver *(1)*. Although orthotopic injection of cell suspensions is an improvement over simple subcutaneous implantation, the technique has several major drawbacks. Orthotopic cell injection so far has been shown to work essentially only with established cell lines, which greatly restricts its utility. The tumors resulting from orthotopic transplantation of cell suspensions often showed relatively low rates of metastasis compared to the original tumor in the patient and to SOI *(2–72)*.

1.3. SOI of Tumor Fragments

The SOI models circumvent the cell disaggregation step used in previous orthotopic models. Instead of injecting cell suspensions into the orthotopic site, we have developed microsurgical technology to transplant tumor fragments orthotopically *(2–72)*. The development of SOI technology led to a profound improvement in the results achieved in that the metastatic rates and sites in the transplanted mice reflect the clinical pattern after SOI. The advantages of SOI appear quite general, having been seen in comparison to orthotopic implantation of cell suspensions for bladder *(3,4)*, lung *(5,10,11,25,27,28)*, stomach *(6,15,19)*, kidney *(134)*, and colon cancers *(2,7,9,17,33,67–71)*.

In a head-to-head comparison of SOI with orthotopic transplantation of cell suspensions, SOI of stomach cancer tissue fragments resulted in metastases in 100% of the nude mice with extensive primary growth. Metastases were found in the regional lymph nodes, liver, and lung, as is characteristic of this cancer *(6)*. In contrast, orthotopic injection of suspensions of stomach cancer cells to the nude mouse stomach resulted in lymph node metastases in only 6.7% of those mice bearing tumors and no distant metastases.

We also compared the metastatic rate of human renal cell carcinoma SN12C in the two orthotopic nude mouse models *(134)*: SOI of tumor tissue and orthotopic injection of cell suspensions in the kidney. The primary tumors resulting from SOI were larger and much more locally invasive than primary tumors resulting from orthotopic transplantation of cell suspensions. SOI generated higher metastatic rates than orthotopic transplantation of cell suspensions. The differences in metastatic rates in the involved organs (lung, liver, and mediastinal lymph nodes) were two- to threefold higher in SOI compared to orthotopic transplantation of cell suspensions ($p < 0.05$). Median survival time in the SOI model was 40 d, which was significantly shorter than that of orthotopic transplantation of cell suspensions (68 d) ($p < 0.001$). Histological observation of the primary tumors from the SOI model demonstrated a much richer vascular network than the orthotopic transplantation of cell suspension model. Lymph node and lung metastases were larger and more cellular in the SOI model compared to the orthotopic transplantation of cell suspension model.

We conclude that the tissue architecture of the implanted tumor tissue in the SOI model plays an important role in the initiation of primary tumor growth, invasion, and distant metastasis. These studies directly demonstrate that the implantation of histologically intact tumor tissue orthotopically allows accurate expression of the clinical features of human renal cancer in nude mice. Experiments showed that distant tumor growths in the SOI models were true time-dependent metastases resulting from clinical-like routes and not due to cells shed in transplantation *(18)*. Thus the SOI models are a significant improvement allowing the full metastatic potential of human tumors to be expressed in a rodent model.

1.4. Development of Patient-Tumor SOI Models

The first model developed with SOI was for colon cancer *(2)*. Indeed, the human patient and human xenograft colon tumors transplanted by SOI resulted in clinically relevant courses such as liver metastasis, lymph node metastasis, and peritoneal carcinomatosis *(2)*. The inital "take" rates for human patient colon tumors transplanted by SOI were > 80%. In a study of colorectal cancer with the University of California, San Diego (UCSD), Department of Surgery, we have successfully transplanted colorectal cancer specimens from 16 patients using SOI. In each case, we have been able to passage the tumor to form large cohorts. The tumors have demonstrated liver metastasis, lymph node metastasis, and other clinically relevant events. Both primary tumors and liver metastasis from patients have been used for SOI (**Table 1**). In a recent study, we have developed an ultrametastatic

Table 1
Human Patient Colon Cancer SOI Models

Case	Site	Stage	Grade
AC 3438	Colon	T3N0M0	Well diff
AC 3445	Right colon	Stage II—T3N0M0	Well diff.
AC 3488	Sigmoid colon	Stage IV—T3N1M1	Poorly diff.
AC 3489	Diffuse met.	—	Poorly diff.
AC 3508	Sigmoid colon	Stage IV—T3N1M1	Mod well diff.
AC 3518	Sigmoid colon	Stage III—T3N1M0	Well diff.
AC 3521	Cecal area	Stage III—T2N1M0	Well diff.
AC 3528	Polyposis coli	Stage IV—T3N2M1 (liver)	Mod diff.
AC 3557	Sigmoid colon	Stage II—T2N0M0	Well diff.
AC 3603	Transverse colon	Stage I—T1N0M0	Well diff.
AC 3609	Rectal	Stage III—T3N1M0	Mod poorly diff.
AC 3612	Ascending colon	Stage II—T3N0M0	Mod diff.
AC 3620	Sigmoid colon	Liver metastasis	Mod diff.
AC 3624	Rectal	Stage II—T3N0M0	Well diff.
AC 3625	Rectal	Stage III—T3N2M0	Mod diff.
AC 3653	Ascending colon	Stage III—T4N2M0	Well diff.

SOI model of human colon cancer with all animals having liver and lymph node metastases by d 10 *(63)*. Banks of patient tumors that are established in the SOI models are being developed for all the major tumor types.

1.5. Establishment and Expansion of SOI Tumor Models

1.5.1. Expanding Quantities of Patient-Like Xenografts Using SOI Models

Patient-derived tumors can be established by SOI with take rates of up to 100% *(2,6,63,67–71)*. It has been shown to be straightforward to expand an SOI tumor population by serial passage to produce large cohorts of 100 or more SOI animals with the tumor phenotype remaining stable. Established tumors can be serially passaged with nearly 100% efficiency *(2,9,63,67–71)*. Such expansion allows the SOI models to serve as an important research and development tool. Making large mouse cohorts with identical tumors available is essential for drug discovery and development and has been achieved *(2,9,63,67–71)*.

The SOI technology is effective with a wide variety of patient cancers. We have constructed SOI models of patient cancers of the colon *(2,9)*, lung *(5,25,27,28)*, head and neck (unpublished data), pancreas *(6)*, stomach *(5)*, ovaries *(16)*, liver *(38)*, and breast *(23)*. Regardless of whether the tumors are passaged subcutaneously or orthotopically, once implanted orthotopically they resemble the donor tissue in detailed morphology, rate and pattern of growth, and metastatic behavior.

The SOI models solve two very major problems in cancer research: provision of animal models that are more representative of clinical cancer for antitumor and anti-metastatic drug discovery and research. The SOI models are also used for producing human primary and metastatic tumor tissue, on demand, with precisely defined characteristics and in large amounts for study of tumor biology, development of diagnostics, and pharmacogenomics studies.

1.6. Validation of the SOI Models

The SOI tumors have demonstrated a close replication of the original tumor. Apparently the analogous mouse host tissue closely replicates the original patient microenvironment that affects tumor progression and chemosensitivity. For example, an orthotopic model of human small cell lung carcinoma demonstrates sensitivity to cisplatin and resistance to mitomycin C, reflecting the clinical situation *(21)*. In contrast, the same tumor xenograft implanted subcutaneously responded to mitomycin and not to cisplatin, thus failing to match clinical behavior for SCLC *(21)*. These data suggest that the orthotopic site is essential to achieve clinically relevant drug response. Other laboratories have observed similar phenomena indicating the effect of the microenvironment on drug sensitivity *(78)*.

To understand further the role of the host organ in tumor progression, we have transplanted into nude mice histologically intact human colon cancer tissue on the serosal layers of the stomach (heterotopic site) and the serosal layers of the colon (orthotopic site) *(32)*. The human colon tumor Co-3, which is well differentiated, and COL-3JCK, which is poorly differentiated, were used for transplantation. After ortbotopic transplantation of the human colon tumors on the nude mouse colon, the growing colon tumors resulted in macroscopically extensive invasive local growth in 4 of 10 mice, serosal spreading in 9 of 10 mice, musclaris propria invasion in 1 of 10 mice, submucosal invasion in 3 of 10 mice, mucosal invasion in 3 of 10 mice, lymphatic duct invasion in 4 of 10 mice, regional lymph node metastasis in 4 of 10 mice, and liver metastasis in 1 of 10 mice. In striking contrast, after heterotopic transplantation of the human colon tumor on the nude mouse stomach, a large growing tumor resulted but with only limited invasive growth and without serosal spreading, lymphatic duct invasion, or regional lymph node metastasis. It has become clear from these studies that the orthotopic site, in particular the serosal and subserosal transplant surface, is critical to the growth, spread, and invasive and metastatic capability of the implanted colon tumor in nude mice. These studies suggest that the original host organ plays a critical role in tumor progression.

Established human colon and stomach tumors were transplanted by SOI to nude mice and tested for response to 5-fluorouracil (5-FU) and Mitomycin-C, the standard treatments for these tumors *(17,19)*. The tumors responded to a dose level that was the mouse equivalent of typical clinical doses. The primary tumors responded as would be expected in the clinic for these agents. The metastases of these tumors were drug insensitive, which replicates the usual clinical situation *(17,19)*. It was demonstrated that antineoplastic agents can exhibit differential activity against metastases vs primary tumors in SOI models for pancreatic *(20)*, colon *(17)*, and stomach cancer *(19)*. Importantly, we have demonstrated that very low passage patient colon tumors transplanted by SOI can respond to 5-FU, the standard drug of treatment for this disease (unpublished data).

A correlative clinical trial was carried out to compare the course of stomach tumors in patients and in SOI models after orthotopic transplantation *(15)*. Of the 20 patient cases whose tumors grew in the nude mice, 6 had clinical peritoneal involvement of their tumor, and of these, 5 resulted in peritoneal metastases in the nude mice. Of the 14 patients without peritoneal involvement whose primary tumors grew locally in the mice, none gave rise to peritoneal involvement in the mice. Of the 20 patient cases, 5 had clinical liver metastases and 15 did not. After SOI of the patients' primary tumors, all 5 primary tumors from the patients with clinical liver metastases gave rise to liver metastases in the nude mice. In contrast, of the 15 primary tumors from patients without liver metastases, only one primary tumor gave rise to liver metastases in the nude mice after SOI. There was a statistical correlation ($p < 0.01$) for both liver metastases and peritoneal involvement between patients and SOI mice. These results indicate that, after surgical orthotopic transplantation of histologically intact gastric cancers from patients to nude mice, the subsequent local and metastatic behavior of the tumor in the mice closely correlated with the course of the tumors in the patients. The histology of both the local and metastatic tumors in the mice closely resembled the original local and metastatic tumors in the patient. These results indicate that the SOI models resemble clinical cancer and correlate with the patient's clinical course and should be useful for drug discovery for both antitumor and antimetastatic agents *(15)*.

1.7. Drug Discovery with SOI Models

The antitumor and antimetastatic efficacy of the following new agents have been demonstrated in SOI models:

1. The metalloproteinase inhibitor Batimastat. Found to be active against an SOI human patient colon tumor model *(29)* including:
   a. inhibition of primary tumor growth
   b. inhibition of metastatic events, and
   c. extension of survival.
2. The metalloproteinase inhibitor CT1746. Found to be active against an SOI human colon tumor xenograft model *(48)* including:
   a. arrest of primary tumor growth
   b. inhibition of metastatic events, and
   c. a large increase in survival.

3. Interferon-γ (IFN-γ). Found to be active against a patient pleural cancer SOI model *(46)* including:
   a. elimination of metastatic events
   b. decrease in cachexia and weight loss, and
   c. extension of survival.
4. Angiogenesis inhibitor TNP-470. Found to be active in patient colon tumor SOI models *(67–71)* including:
   a. inhibition of liver metastasis in colon cancer
   b. minimal or no effect on primary tumor

Feasibility for the drug discovery in the SOI models has been demonstrated with colon, pancreatic, stomach, and lung cancer, the chemotherapy for which has resulted in dose–response, differential sensitivity of primary and metastatic tumors, reproducibility, and correlation to historical clinical activity of the drugs *(17,19–21,23–27,29,67–72)*. SOI models are appropriate for investigating the antitumor and antimetastatic efficacy of new agents and combinations with different mechanisms *(73,80–82,130–133)*.

1.8. Discovery of Basic Aspects of Metastasis and Possible New Therapeutic Targets

It was shown with the SOI colon cancer models that liver colonization is the governing process of colon cancer liver metastasis *(33,35)*. This study further confirmed Paget's seed and soil hypothesis and demonstrated that the liver colonization event is a potential therapeutic target to prevent metastasis.

1.9. Bone Metastasis in SOI Models

1.9.1. Breast Cancer

The mechanisms of breast cancer metastasizing to bone have been extensively studied *(88–90)*, but remain poorly understood. One of the major impediments is the lack of an accurate animal model *(91,118)*. Although human breast cancer cells injected into the mammary fat pad of nude mice can metastasize to the soft tissue organs such as the lung and lymph nodes, spontaneous metastasis of nonselected tumor cell lines to bone has not been reported *(92–96)*. Bone metastasis thus far has been achieved by injecting breast cancer cells into the left ventricle *(97–101)* or directly into the bone of nude mice *(102)*. Although such a model of experimental bone metastasis of human breast cancer provides a tool for testing novel therapeutic agents against bone metastasis, it is not clinically accurate. An orthotopic cell suspension model of a FGF-transformed MCF-7 human breast cancer cell line demonstrated some bone metastasis *(95)*.

We have developed a spontaneous, highly metastatic nude mice model of human breast cancer MDA-MB-435, with SOI. Histologically intact MDA-MB-435 tumor tissues were implanted into the mammary fat pads of female nude mice. The results showed extensive metastasis to numerous soft organs and throughout the skeletal system in every transplanted animal. Orthotopic tumor growth and metastasis occurred throughout the axial skeleton at very high incidence (vertebra, 96%; femur, 88%; tibia, 88%; fibula, 64%; humerus, 88%; sternum, 76%; scapula, 40%; skull, 24%; rib, 44%; pelvis, 24%; and maxillofacial region, 20%) in the SOI animals. Bone metastasis occurred in 25 of 25 transplanted animals. Extensive metastasis also involved numerous visceral organs including lung, lymph node, heart, spleen, diaphragm, adrenal gland, spinal cord, skeletal muscles, parietal pleural membrane, peritoneal cavity, pancreas, liver, and kidney. Histologically, the involved bones had obvious osteolytic changes, mimicking clinical bone metastasis in breast cancer. To our knowledge, this is the first report demonstrating extensive spontaneous bone metastasis of human breast cancer from the orthotopic site in nude mice. This clinically accurate model of human estrogen-receptor-negative, advanced breast cancer should be of significant value for the study and development of effective treatment of bone *(113–117)* and other metastasis of human breast cancer (An, Z. and Hoffman, R. M., unpublished data).

1.9.2. Prostate Cancer

Prostate cancer has become the most prevalent cancer diagnosed and the second cause of cancer death for North American men *(103)*. In spite of improvement in early detection, more refined diagnostic modalities, and a better understanding of the natural history of the disease, metastatic prostate cancer, which almost always involves highly painful bone lesions, remains largely untreatable *(104)*. Therefore, to gain further insight into and develop new therapeutics for human prostate cancer progression and bone metastasis in particular, an accurate in vivo model is essential.

In previous models of the androgen-independent PC-3 human prostate cancer cell line, which originated from a bone metastasis *(105)*, osseous metastasis could be induced in nude mice by injecting tumor cells intravenously with concomitant occlusion of the inferior cava or by intracardiac implantation *(106–108)*.

In orthotopic transplant models of human prostate cancer, Maeda et al. *(79)*, Hillman et al. *(87)*, Stephenson et al. *(109)*, Fu et al. *(12)*, Pettaway et al. *(107)*, Sato et al. *(110)*, Rembrink et al. *(111)*, An et al. *(59)*, and Wang et al. *(66)* have observed prostate cancer metastasis but only in the lymph nodes and the lung. Thalmann et al. reported a spontaneous bone metastasis model of androgen-independent human prostate cancer LNCaP-derived sublines. The animals developed bone metastasis in 10% and 21.5% of intact and castrated hosts, respectively, after orthotopic injection of cell suspensions *(112)*. These results provided some useful information on the biological behavior of prostate cancer.

We have developed new models of human and animal cancer by transfer of the *Aequorea victoria* jellyfish green fluorescent protein (GFP) gene to tumor cells that enabled visualization of fluorescent tumors and metastases at the microscopic level in fresh viable tissue after transplantation *(50,52–54,56,62)*. The methodology for this is described in Chapter 25 by this author. We have now developed a fluorescent spontaneous bone metastatic model of human prostate cancer SOI of GFP-expressing prostate cancer tissue. Human prostate cancer PC-3 cells were transduced with the pLEIN expression retroviral vector containing the enhanced green fluorescent protein (EGFP) and neomycin resistance genes. Stable GFP high-expression PC-3 clones were selected in vitro with G418 which were then combined and injected subcutaneously in nude mice. To utilize GFP expression for metastasis studies, fragments of a single highly fluorescent subcutaneously growing tumor were implanted by SOI in the prostate of a series of nude mice. Subsequent micrometastases and metastases were visualized by GFP fluorescence throughout the skeleton including the skull, rib, pelvis, femur, and tibia. The central nervous system was also involved with tumor, including the brain and spinal cord, as visualized by GFP fluorescence. Systemic organs including the lung, plural membrane, liver, kidney, and adrenal gland also had fluorescent metastases. The metastasis pattern in this model accurately reflects the bone and other metastatic sites of human prostate cancer *(65)*.

1.10. Ultrametastatic SOI Model of Colon Cancer

An ultrahigh metastatic SOI model of human colon cancer was established from a histologically intact liver metastasis fragment derived from a surgical specimen of a patient with metastatic colon cancer *(63)*. The stably ultrametastatic SOI model is termed AC3488UM. One hundred percent of mice transplanted with AC3488UM with SOI to the colon exhibited local growth, regional invasion, and spontaneous metastasis to the liver and lymph nodes. Liver metastases were detected by the tenth day after transplantation in all animals. Half the animals died of metastatic tumor 25 d after transplantation. Histological characteristics of AC3488UM tumor were poorly differentiated adenocarcinoma of colon. Mutant p53 is expressed heterogeneously in the primary tumor and more homogeneously in the liver metastasis, suggesting a possible role of p53 in the liver metastasis. The human origin of AC3488UM was confirmed by positive fluorescence staining for *in situ* hybridization of human DNA. The AC3488 human colon tumor model with its ultrahigh metastatic capability in each transplanted animal, short latency, and a short median survival period is different from any known human colon cancer model and will be an important tool for the study of and development of new therapy for highly metastatic human colon cancer *(63)*.

1.11. Transgenic Mouse Models of Cancer

Detailed methodology for transgenic animal models is given in Chapter 22 by Guy and Cardoso. Examples of transgenic mouse cancer models are outlined in the following subheadings for comparison with SOI models.

1.11.1. Breast Cancer

Stewart et al. *(119)* and Sinn et al. *(120)* developed transgenic mice in which expression of the c-*myc* or v-Ha-*ras* oncogenes or both were targeted to mammary tissue using the MMTV (mouse mammary tumor virus) long terminal repeat promotor. Both lines of mice, MMTV-*myc* *(119,120)* and MMTV-*ras* *(120)*, were found to have mammary tumors after several months of life. In lines with both oncogenes, tumors developed more rapidly than either of the single transgenic lines *(120)*. In one strain, all surviving F1 female progeny that inherited the MTV/*myc* fusion gene developed breast tumors at 5–6 mo of age during their second or third pregnancies *(119)*. The tumors in the double transgenics arose in a stochastic fashion, as solitary adenocarcinomas or as monoclonal B cell lymphomas *(120)*.

Mice expressing the polyomavirus middle T-antigen (MTAg) under the control of the MMTV promoter/enhancer (MMTV-MTAg mice) had synchronous multifocal mammary adenocarcinoma with a short latency period and a high rate of metastasis to lung *(121)*. Not all tumors in MMTV-MTAg mice are uniform or synchronous. All mice with established primary mammary tumors did not have metastatic disease *(123)*.

MMTV-*neu* transgenic mice overexpress *neu* in the mammary epithelium and develop focal, frequently metastatic mammary adenocarcinoma after a relatively long latency period *(122)*.

A transgenic mouse strain was constructed with the mammary tumor virus LTR/c-*myc* fusion gene. The glucocorticoid inducible c-*myc* transgene led to an increased incidence of breast, testicular, and lymphocytic (B cell and T cell), and mast cell tumors *(124)*.

1.11.2. Prostate Cancer

A recombinant probasin (PB)-SV40 Tag (T antigen) transgenic mouse was developed *(125,126)*. These transgenic animals were termed TRAMP (transgenic adenocarcinoma mouse prostate) *(125,126)*. In TRAMP mice, expression of the PB-Tag transgene is restricted to the dorsolateral lobes of the prostate. TRAMP mice have high-grade PIN (prostatic intraepithelial neoplasia) and/or well-differentiated prostate cancer by the age of 10–12 wk *(127)*. TRAMP mice spontaneously develop invasive primary tumors that routinely metastasize to the lymph nodes and lungs and less frequently metastasize to the spinal column, kidneys, and adrenal glands *(126)*. Hind limb paraplegia was observed in a single TRAMP mouse at the age of 22 wk. Histological examination of decalcified sections of the spine at the level of the thoracolumbar vertebrae demonstrated that the spinal canal was filled with metastatic tumor. The tumor appeared to have destroyed the spinal cord through pressure atrophy rather than invasion and destruction of the adjacent vertebral bone, as typically seen with osteolytic metastatic tumors

(126). Lymph node metastasis were found in 31% (5 of 16) of TRAMP mice between 18 and 24 wk of age. Pulmonary metastases were found in 4 of 11 (36%) animals by 24 wk. A metastasis in the kidney has been found in one mouse at 12 wk. Two metastases to the adrenal gland were found *(126)*. At 30–36 wk of age, 100% of TRAMP animals have primary tumors and metastatic disease *(127)*.

1.11.3. Colon Cancer

The *Smad3* gene was inactivated in mice by homologous recombination. Homozygous mutants were viable and spontaneously form colorectal adenocarcinomas *(128)*. Between 4 and 6 mo of age, the *Smad3* mutant mice become moribund with the colorectal adenocarcinomas. The colorectal cancers penetrated through all layers of the intestinal wall and metastasized to lymph nodes *(128)*.

1.11.4. p53 Knockouts

Homozygous *p53*-deficient mice and normal littermates (with wild-type *p53* genes) were monitored for spontaneous neoplasms *(129)*. Wild-type mice (95 animals) by the age of 9 mo did not develop tumor. By 9 mo, only 2 of 96 heterozygous animals developed tumors. One heterozygous mouse developed an embryonal carcinoma of the testis at 5 mo and another developed a malignant lymphoma at the age of 9 mo *(129)*. Of 35 homozygous animals, 26 (74%) developed neoplasms by 6 mo of age. Some tumors appeared before 10 wk of age, and tumor occurrence increased rapidly between 15 and 25 wk of age *(129)*. Multiple primary neoplasms of different origin were observed in 9 of the 26 homozygous mice with tumors. Malignant lymphomas were found in 20 of 26 animals, but sarcomas also occurred with some frequency. There were seven hemangiosarcomas, three undifferentiated sarcomas, and one osteosarcoma. Only one female mouse developed a mammary adenocarcinoma *(129)*.

It can be clearly seen that the transgenic mouse models of breast, prostate, and colon cancer do not reflect human clinical cancer as do the SOI models. For example, the transgenic breast cancer models did not metastasize to the bone, the prostate cancer transgenic model metastasized to the bone in only one reported animal, the colon cancer transgenic model did not metastasize to the liver, and in the *p53* knockout models only one animal had breast cancer. The SOI models thus offer unique and critically important features for antitumor and antimetastatic drug discovery.

2. Methods

2.1. General Construction of Models

2.1.1. Mice

Four-to-six week-old outbred *nu/nu* mice of both sexes are used for the orthotopic transplantation. All the mice are maintained in a pathogen-free environment. Cages, bedding, food, and water are autoclaved and changed regularly. All the mice are maintained in a daily cycle of 12-h periods of light and darkness. Bethaprim Pediatric Suspension (containing sulfamethoxazole and trimethoprim) is added to the drinking water. Mice are periodically sent to the University of Missouri to test for pathogens.

2.1.2. Specimens

Fresh surgical specimens are kept in Earle's minimum essential medium at 4°C and obtained as soon as possible from hospitals. Before transplantation, each specimen is inspected, and all necrotic and suspected necrotic tumor tissue is removed. To take into account tumor heterogeneity, each specimen is equally divided into five parts, separated, and each part is subsequently cut into small pieces of about 1 mm^3 size. Tumor pieces for each transplantation are taken from five parts of each specimen equally. In our experience, a typical colon tumor specimen of 1–2 g provides sufficient material for initial surgical orthotopic implantation of more than 20 mice. Additional SOI models of this same tumor can subsequently be generated by a single passage using SOI. It should be noted that patient tumors are routinely passaged orthotopically to produce large cohorts. One hundred or more mice can be readily transplanted in the first passage, which are more than sufficient for treatment studies.

2.2. Surgical Orthotopic Implantation

2.2.1. Colon Cancer

2.2.1.1. Colonic Transplantation

For transplantation, nude mice are anesthetized, and the abdomen sterilized with iodine and alcohol swabs. A small midline incision is made and the colocecal part of the intestine is exteriorized. Serosa of the site where tumor pieces are to be implanted is removed. Eight pieces of 1 mm^3 size tumor are implanted on the top of the animal intestine. An 8-0 surgical suture is used to penetrate these small tumor pieces and suture them on the wall of the intestine. The intestine is returned to the abdominal cavity, and the abdominal wall is closed with 7-0 surgical sutures. Animals are kept in a sterile environment. Tumors of all stages and grades can be utilized (2).

2.2.1.2. Intrahepatic Transplantation

Nude mice are anesthetized with isoflurance (Forane) inhalation. An incision is made through the left upper abdominal pararectal line and peritoneum. The left lobe of the liver is carefully exposed and the liver is cut about 3 mm with scissors. Two to three pieces of 1–2 mm^3 size are put on the nude mouse liver and attached immediately with double sutures using 8-0 nylon with an atraumatic needle. After confirmation that no bleeding is occurring, the liver is returned to the peritoneal cavity. The abdominal wall and skin are then closed with 6-0 back silk sutures (31).

2.2.2. Breast Cancer

Mice are anesthetized with isoflurane inhalation and put in a supine position. The right second mammary gland is chosen for orthotopic implantation. A small incision is made along the medial side of the nipple. The mammary fat pad is exposed through blunt dissection. A small cut is made on the fat pad and then bluntly expanded to form a small pocket. Four pieces of tumor tissue, previously prepared as described earlier, are inserted into the pocket. An 8-0 nylon suture is used to close the pocket. The skin is closed with a 6-0 silk suture. All procedures are carried out under a ×5 dissecting microscope *(23)*.

2.2.3. Prostate Cancer

Tumor fragments are prepared as for colon and breast tumors. Two tumor fragments (1 mm³) from a subcutaneous tumor are implanted by SOI in the dorsolateral lobe of the prostate in each of five nude mice. After proper exposure of the bladder and prostate following a lower midline abdominal incision, the capsule of the prostate is opened and the two tumor fragments are inserted into the capsule. The capsule is then closed with an 8-0 surgical suture. The incision in the abdominal wall is closed with a 6-0 surgical suture in one layer *(12,66)*. The animals are kept under isoflurane anesthesia during surgery *(65)*.

2.2.4. Lung Cancer

The mice are anesthetized by isoflurane inhalation. The animals are put in a position of right lateral decubitus, with four limbs restrained. A 0.8-cm transverse incision of skin is made in the left chest wall. Chest muscles are separated by sharp dissection and costal and intercostal muscles are exposed. A 0.4–0.5 cm intercostal incision between the third and fourth rib on the chest wall is made and the chest wall is opened. The left lung is taken up by a forceps and tumor fragments are sewn promptly into the upper lung by one suture. The lung is then returned into the chest cavity. The incision in the chest wall is closed by a 6-0 surgical suture. The closed condition of the chest wall is examined immediately and, if a leak exists, it is closed by additional sutures. After closing the chest wall, an intrathoracic puncture is made by using a 3-mL syringe and 25G 1/2 needle to withdraw the remaining air in the chest cavity. After the withdrawal of air, a completely inflated lung can be seen through the thin chest wall of the mouse. Then the skin and chest muscle are closed with a 6-0 surgical suture in one layer *(62)*.

2.2.5. Kidney Cancer

Mice are anesthetized by isoflurane and positioned laterally. A small incision is made along the left flank of the mice. The kidney is exposed with a small retractor. A small cut is made on the renal subcapsule. One piece of tumor tissue is inserted into the capsule. The cut is covered with surrounding soft tissue using an 8-0 nylon suture. The abdomen is closed with a 6-0 silk suture. All procedures are carried out under a ×5-dissection microscope *(134)*.

2.2.6. Liver Cancer

A left upper abdominal pararectal incision is made under anesthesia; the left lobe of the liver is exposed and a part of the liver surface mechanically injured with scissors. Tumor pieces are sutured within the liver tissue. The liver is returned to the peritoneal cavity and the abdominal wall closed *(38)*.

2.2.7. Ovarian Cancer

The mice are anesthetized with nembutal, and a right lateral dorsal incision is made. The retroperitoneum is then opened, and part of the right ovary is well exposed. One tissue block is implanted on the ovarian capsule with a 7-0 surgical suture. The retroperitoneum and skin are then closed with a 7-0 surgical suture *(64)*.

2.2.8. Pancreatic Cancer

Mice are anesthetized and an incision is then made through the left upper abdominal pararectal line and peritoneum. The pancreas is carefully exposed and a tumor piece is transplanted on the middle of the pancreas with a 6-0 suture. The pancreas is then returned into the peritoneal cavity, and the abdominal wall and the skin closed with 6-0 sutures *(20)*.

Alternatively, a retractor is used to expose the pancreas. Approximately 10 pieces of tumor tissue are then transplanted on the tail of the pancreas near the spleen using 8-0 sutures. The abdominal wall and skin are closed with 6-0 sutures *(39)*.

2.2.9. Bladder Cancer

The nude mice are anesthetized by isofluorene inhalation and the lower abdomen is sterilized with iodine and ethanol swabs. A small midline incision is made and the urinary bladder is exposed. The surgical adhesive 2-cyanoacrylic acid ester is applied on one side of the 2-mm^3 tumor xenograft tissue. Five pieces of tumor are glued on the serosa of the urinary bladder. The abdominal incision is closed with 7-0 silk surgical sutures in one layer *(57)*.

2.2.10. Stomach Cancer

Mice are anesthetized with 2.5% Avertin. An incision is made through the left upper abdominal pararectal line and peritoneum. The stomach wall is carefully exposed and a part of the serosal membrane, about 3 mm in diameter, in the middle of the greater curvature of the glandular stomach is mechanically injured using scissors. A tumor piece of 150 mg is then fixed on each injured site of the serosal surface with a 4-0 suture. The stomach is then returned to the peritoneal cavity, and the abdominal wall and skin are closed with 4-0 sutures *(14)*.

In another approach, tumor tissue is cut into smaller pieces of about 1 mm³. Eight to 15 pieces of 1 mm³ tumor fragments are implanted on the top of the nude mouse stomach where the serosa has been injured. An 8-0 surgical suture is used to penetrate these small tumor pieces and suture them on the wall of the stomach. Then the abdominal wall and the skin are closed as described above *(14)*.

2.3. Cohorts of Tranplanted Animals for Treatment

Cohorts of more than 100 SOI models have been constructed from many SOI models. The "take rate" for tranplantation after the first passage is generally 100%. Cohorts of 100 mice per case can be easily constructed *(63)*.

2.4. Determination and Characterization of Xenografted Tumors

Complete autopsy with histological examination *(86)* is performed on all mice at time of death. All of the major organs are examined carefully and routinely sampled, along with any tissues showing gross abnormalities.

2.5. Histological Evaluation

An important part of the process of the SOI model validation involves comparison of tumor histology between the original clinical tumor specimen and the SOI models xenograft formed from this specimen. Tissue is first placed into a histology specimen cassette and fixed in 10% neutral buffered formalin (NBF), dehydrated with 95% ethanol, 100% ethanol, and Clearite-3 and rinsed with paraffin. After opening the cassette, the specimen is placed in a metal mold and embedded in paraffin. After cooling and trimming, the specimen block is sectioned at a thickness of 5 µm with sections placed in a water bath. The resulting ribbon is carefully separated so that two to five sections of the specimen can be placed on each glass slide. The slides are then heated in an oven at 60°C for at least 4 h, and deparaffinized by rinsing with Clearite-3, 100% ethanol, 95% ethanol, and then water. Slides are evaluated microscopically following hematoxylin/eosin staining. For each implanted tumor, pairs of slides are prepared, consisting of a section of the original tumor, a section of the transplanted primary growing tumor, and any resulting metastases. Clinical/xenograft pairs, and pairs of slides derived entirely from the parent tumor (clinical/clinical), are evaluated.

To assess the extent of metastasis, relevant tissues are sectioned for histological evaluation of tumor formation. Sufficient slides are made to completely section each organ, to ensure that any metastatic loci will be observed. We have a large experience with determination of measurement of primary tumor, lymph node metastases, peritoneal seeding, and distant metastases in the liver, lung, and elsewhere resulting from colon cancer in the SOI models *(2,9,17,18, 22,29,73)*; please *see* **Subheading 2.6.**

2.6. Evaluation of Growth and Metastasis of Orthotopically Transplanted Tumors

The mice are autopsied and analyzed histologically for the presence of local growth and metastases upon sacrifice after they become moribund. Mice are killed if they develop signs of distress. For example, in the colon tumor models the distress symptoms include a decline in performance status and weight loss due to cachexia or drug treatment. At autopsy, the colon and all peritoneal organs, lymph nodes, liver, and lungs are resected and processed for routine histological examination for tumors. Metastases are considered to have occurred if at least one microscopic metastatic lesion is found in any of the animals. The growth of locally growing tumors is determined by caliper measurement of the locally growing tumor which is possible, since the body wall is so thin, and by weighing the tumors that are removed at autopsy. Caliper measurements of the primary tumor can also allow determination of tumor regression. The primary tumor is weighed at autopsy.

References

1. Fidler, I. J. (1990) Critical factors in the biology of human cancer metastases: twenty eighth G.H.A. Clowes Memorial Lecture. *Cancer Res.* **50,** 6130–6138.
2. Fu, X., Besterman, J. M., Monosov, A., and Hoffman, R. M. (1991) Models of human metastatic colon cancer in nude mice orthotopically constructed by using histologically-intact patient specimens. *Proc. Natl. Acad. Sci. USA* **88,** 9345–9349.
3. Fu, X., Theodorescu, D., Kerbel, R. S., and Hoffman, R. M. (1991) Extensive multi-organ metastasis following orthotopic onplantation of histologically-intact human bladder carcinoma tissue in nude mice. *Int. J. Cancer* **49,** 938–939.
4. Fu, X. and Hoffman, R. M. (1992) Human RT-4 bladder carcinoma is highly metastatic in nude mice and comparable to ras-H-transformed RT-4 when orthotopically onplanted as histologically-intact tissue. *Int. J. Cancer* **51,** 989–991.
5. Wang, X., Fu, X., and Hoffman, R. M. (1992) A new patient-like metastatic model of human lung cancer constructed orthotopically with intact tissue via thoracotomy in immunodeficient mice. *Int. J. Cancer* **51,** 992–995.
6. Fu, X., Guadagni, F., and Hoffman, R. M. (1992) A metastatic nude-mouse model of human pancreatic cancer constructed orthotopically from histologically-intact patient specimens. *Proc. Natl. Acad. Sci. USA* **89,** 5645–5649.
7. Hoffman, R.M. (1992) Patient-like models of human cancer in mice. *Curr. Perspect. Mol. Cell. Oncol.* **1(B),** 311–326.
8. Kuo, T-H, Kubota, T., Watanabe, M., Furukawa, T., Kase, S., Tanino, H., et al. (1992) Orthotopic reconstitution of human small-cell lung carcinoma after intravenous transplantation in SCID mice. *Anticancer Res.* **12,** 1407–1410.

9. Fu, X., Herrera, H., Kubota, T. and Hoffman, R. M. (1992) Extensive liver metastasis from human colon cancer in nude and scid mice after orthotopic onplantation of histologically-intact human colon carcinoma tissue. *Anticancer Res.* **12,** 1395–1398.

10. Wang, X., Fu, X., and Hoffman, R. M. (1992) A patient-like metastasizing model of human lung adenocarcinoma constructed via thoracotomy in nude mice. *Anticancer Res.* **12,** 1399–1402.

11. Wang, X., Fu, X., Kubota, T., and Hoffman, R. M. (1992) A new patient-like metastatic model of human small-cell lung cancer constructed orthotopically with intact tissue via thoracotomy in nude mice. *Anticancer Res.* **12,** 1403–1406.

12. Fu, X., Herrera, H., and Hoffman, R. M. (1992) Orthotopic growth and metastasis of human prostate carcinoma in nude mice after transplantation of histologically intact tissue. *Int. J. Cancer* **52,** 987–990.

13. Hoffman, R. M. (1992) Histoculture and the immunodeficient mouse come to the cancer clinic: rational approaches to individualizing cancer therapy and new drug evaluation (Review). *Int. J. Oncol.* **1,** 467–474.

14. Furukawa T., Fu X., Kubota T., Watanabe M., Kitajima M., and Hoffman R. M. (1993) Nude mouse metastatic models of human stomach cancer constructed using orthotopic implantation of histologically-intact tissue. *Cancer Res.* **53,** 1204–1208.

15. Furukawa, T., Kubota, T., Watanabe, M., Kitajima, M., and Hoffman, R. M. (1993) Orthotopic transplantation of histologically-intact clinical specimens of stomach cancer to nude mice: correlation of metastatic sites in mouse and individual patient donors. *Int. J. Cancer* **53,** 608–612.

16. Fu, X. and Hoffman, R. M. (1993) Human ovarian carcinoma metastatic models constructed in nude mice by orthotopic transplantation of histologically-intact patient specimens. *Anticancer Res.* **13,** 283–286.

17. Furukawa, T., Kubota, T., Watanabe, M., Kuo, P. H., Kase, S., Saikawa, Y., et al. (1993) Immunochemotherapy prevents human colon cancer metastasis after orthotopic onplantation of histologically-intact tumor tissue in nude mice. *Anticancer Res.* **13,** 287–291.

18. Kuo, T.-H., Kubota, T., Watanabe, M., Fujita, S., Furukawa, T., Teramoto, T., et al. (1993) Early resection of primary orthotopically-growing human colon tumor in nude mouse prevents liver metastasis: further evidence for patient-like hematogenous metastatic route. *Anticancer Res.* **13,** 293–298.

19. Furukawa, T., Kubota, T., Watanabe, M., Kitajima, M., and Hoffman, R. M. (1993) Differential chemosensitivity of local and metastatic human stomach cancer after orthotopic transplantation of histologically-intact tumor tissue in nude mice. *Int. J. Cancer* **54,** 397–401.

20. Furukawa, T., Kubota, T., Watanabe, M., Kitajima, M., and Hoffman, R. M. (1993) A novel "patient-like" treatment model of human pancreatic cancer constructed using orthotopic transplantation of histologically-intact human tumor-tissue in nude mice. *Cancer Res.* **53,** 3070–3072.

21. Kuo, T.-H., Kubota, T., Watanabe, M., Furukawa, T., Kase, S., Tanino, H., et al. (1993) Site-specific chemosensitivity of human small-cell lung carcinoma growing orthotopically compared to subcutaneously in SCID mice: The importance of orthotopic models to obtain relevant drug evaluation data. *Anticancer Res.* **13,** 627–630.

22. Furukawa, T., Kubota, T., Watanabe, M., Kuo, T.-H, Nishibori, H., Kase, S., et al. (1993) A metastatic model of human colon cancer constructed using cecal implantation of cancer tissue in nude mice. *Jpn. J. Surg.* **23,** 420–423.

23. Fu, X., Le, P., and Hoffman, R. M. (1993) A metastatic orthotopic transplant nude-mouse model of human patient breast cancer. *Anticancer Res.* **13,** 901–904.

24. Astoul, P. Colt, H. G., Wang, X., and Hoffman, R. M. (1993) Metastatic human pleural ovarian cancer model constructed by orthotopic implantation of fresh histologically-intact patient carcinoma in nude and SCID-mice. *Anticancer Res.* **13,** 1999–2002.

25. Astoul, P., Wang, X., and Hoffman, R. M. (1993) "Patient-Like" nude and SCID mouse models of human lung and pleural cancer (Review). *Int. J. Oncol.* **3,** 713–718.

26. Kubota, T., Inoue, S., Furukawa, T., Ishibiki, K., Kitajima, M., Kawamura, E., and Hoffman, R. M. (1993) Similarity of serum–tumor pharmacokinetics of antitumor agents in man and nude mice. *Anticancer Res.* **13,** 1481–1484.

27. Astoul, P., Colt, H. G., Wang, X., and Hoffman, R. M. (1994) A "patient-like" nude mouse model of parietal pleural human lung adenocarcinoma. *Anticancer Res.* **14,** 85–92.

28. Astoul, P., Colt, H. G., Wang, X., Boutin, C., and Hoffman, R. M. (1994) " A "patient-like" nude mouse metastatic model of advanced human pleural cancer." *J. Cell Biochem.* **56,** 9–15.

29. Wang, X., Fu, X., Brown, P. D., Crimmin, M. J., and Hoffman, R. M. (1994) Matrix metalloproteinase inhibitor BB-95 (Batimastat) inhibits human colon tumor growth and spread in a patient-like orthotopic model in nude mice. *Cancer Res* **54,** 4726–4728.

30. Hoffman, R. M. (1994) Orthotopic is orthodox: why are orthotopic-transplant metastatic models different from all other models? *J. Cell Biochem.* **56,** 1–3.

31. Togo, S., Shimada, H., Kubota, T., Moossa, A. R., and Hoffman, R.M. (1995) Seed to soil is a return trip in metastasis. *Anticancer Res.* **15,** 791–794.

32. Togo, S., Shimada, H., Kubota, T., Moossa, A. R., and Hoffman, R. M. (1995) Host organ specifically determines cancer progression. *Cancer Res.* **55,** 681–684.

33. Kuo, T.-H., Kubota, T., Watanbe, M., Furukawa, T., Teramoto, T., Ishibiki, K., et al. (1995) Liver colonization competence governs colon cancer metastasis. *Proc. Natl. Acad. Sci. USA* **92,** 12085–12089.

34. Togo, S., Wang, X., Shimada, H., Moossa, A. R., and Hoffman, R. M. (1995) Cancer seed and soil can be highly selective: human-patient colon tumor lung metastasis grows in nude mouse lung but not colon or subcutis. *Anticancer Res.* **15,** 795–798.

35. Dutton, G. (1996) AntiCancer Inc. scientists identify a key governing step in the metastasis of cancer. *Genet. Engng. News* **16,** January 15.

36. Holzman, D. (1996) Of mice and metastasis: a new for-profit model emerges. *J. Natl. Cancer Inst.* **88,** 396–397.

37. Leff, D. N. (1996) MetaMouse models colon cancer metastasis with clinical potential. *BioWorld Today* **7,** January 8.

38. Sun, F. X., Tang, Z. Y., Liu, K. D., Ye, S. L., Xue, Q., Gao, D. M., and Ma, Z. C. (1996) Establishment of a metastatic model of human hepatocellular carcinoma in nude mice via orthotopic implantation of histologically intact tissues. *Int. J. Cancer* **66**, 239–243.

39. An, Z., Wang, X., Kubota, T., Moossa, A. R., and Hoffman, R. M. (1996) A clinical nude mouse metastatic model for highly malignant human pancreatic cancer. *Anticancer Res.* **16**, 627–632.

40. Riordan, T. (1996) A technique is said to ease attachment of tumors to mice, making them "little cancer patients." *New York Times*, "Patents" Column, March 4.

41. Murray, G., Duncan, M., O'Neil, P., Melvin, W., and Fothergill, J. (1996) Matrix metalloproteinase-1 is associated with poor prognosis in colorectal cancer. *Nat. Med.* **2**, 461–462.

42. Hoffman, R. M. (1996) Fertile seed and rich soil: development of patient-like models of human cancer by surgical orthotopic implantation of intact tissue, in *Update Series: Comprehensive Textbook of Oncology,* Vol. 3, Schimpff, S. C. et al. (eds.), Williams & Wilkins, Baltimore, pp. 1–10.

43. Sun, F-X., Tang, Z-Y., Liu, K-D., Xue, Q., Gao, D-M., Yu, Y-Q., et al. (1996) Metastatic models of human liver cancer in nude mice orthotopically constructed by using histologically intact patient specimens. *J. Cancer Res. Clin. Oncol.* **122**, 397–402.

44. Astoul, P., Wang, X., Colt, H. G., Boutin, C., and Hoffman, R. M. (1996) A patient-like human malignant pleural mesothelioma nude-mouse model. *Oncol. Rep.* **3**, 483–487.

45. Colt, H. G., Astoul, P., Wang, X., Yi, E. S., Boutin, C., and Hoffman, R. M. (1996) Clinical course of human epithelial-type malignant pleural mesothelioma replicated in an orthotopic-transplant nude mouse model. *Anticancer Res.* **16**, 633–640.

46. An, Z., Wang, X., Astoul, P., Danays, T., and Hoffman, R. M. (1996) Interferon gamma is higly effective against orthotopically-implanted human pleural adenocarcinoma in nude mice. *Anticancer Res.* **16**, 2545–2551.

47. Olbina, G., Cieslak, D., Ruzdijic, S., Esler, C., An, Z., Wang, X., et al. (1996) Reversible inhibition of IL-8 receptor B mRNA expression and proliferation in non-small cell lung cancer by antisense oligonucleotides. *Anticancer Res.* **16**, 3525–3530.

48. An, Z., Wang, X., Willmott, N., Chander, S. K., Tickle, S., Docherty, A. J. P., et al. (1997) Conversion of highly malignant colon cancer from an aggressive to a controlled disease by oral administration of a metalloproteinase inhibitor. *Clin. Exp. Metast.* **15**, 184–195.

49. Hoffman, R. M. (1997) Fertile seed and rich soil: the development of clinically relevant models of human cancer by surgical orthotopic implantation of intact tissue, in *Anticancer Drug Development Guide: Preclinical Screening, Clinical Trials, and Approval,* Teicher, B. (ed.), Humana Press, Totowa, NJ, pp. 127–144.

50. Chishima, T., Miyagi, Y., Wang, X., Yamaoka, H., Shimada, H., Moossa, A. R., and Hoffman, R. M. (1997) Cancer invasion and micrometastasis visualized in live tissue by green fluorescent protein expression. *Cancer Res.* **57**, 2042–2047.

51. Inada, T., Ichikawa, A., Kubota, T., Ogata, Y., Moossa, A. R., and Hoffman, R. M. (1997) 5-FU-induced apoptosis correlates with efficacy against human gastric and colon cancer xenografts in nude mice. *Anticancer Res.* **17**, 1965–1972.

52. Chishima, T., Miyagi, Y., Wang, X., Baranov, E., Tan, Y., Shimada, H., et al. (1997) Metastatic patterns of lung cancer visualized live and in process by green fluorescent protein expression. *Clin. Exp. Metast.* **15,** 547–552.

53. Chishima, T., Miyagi, Y., Wang, X., Tan, Y., Shimada, H., Moossa, A. R., and Hoffman, R. M. (1997) Visualization of the metastatic process by green fluorescent protein expression. *Anticancer Res.* **17,** 2377–2384.

54. Chishima, T., Yang, M., Miyagi, Y., Li, L., Tan, Y., Baranov, E., et al. (1997) Governing step of metastasis visualized *in vitro. Proc. Natl. Acad. Sci. USA* **94,** 11,573–11576.

55. Tomikaw,a, M., Kubota, T., Matsuzaki, S.W., Takahasi, S., Kitajima, M., Moossa, A. R., and Hoffman, R. M. (1997) Mitomycin C and cisplatin increase survival in a human pancreatic cancer metastatic model. *Anticancer Res.* **17,** 3623–3626.

56. Chishima, T., Miyagi, Y., Li, L., Tan, Y., Baranov, E., Yang, M., et al. (1997) The use of histoculture and green fluorescent protein to visualize tumor cell host interaction. *In Vitro Cell. Dev. Biol.* **33,** 745–747.

57. Chang, S-G., Kim, J.I., Jung, J-C., Rho, Y-S., Lee, K-T., An, Z., Wang, X., and Hoffman, R. M. (1997) Antimetastatic activity of the new platinum analog {Pt(cis-dach)(DPPE)·2NO$_3$} in a metastatic model of human bladder cancer. *Anticancer Res.* **17,** 3239–3242.

58. Dev, S. B., Nanda, G. S., An, Z., Wang, X., Hoffman, R. M., and Hofmann, G. A. (1997) Effective electroporation therapy of human pancreatic tumors implanted in nude mice. *Drug Delivery* **4,** 293–299.

59. An, Z., Wang, X., Geller, J., Moossa, A. R., and Hoffman, R. M. (1998) Surgical orthotopic implantation allows high lung and lymph node metastatic expression of human prostate carcinoma cell line PC-3 in nude mice. *Prostate* **34,** 169–174.

60. Nanda, G. S., Sun, F. X., Hofmann, G. A., Hoffman, R. M., and Dev, S. B. (1998) Electroporation therapy of human larynx tumors HEp-2 implanted in nude mice. *Anticancer Res.* **18,** 999–1004.

61. Nanda, G. S., Sun, F. X., Hofmann, G. A., Hoffman, R. M., and Dev, S. B. (1998) Electroporation enhances therapeutic efficacy of anticancer drugs: Treatment of human pancreatic tumor in animal model. *Anticancer Res.* **18,** 1361–1366.

62. Yang, M., Hasegawa, S., Jiang, P., Wang, X., Tan, Y., Chishima, T., et al. (1998) Widespread skeletal metastatic potential of human lung cancer revealed by green fluorescent protein expression. *Cancer Res.* **58,** 4217–4221.

63. Sun, F-X., Sasson, A. R., Jiang, R., An, Z., Gamagami, R., Li, L., Moossa, A. R., and Hoffman, R. H. (1999) An ultra-metastatic model of human colon cancer in nude mice. *Clin. Exp. Metast.* **17,** 41–48.

64. Kiguchi, K., Kubota, T., Aoki, D., Udagawa, Y., Tamanouchi, S., Saga, M., et al. (1998) A patient-like orthotopic implantation nude mouse model of highly metastatic human ovarian cancer. *Clin. Exp. Metast.* **16,** 751–756.

65. Yang, M., Jiang, P., Sun, F. X., Hasegawa, S., Baranov, E., Chishima, T., et al. (1999) A fluorescent orthotopic bone metastasis model of human prostate cancer. *Cancer Res.* **59,** 781–786.

66. Wang, X., An, Z., Geller, J., and Hoffman, R. M. (1999) A high malignancy orthotopic nude mouse model of the human prostate cancer LNCaP. *Prostate* **39**, 182–186.

67. Kanai, T., Konno, H., Tanaka, T., Matsumoto, K., Baba, M., Nakamura, S., and Baba, S.(1997) Effect of angiogenesis inhibitor TNP-470 on the progression of human gastric cancer xenotransplanted into nude mice. *Int. J. Cancer* **71**, 838–841.

68. Konno, H., Tanaka, T., Kanai, T., Maruyama, K., Nakamura, S., and Baba,S. (1996) Efficacy of an angiogenesis inhibitor, TNP-470, in xenotransplanted colorectal cancer with high metastatic potential. *Cancer* **77**, 1736–1740.

69. Konno, H., Tanaka, T., Matsuda, I., Kanai, T., Maruo, Y., Nishino, N., et al. (1995) Comparison of the inhibitory effect of the angiogenesis inhibitor, TNP-470 and mitomycin C on the growth and liver metastasis of human colon cancer. *Int. J. Cancer* **61**, 268–271.

70. Konno, H., Tanaka, T., Baba, M., Matsumoto, K., Kamiya, K., Nakamura, S., et al. (1997) Antitumor effect of angiogenesis inhibitors on colon cancer. *Biotherapy* **11**, 993–996.

71. Tanaka, T., Konno, H., Matsuda, I., Nakamura, S., and Baba, S. (1995) Prevention of hepatic metastasis of human colon cancer by angiogenesis inhibitor TNP-470. *Cancer Res.* **55**, 836–839.

72. Konno, H., Arai, T., Tanaka, T., Baba, M., Matsumoto, K., Kanai, T., et al. (1998) Antitumor effect of neutralizing antibody to vascular endothelial growth factor on liver metastasis of endocrine neoplasm. *Jpn. J. Cancer Res.* **89**, 933–939.

73. Tanizawa, A., Fujimori, A., Fujimori, Y., and Pommier, Y. (1994) Comparison of topoisomerase I inhibition, DNA damage, and cytotoxicity of camptothecin derivatives presently in clinical trials. *J. Natl. Cancer Inst.* **86**, 836–842.

74. Schabel, F. M. (1975) animal models as predictive systems. In *Cancer Chemotherapy Fundamental Concepts and Recent Advances*, Year Book Publishers, pp. 323–355.

75. Goldin, A., Serpick, A. A., and Mantel, N. (1966) A commentary. Experimental procedures and clinical predictability value. *Cancer Chemother. Rep.* **50**, 173–218.

76. Rygaard, J. and Poulsen, C. O. (1969) Heterotransplantation of a human malignant tumor to nude mice. *Acta Pathol. Microbiol. Scand.* **77**, 758–760.

77. Ovejera, A. (1987) The use of human tumor xenografts in large-scale drug screening, in *Rodent Tumor Model in Experimental Cancer Therapy*, Pergamon Press, Kalimann, R. F. (ed.), New York, pp. 218–220.

78. Wilmanns, C., Fan, D., O'Brian, C. A., Bucana, C. D., and Fidler, I. J. (1992) Orthotopic and ectopic organ environments differentially influence the sensitivity of murine colon carcinoma cells to doxorubicin and 5-fluorouracil. *Int. J. Cancer* **52**, 98–104.

79. Maeda, H., Segawa, T., Kamoto, T., Yoshida, H., Kakizuka, A., Ogawa, O., and Kakehi, Y. (2000) Rapid detection of candidate metastatic foci in the orthotopic inoculation model of androgen-sensitive prostate cancer cells introduced with green fluorescent protein. *Prostate* **45**, 335–340.

80. Rougier, R., Bugat, R., Douillard, J. Y., Culine, S., Suc, E., Brunet, P., et al. (1997) Phase II study of irinotecan in the treatment of advanced colorectal cancer in chemotherapy-naïve patients and patients pretreated with fluorouracil-based chemotherapy. *J. Clin. Oncol.*, **15**, 251–260.

81. Bissery, M-C., Vrignaud, P., and Lavelle, F. (1995) Preclinical Profile of Docetaxel (Taxotere): efficacy as a single agent and in combination. *Semin. Oncol.* **22, Suppl. 13,** 3–16.

82. Bissery, M-C., Guénard, D., Guéritte-Voegelein, F., and Lavelle, F. (1991) Experimental antitumor activity of Taxotere (RP 56976, NSC 628503), a taxol analogue. *Cancer Res.* **51,** 4845–4852.

83. Nomura, T., Sakurai, Y., and Inaba, M. (1996) *The Nude Mouse and Anticancer Drug Evaluation.* Central Institute for Experimental Animals, Kawasaki, Japan, 1996.

84. Plowman, J., Camalier, R., Alley, M., Sausville, E., and Schepartz, E. (1999) US-NCI testing procedures, in *Relevance of Tumor Models for Anticancer Drug Development,* Karger, pp. 121–136.

85. Double, J. A. (1999) A pharmacological approach for the selection of potential anticancer agents, in *Relevance of Tumor Models for Anticancer Drug Development,* Karger, pp. 137–144.

86. Culling, C. F. A., ed. (1963) *Handbook of Histopathological Techniques,* 2nd edit., Butterworth, London.

87. Hillman, G. G., Maughn, R. L., Grignon, D. J., Yudelev, M., Rubio, J., Tekyi-Mensah, S., et al. (2001) Neutron or photon irradiation for prostate tumors: enhancement of cytokine therapy in a metastatic tumor model. *Clin. Cancer Res.* **7,** 136–144.

88. Cifuentes, N. and Pickren, J. W. (1979) Metastasis from carcinoma of mammary gland: an autopsy study. *J. Surg. Oncol.* **11,** 193–205.

89. Mundy, G. R. and Yoneda, T. (1995) Facilitation and suppression of bone metastasis. *Clin. Orthop.* **312,** 34–44.

90. Guise, T. A. (1997) Parathyroid hormone-related protein and bone metastases. *Cancer* **80,** 1572–1580.

91. Olden, K. (1990) Human tumor bone metastasis model in athymic nude rats. *J. Natl. Cancer Inst.* **82,** 340–341.

92. Price, J. E., Polyzos, A., Zhang, R. D., and Daniels, L. M. (1990) Tumorigenicity and metastasis of human breast carcinoma cell lines in nude mice. *Cancer Res.* **50,** 717–721.

93. Jia, T., Liu, Y. E., Liu, J., and Shi, Y. E. (1999) Stimulation of breast cancer invasion and metastasis by synuclein-γ. *Cancer Res.* **59,** 742–747.

94. Bagheri-Yarmand, R., Kourbali, Y., Rath, A. M., Vassy, R., Martin, A., Jozefonvicz, J., et al. (1999) Carboxymethyl benzylamide dextran blocks angiogenesis of MDA-MB435 breast carcinoma xenograft in fat pad and its lung metastases in nude mice. *Cancer Res.* **59,** 507–510.

95. Kurebayashi, J., Nukatsuka, M., Fujioka, A., Saito, H., Takeda, S., Unemi, N., et al. (1997) Postsurgical oral administration of uracil and tegafur inhibits progression of micrometastasis of human breast cancer cells in nude mice. *Clin. Cancer Res.* **3,** 653–659.

96. Thompson, E. W., Brunner, N., Torri, J., Johnson, M. D., Boulay, V., Wright, A., et al. (1993) The invasive and metastatic properties of hormone-independent but hormone-responsive variants of MCF-7 human breast cancer cells. *Clin. Exp. Metast.* **11,** 15–26.

97. Arguello, F. B., Baggs, R. B., and Frantz, C. N. (1988) A murine model of experimental metastasis to bone and bone marrow. *Cancer Res.* **48,** 6876–6881.

98. Sasaki, A., Boyce, B. F., Story, B., Wright, K. R., Chapman, M., Boyce, R., et al. (1995) Bisphosphonate risedronate reduces metastatic human breast cancer burden in bone in nude mice. *Cancer Res.* **55,** 3551–3557.

99. Morinaga, Y., Fujita, N., Ohishi, K., and Tsuruo, T. (1997) Stimulation of interleukin-11 production from osteoblast-like cells by transforming growth factor-β and tumor cell factors. *Int. J. Cancer* **71,** 422–428.

100. Guise, T. A., Yin, J. J., Taylor, S. D., Kumagai, Y., Dallas, M., Boyce, B. F., et al. (1996) Evidence for a causal role of parathyroid hormone-related protein in the pathogenesis of human breast cancer-mediated osteolysis. *J. Clin. Invest.* **98,** 1544–1549.

101. Sung, V., Gilles, C., Murray, A., Clarke, R., Aaron, A. D., Azumi, N., and Thompson, E. W. (1998) The LCC15-MB human breast cancer cell line expresses osteopontin and exhibits an invasive and metastatic phenotype. *Exp. Cell Res.* **241,** 273–284.

102. Wang, C. Y. and Chang, Y. W. (1997) A model for osseous metastasis of human breast cancer established by intrafemur injection of the MDA-MB-435 cells in nude mice. *Anticancer Res.* **17,** 2471–2474.

103. Boring, C. C., Squines, T. S., Tong, T., and Montgomery, S. (1994) *Cancer Statistics CA.* **44,** 7–26.

104. Lepor, H., Ross, A., and Walsh, P. C. (1982) The influence of hormonal therapy on survival of men with advanced prostatic cancer. *J. Urol.* **128,** 335–340.

105. Kaighn, M. E., Narayan, K. S., Ohnuki, Y., Lechner, J. F., and Jones, L. W. (1979) Establishment and characterization of a human prostate carcinoma cell line (PC-3). *Invest. Urol.* **17,** 16–23.

106. Shevrin, D. H., Kukreja, S. C., Ghosh, L., and Lad, T. E. (1988) Development of skeletal metastasis by human prostate cancer in athymic nude mice. *Clin. Exp. Metast.* **6,** 401–409.

107. Pettaway, C. A., Pathak, S., Greene, G., Ramirez, E., Wilson, M. R., Killion, J. J., and Fidler, I. J. (1996) Selection of highly metastatic variants of different human prostatic carcinomas using orthotopic implantation in nude mice. *Clin. Cancer Res.* **2,** 1627–1636.

108. Wu, T. T., Sike, R. A., Cui, Q., Thalmann, G. N., Kao, C., Murphy, C. F., et al. (1998) Establishing human prostate cancer cell xenografts in bone: induction of osteoblastic reaction by prostate-specific antigen-producing tumors in athymic and SCID/bg mice using LNCaP and lineage-derived metastatic sublines. *Int. J. Cancer* **77,** 887–894.

109. Stephenson, R. A., Dinney, C. P. N., Gohji, K., Ordonez, N. G., Kilion, J. J., and Fidler, I. J. (1992) Metastasis model for human prostate cancer using orthotopic implantation in nude mice. *J. Natl. Cancer Inst.* **84,** 951–957.

110. Sato, N., Gleave, M. E., Bruchovshy, N., Rennie, P. S., Beraldi, E., and Sullivan, L. D. (1997) A metastatic and androgen-sensitive human prostate cancer model using intraprostatic inoculation of LNCaP cells in SCID mice. *Cancer Res.* **57,** 1584–1589.

111. Rembrink, K., Romijn, J. C., van der Kwast, T. H., Rubben, H., and Schroder, F. H. (1997) Orthotopic implantation of human prostate cancer cell lines: a clinically-relevant animal model for metastatic prostate cancer. *Prostate* **31,** 168–174.

112. Thalmann, G. N., Anezinis, P. E., Chang, S. M., Zhau, H. E., Kim, E. E., Hopwood, V. L., et al. (1994) Androgen-independent cancer progression and bone metastasis in the LNCaP model of human prostate cancer. *Cancer Res.* **54,** 2577–2581.

113. Fleisch, H. (1991) Biphosphonates. Pharmacology and use in the treatment of tumour-induced hypercalcaemic and metastatic bone disease. *Drugs* **42,** 919–944.

114. Diel, I. J., Solomayer, E-F., Costa, S. D., Gollan, C., Goerner, R., Wallwiener, D., et al. (1998) Reduction in new metastasis in breast cancer with adjuvant clodronate treatment. *N. Engl. J. Med.* **339,** 357–363.

115. Hortobagyi, G. N., Theriault, R. L., Porter, L., et al. (1996) Efficacy of pamidronate in reducing skeletal complications in patients with breast cancer and lytic bone metastases. *N. Engl. J. Med.* **335,** 1785–1791.

116. O'Rourke, N., McCloskey, E., Houghton, F., Huss, H., and Kanis, J. A. (1995) Double-blind, placebo-controlled, dose-response trial of oral clodronate in patients with bone metastases. *J. Clin. Oncol.* **13,** 929–934.

117. Kanis, J. A., Powles, T., Paterson, A. H. G., McCloskey, E. V., and Ashley S. (1996) Clodronate decreases the frequency of skeletal metastases in women with breast cancer. *Bone* **19,** 663–667.

118. Sasaki, A., Yoneda, T., Terakado, N., Alcalde, R. E., Suzuki, A., and Matsumura, T. (1998) Experimental bone metastasis model of the oral maxillofacial region. *Anticancer Res.* **18,** 1579–1584.

119. Stewart, T. A., Pattengale, P. K., and Leder, P. (1984) Spontaneous mammary adenocarcinomas in transgenic mice that carry and express MTV/myc fusion genes. *Cell* **38,** 627–637.

120. Sinn, E., Muller, W., Pattengale, P., Tepler, I., Wallace, R., and Leder, P. (1987) Coexpression of MMTV/v-Ha-ras and MMTV/c-myc genes in transgenic mice: synergistic action of oncogenes *in vivo. Cell* **49,** 465–475.

121. Guy, C. T., Cardiff, R. D., and Muller, W. J. (1992) Induction of mammary tumors by expression of polyomavirus middle T oncogene: a transgenic mouse model for metastatic disease. *Mol. Cell. Biol.* **12,** 954–961.

122. Guy, C. T., Webster, M. A., Schaller, M., Parsons, T. J., Cardiff, R. D., and Muller, W. J. (1992) Expression of the *neu* protooncogene in the mammary epithelium of transgenic mice induces metastatic disease. *Proc. Natl. Acad. Sci. USA* **89,** 10578–10582.

123. Ritland, S. R., Rowse, G. J., Chang, Y., and Gendler, S. J. (1997) Loss of heterozygosity analysis in primary mammary tumors and lung metastases of MMTV-MTAg and MMTV-*neu* transgenic mice. *Cancer Res.* **57,** 3520–3525.

124. Leder, A., Pattengale, P. K., Kuo, A., Stewart, T. A., and Leder, P. (1986) Consequences of widespread deregulation of the c-*myc* gene in transgenic mice: multiple neoplasma and normal development. *Cell* **45,** 485–495.

125. Greenberg, N. M., DeMayo, F., Finegold, M. J., Medina, D., Tilley, W. D., Aspinall, J. O., et al. (1995) Prostate cancer in a transgenic mouse. *Proc. Natl. Acad., Sci. USA* **92,** 3439–3443.

126. Gingrich, J. R., Barrios, R. J., Morton, R. A., Boyce, B. F., DeMayo, F. J., Finegold, M. J., et al. (1996) Metastatic prostate cancer in a transgenic mouse. *Cancer Res.* **56,** 4096–4102.

127. Gingrich, J. R., Barrios, R. J., Kattan, M. W., Nahm, H. S., Finegold, M. J., and Greenberg, N. M. (1997) Androgen-independent Prostate Cancer Progression in the TRAMP Model. *Cancer Res.* **57,** 4687–4691.

128. Zhu, Y., Richardson, J. A., Parada, L. F., and Graff, J. M. (1998) Smad3 Mutant Mice Develop Metastatic Colorectal Cancer. *Cell* **94,** 703–714.

129. Donehower, L. A., Harvey, M., Slagle, B. L., McArthur, M. J., Montgomery Jr., C. A., Butel, J. S., and Bradley, A. (1992) Mice deficient for p53 are developmentally normal but susceptible to spontaneous tumors. *Nature* **356,** 215–221.

130. Advanced Colorectal Cancer Meta-Analysis Project (1992) Modulation of fluorouracil by leucovorin in patients with advanced colorectal cancer: evidence in terms of response rate. *J. Clin. Oncol.* **10,** 896–903.

131. De Gramont, A., Bosset, J. F., Milan, C., et al. (1995) A prospectively randomized trial comparing 5-FU bolus with low dose folinic acid (FUFOL1d) and 5-FU bolus plus continuous infusion with high dose folinic acid (LV5FU2) for advanced colorectal cancer. *Proc. Am. Soc. Clin. Oncol.* **14,** 455 (Abstr).

132. Creemer, G. J., Lund, B., and Verweij, J. (1994) Topoisomerase I inhibitors: topotecan and irinotecan. *Cancer Treat. Rev.* **20,** 73–96.

133. Hsiang, Y. H., Lihou, M. G., and Liu, L. F. (1989) Arrest of replication forks by drug-stabilized topoisomerase I-DNA cleavable complexes as a mechanism of cell killing by camptothecin. *Cancer Res.* **49,** 5077–5082.

134. An, Z., Jiang, P., Wang, X., Moossa, A. R., and Hoffman, R. M. (1999) Development of a high metastatic orthotopic model of human renal cell carcinoma in nude mice: benefits of fragment implantation compared to cell-suspension injection. *Clin. Exp. Metast.* **17,** 265–270.

24

Dissection of Tumor and Host Cells from Metastasized Organs for Testing Gene Expression Directly Ex Vivo

Marian Rocha, Volker Schirrmacher, and Victor Umansky

1. Introduction

The interaction between tumor and host cells determines to a large extent the outcome, namely tumor growth and progression toward metastases or tumor arrest, dormancy, or rejection. Most of the studies published so far on interactions of tumor cells and host cells were made in vitro and dealt with aspects such as cell adhesion, proliferation, invasiveness, cytotoxicity, or cytokine production. As the microenvironment in tissue culture differs in many respects from that in vivo, new approaches for in vivo studies of tumor–host cell interactions is of utmost importance in cancer research. To elucidate the metastatic phenotype, approaches have been made to relate, for instance, cell surface molecules expressed on the tumor cell lines from tissue culture to their propensity to generate metastases in vivo (1). Several authors have reported that certain steps of the metastatic cascade are rate limiting (2–6). To produce metastases, tumor cells must complete each of the sequential steps in the pathogenesis of cancer metastasis. Each discrete step appears to depend on the interaction between tumor cells and multiple host factors (i.e., the microenvironment of the tumor) and to be regulated by transient or permanent changes in multiple genes at the level of DNA, RNA, or protein. On this background, the need for comprehensive in vivo/ex vivo studies on tumor–host interactions and their kinetics in relevant model systems becomes obvious.

The processes of tumor metastasis formation and its interplay with the host immune system have been extensively studied in the murine lymphoma system Eb/ESb/ESb-MP (7–12). The spontaneous highly metastatic lymphoma variant ESbL is able to kill syngeneic animals in <12 d following subcutaneous inoculation of 10^5 cells, whereby the metastatic spread involves several visceral organs, in

From: *Methods in Molecular Medicine, vol. 58:*
Metastasis Research Protocols, Vol. 2: Cell Behavior In Vitro and In Vivo
Edited by: S. A. Brooks and U. Schumacher © Humana Press Inc., Totowa, NJ

particular the liver. Detection of micrometastasis and also of low levels of dormant tumor cells *(7)* has only recently been possible in this model by genetically tagging the tumor line with the bacterial *lacZ* gene. This foreign gene codes for β-D-galactosidase (β-gal), whose enzymatic activity can be detected by staining with the chromogenic substrate X-gal. This results in a precipitate of an indigo blue reaction product that allows single ESb *lacZ*-tumor cells to be detected in infiltrated organs such as lymph nodes, bone marrow, or liver *(13)*. Despite expression of the *lacZ* gene, the tumor cells were still tumorigenic, highly metastastatic, unchanged in phenotype, and therefore comparable to the parental ESb cells. After spontaneous metastasis, whole organ staining revealed metastatic foci at the surface of the liver, while X-gal staining of frozen tissue sections revealed micrometastasis in the form of clusters and diffusely disseminated single cells *(14)*. It was also possible to re-isolate cells from metastases and to quantify all cells per organ that have metastasized into it via hypotonic shock mediated loading with the β-gal substrate fluorescein β-D-galactopyranoside (FDG), which allowed live tumor ESb-lacZ cell staining and quantitative FACScan analysis. In a typical experiment, 28 d after intradermal tumor cell inoculation, 55% of the reisolated cells from the liver and 13% of the cells from the spleen were tumor cells *(15)*.

Using the liver derived ESbL lymphoma line transduced with the *lacZ* gene we have established a new method allowing the ex vivo isolation of tumor and host cells (tumor microenvironment) at any time point during the metastatic process and without any further in vitro culture. It allows the direct ex vivo analysis of gene expression at the RNA or protein level in tumor and host cells at any time point during tumor growth and metastasis *(16,17)*. This methodology involves the use of different techniques such as (1) liver perfusion and metrizamide gradient centrifugation for isolation of tumor and sinusoidal cells from the liver, (2) differential adhesion to isolate endothelial and Kupffer cells, (3) FDG staining and sorting to separate tumor cells and lymphocytes, (4) antibody staining and FACS analysis to evaluate the purity of the obtained populations and to study the changes at the protein level in both tumor and host cells during tumor growth and metastasis (FACS analysis is also covered by Chapter 1 by Davies), (5) RNA preparation and dot or Northern blot analysis to study the same parameters at the RNA level (RNA preparation techniques are also described in Chapter 16 by Jones et al. and Chapter 17 by Tennant et al., and Northern blot analysis is also described in detail by Tennant et al., all in the companion volume).

2. Materials

1. Mice: DBA/2 mice were obtained from Iffa Credo (Lyon, France) and used at 6–12 wk of age.
2. *lacZ* transduced ESbL cells (clone L-CI.5s) were cultured as described in **ref. *13***. Cells were washed in phosphate-buffered saline (PBS) and adjusted to the

appropriate concentration. For standard intradermal injection, 2×10^5 cells were injected into the animal's cutis at the shaved flank of anesthesized (Rompun [0.1%]—Ketanest [0.25%]–PBS diluted 1:1:3 [by vol]) animals.

3. α-Modified Eagle medium (α-MEM) containing 15 mM HEPES (2.4 g/L); FACS buffer consisting of PBS and 5% fetal calf serum (FCS).

4. Enzymes: Pronase E (Boehringer Mannheim), collagenase A (from *Clostridium hystolyticum*, Boehringer Mannheim) and DNase (Sigma Chemical, US) were dissolved at 0.5%, 1%, and 0.005% w/v, respectively, in α-MEM–HEPES and stored at –20°C.

5. 2-(3-Acetoamyde-5-methylacetamido-2,4,6-triodobenzamido)2-deoxyglucose (Metrizamide) (Sigma) was prepared as a continuous gradient at stock concentration of 30% w/v in α-MEM–HEPES, pH 7.4, and was stored at 4°C.

6. Type I Collagen (Biochrom) was dissolved at 1% w/v in a α-MEM–HEPES and stored at 4°C.

7. Fluorescein-di-β-galactopyranoside (FDG) (Molecular Probes, Inc., Eugene, OR) was dissolved in distilled water (1:20).

8. Glutaraldehyde (Merck, Germany) was prepared at 2.5% w/v in PBS.

9. For RNA isolation: RNA-Clean (Angewandte Gentechnologie System, Heidelberg, Germany), 20X saline sodium citrate (SSC), 1% v/v sodium dodecyl sulfate (SDS). Oligolabeling kit (Pharmacia, Sweden) and O-MAT films (Kodak, Germany) were used.

3. Methods

A draft of the overall procedure is represented schematically in **Fig. 1**.

3.1. Simultaneous Ex Vivo Isolation of Tumor Cells and Host Cells from the Target Organs of Metastases by Liver Perfusion and Metrizamide Gradient Centrifugation

1. Kill the mice, open the abdominal cavity, and insert a thread under the portal vein (*see* **Note 1**).

2. Insert the needle (25-gauge) into the portal vein, close tightly the thread around the needle, and perfuse at 37°C with 10 mL of α-MEM containing 15 mM HEPES at a flow rate of 3 mL/min.

3. Digest the tissue by perfusion with 10 mL of α-MEM–HEPES containing 0.05% pronase E at 1 mL/min and then with 15 mL of the same medium containing 0.03% pronase E, 0.04% collagenase A (final concentrations) (*see* **Note 2**).

4. After perfusion, mince the livers and stir in 13 mL of α-MEM–HEPES containing 0.04% w/v pronase E, 0.04% w/v collagenase, and 0.0004% w/v DNase (final concentrations) at 37°C for 10 min.

5. Filter the cell suspension through a nylon gauze and centrifuge at 300g for 10 min.

6. To remove cell debris and erythrocytes, centrifuge the cell pellet at 1400g for 15 min in α-MEM–HEPES containing 17.5% w/v metrizamide.

7. Take the interphase with a Pasteur pipet and wash with α-MEM–HEPES at 300g for 10 min. Count cells (*see* **Note 3**).

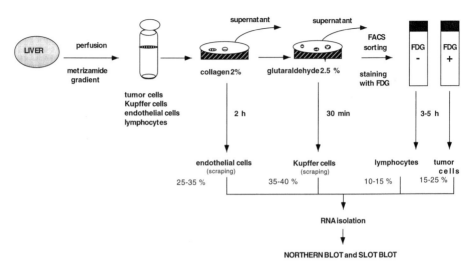

Fig. 1. Method of ex vivo separation of cells from a metastasized liver for preparation of total RNA. Sinusoidal cells and tumor cells from metastatic livers were fractionated into subpopulations by differential adhesion (endothelial and Kupffer cells) and by FACS (lymphocytes and tumor cells). Numbers indicate the range in percentage of cells obtained in each purification step relative to the total number of live recovered cells.

3.2. Isolation of Liver Endothelial Cells by Differential Adhesion

1. Culture the liver sinusoidal and tumor cells obtained in **Subheading 3.1.** on type 1 collagen-coated plastic Petri dishes in α-MEM supplemented with 10% FCS at 37°C in an incubator under 5% CO_2.
2. Two hours later, collect supernatants for further experiment and scrape off adherent cells (endothelial cells) with a rubber spatula.
3. Count cells, pellet them, snap freeze in liquid nitrogen, and keep at –70°C for RNA studies.

3.3. Isolation of Kupffer Cells from Metastatic Livers by Differential Adhesion

1. Treat plastic culture dishes with 2.5% glutaraldehyde in PBS for 2 h at 4°C.
2. Wash 10× with cold PBS.
3. Culture collected supernatants from **Subheading 3.2.** on the treated Petri dishes for 30 min at 37°C in 5% CO_2 (*see* **Note 4**).
4. Remove adherent cells (Kupffer cells) with a rubber spatula, count cells, pellet them, snap freeze in liquid nitrogen, and keep at –70°C for RNA studies.

3.4. Isolation of Lymphocytes and Tumor Cells from Metastatic Livers by FDG Staining and Sorting

1. Prepare Eppendorf tubes containing 5×10^6 cells of isolated tumor and lymphoid cells that remained after the two adhesion steps described previously.

2. Wash them in FACS buffer and incubate in 100 μL of FACS buffer at 37°C for 10 min.
3. Add 100 μL of prewarmed FDG in distilled water to the cell suspension and incubate for 4 min at 37°C (hypotonic shock).
4. Add 1.8 mL of cold 5% FCS–PBS, keep cells for 10 min on ice, and stain them with 1.5 μ*M* propidium iodide (final concentration).
5. Define a window for sorting in the FDG-positive cells (tumor cells) excluding dead cells and debris with propidium iodide.
6. Use a flow rate of 3000–5000 cells/s.
7. Collect sorted cells in sterile tubes containing RPMI with 20% FCS.
8. After centrifugation of the total collected fractions, tumor cells, and lymphocytes, pellet cells, snap freeze them in liquid nitrogren, and keep at –70°C until use for RNA extraction.

3.5. Flow Cytometry Analysis of Tumor and Host Cells
3.5.1. Antibody Staining of Tumor and Sinusoidal Cells

1. Wash 1×10^6 cells in FACS buffer and incubate at 4°C for 10 min with first antibodies. The following rat anti-mouse monoclonal antibodies are used as culture supernatants to evaluate the purity of the isolated populations: anti-CD4 (clone GK 1.5); E-selectin (clone 21KC10), specific for endothelial cells; antimacrophage antibody (F4/80).
2. After washing, incubate cells with the second antibody (F(ab')$_2$ goat anti-rat, mouse Ig absorbed, R-Phycoerythrin conjugated (Gibco BRL).
3. Incubate the control cells with FACS buffer instead of the antibody, prior to staining with the second antibody.

3.5.2. FDG Staining and FACS Analysis of Tumor and Host Cells

1. After antibody staining, wash sinusoidal and tumor cells with FACS buffer and incubate in 100 μL FACS buffer at 37°C for 10 min.
2. For quantification of liver metastases at the single cell level perform the loading and staining with FDG as described in **Subheading 3.4.**
3. Measure 30,000 cells/sample simultaneously for FSC and integrated side scatter (SSC) as well as green (FL1) and red (FL2 and FL3) fluorescences (expressed as logarithm of the integrated fluorescence light) only on propidium iodide negative (viable) cells of the red (FL3) fluorescence, excluding aggregates whose FSCs are out of range.
4. Analyze ex vivo expression of cell surface molecules by histograms of red fluorescence (FL2) distribution plotted as number of cells (*y*-axis) vs fluorescence intensitiy (*x*-axis) for the different tumor and sinusoidal cell populations.

3.6. RNA Extraction, Hybridization, and Densitometric Quantitation

1. Homogenize cell pellets (corresponding to 1×10^6 cells) with 0.2 mL of RNA-Clean™.
2. Perform RNA extraction by10% v/v chloroform.

3. Precipitate the extracted RNA with isopropanol, wash pellet in ethanol, dry under vacuum, and resuspend in diethyl pyrocarbonate (DEPC)–water. Measure quantity of RNA by absorbance at 260 nm.

4. Denature total isolated RNA and spot onto a nitrocellulose filter using a dot blot apparatus and fix by UV cross-linking with vacuum.

5. Prehybridize membranes for 2 h at 42°C in solution containing 1% formamide, 20X SSC, and 1% SDS.

6. Hybridize in the same solution for 24–48 h at 42°C with the cDNA probes. cDNA inserts are labeled with ^{32}P to a specific activity of about 2×10^8 cpm/mg of DNA by an oligolabeling kit.

7. After hybridization, wash filters 3× for 30 min with SSC and SDS at 68°C.

8. Expose membranes to O-MAT films at –70°C.

9. Quantify expression of the mRNA by densitometry of autoradiograms using the Adobe Photoshop program and the SCAN analysis program from Macintosh. The RNA expression is calculated from the ratio between the average areas of the specific mRNA transcripts and of the β-actin mRNA transcripts.

3.7. Conclusions

Constant interactions of tumor cells with host cells eventually determine the fate of the affected host. Interactions between tumor and host cells contribute to angiogenesis, invasion, migration, tumor cell survival in the bloodstream, adhesion and again invasion, migration, and growth at a distant site. The molecular basis of these different steps of the metastatic cascade has been studied extensively, although mostly in vitro. The conditions provided in the tissue culture experiments do not resemble the in vivo microenvironment where complex relationships between tumor and host cells, secreted molecules, and extracellular matrix structures have key functions. Therefore, the approach for direct ex vivo analyses of tumor and host cells is an important methodological improvement for cancer research in the future.

The described techniques provide new possibilities of using ex vivo isolated cells for different purposes. Ex vivo isolated metastasized tumor cells can be used for cell–cell interaction studies with different host cells, for investigation of cytokine and growth factor production, and as target cells in cytotoxicity assays with ex vivo isolated lymphocytes or macrophages. Endothelial and Kupffer cells provide a tool for adhesion studies with tumor cells and for evaluation of the production of different cytokines and cytotoxic molecules, for instance, nitric oxide (NO) *(18,19)*. Lymphocytes can be used for the investigation of cytokine production, in proliferation assays, and as a tool for different therapeutical interventions.

This experimental approach opens up a broad possibility for studies of basic mechanisms of tumor development, for example: (1) evaluation of vaccination effects in target organs; (2) determination of the right window in time for cancer therapy; (3) investigation of the effects of transferred immune cells, tissues, or organs on the host, for instance, in the processes of graft vs leukemia and graft vs host disease *(20,21)*.

4. Notes

1. It is crucial to perfuse the livers immediately after killing the animals; otherwise blood coagulation will hamper the washing of the liver.
2. The enzymatic solutions have to be maintained in the right temperature for their optimal activity. Therefore, tubes containing the enzymes should stay in a water bath at approx 42°C during the whole perfusion process.
3. The number of sinusoidal cells obtained per mouse liver is $5-8 \times 10^6$ depending on the factors such as age and weight of the mice and size of the liver. In the case of metastatic livers, the total amount of sinusoidal and tumor cells is $20-25 \times 10^6$ per mouse. Viability is higher than 93% in both cases. Numbers of every single isolated population are shown in **Fig. 1**.
4. Incubation of Kupffer cells in glutaraldehyde-pretreated Petri dishes for more than 30 min can decrease the viability and the number of the obtained cells.

Acknowlegment

This work was partially supported by Dr. Mildred Scheel Stiftung (V.U.).

References

1. Nicolson, G. L. (1987) Tumor cell instability, diversification and progression to the metastatic phenotype: from oncogene and oncofetal expression. *Cancer Res.* **47**, 1473–1487.
2. Hart, I. R., Goode, N. T., and Wilson, R. E. (1989) Molecular aspects of the metastatic cascade. *Biochim. Biophys. Acta* **989**, 65–84.
3. Fidler, I. J. (1990) Critical factors in the biology of human cancer metastasis: twenty-eight GHA Clowes Memorial Award Lecture. *Cancer Res.* **50**, 6130–6138.
4. Fidler, I. J. and Radinsky, R. (1990) Genetic control of cancer metastasis. *J. Natl. Cancer Inst.* **82**, 166–168.
5. Kerbel, R. S. (1990) Growth dominance of the metastatic cancer cell: cellular and molecular aspects. *Adv. Cancer Res.* **55**, 87–132.
6. Fodstad, O. (1993) Metastatic ability of cancer cells: pheno- and genotypic characteristics and role of the micro-environment, in *New Frontiers in Cancer Causation* (Iversen, O. H., ed.), Taylor & Francis, Washington, DC, pp. 349–358.
7. Schirrmacher, V., Landolof, A., Zawatzky, R., and Kirchner, H. (1981) Immunogenetic studies of mice to highly metastatic DBA/2 tumor cell variants: II. Influence of minor histocompatibility antigens on tumor resistance, gamma interferon induction and cytotoxic response. *Invas. Metast.* **1**, 175–194.
8. Schirrmacher, V., Fogel, M., Russmann, E., Bosslet, K., Altevogt, P., and Beck, L. (1982) Antigenic variation in cancer metastasis: immune escape versus immune control. *Cancer Metast. Rev.* **1**, 241–274.

9. Schirrmacher, V., Schild, H. J., Gückel, B., and von Hoegen, P. (1992) Tumour-specific CTL response requiring interactions of four different cell types and recognition of MHC class I and class II restricted tumour antigens. *Immunol. Cell Biol.* **71**, 311–326.

10. Altevogt, P., Leidig, S., and Heckl-Oestreicher, B. (1984) Resistance of metastatic tumor variants to tumor-specific cytotoxic T-lymphocytes not due to defects in expression of restricting major histocompatibility complex molecules in murine cells. *Cancer Res.* **44**, 5305–5313.

11. Schirrmacher, V. and Barz, D. (1986) Characterization of cellular and extracellular plasma membrane vesicles from a low metastatic lymphoma (Eb) and its high metastatic variant (ESb): inhibitory capacity in cell–cell interaction systems. *Biochim. Biophys. Acta* **860**, 236–242.

12. von Hoegen, P., Altevogt, P., and Schirrmacher, V. (1987) New antigens presented on tumor cells can cause immune rejection without influencing the frequency of tumor-specific cytolytic T cells. *Cell. Immunol.* **109**, 333–348.

13. Krüger, A., Schirrmacher, V., and von Hoegen P. (1994a) Scattered micrometastais visualized at the single cell level: detection and re-isolation of lacZ labeled metastasized lymphoma cells. *Int. J. Cancer* **58**, 275–284.

14. Krüger, A., Umansky, V., Rocha, M., Hacker, H.J., Schirrmacher, V., and von Hoegen P. (1994b) Pattern and load of spontaneous liver metastasis dependent on host immune status studied with a lacZ transduced lymphoma. *Blood* **84**, 3166–3174.

15. Schirrmacher, V., Beckhove, P., Krüger, A., Rocha, M., Umansky, V., Fichtner, K. P., et al. (1995) Effective immune rejection of advanced metastasized cancer. *Int. J. Oncol.* **6**, 505–521.

16. Rocha, M., Hexel, K., Bucur, M., Schirrmacher, V., and Umansky, V. (1996a) Dissection of tumor and host cells from a metastasized organ for testing gene expression directly ex vivo. *Br. J. Cancer* **74**, 1216–1222.

17. Rocha M., Krüger, A., Umansky, V., von Hoegen, P., Naor, D., and Schirrmacher, V. (1996b) Dynamic expression changes in vivo of adhesion and costimulatory molecules determine load and pattern of lymphoma liver metastasis. *Clin. Cancer Res.* **2**, 811–820.

18. Rocha, M., Krüger, A., Van Rooijen, N., Schirrmacher, V., and Umansky, V. (1995) Liver endothelial cells particiapte in T-cell dependent host resistance to lymphoma metastasis by production of nitric oxide in vivo. *Int. J. Cancer* **63**, 405–411.

19. Umansky, V., Rocha, M., Krüger, A., von Hoegen, P., and Schirrmacher, V. (1995) In situ activated macrophages are involved in host resistance to lymphoma metastasis by production of nitric oxide. *Int. J. Oncol.* **7**, 33–40.

20. Schirrmacher, V., von Hoegen, P., Griesbach, A., Schild, H. J., and Zangemeister-Wittke, U. (1991) Specific eradication of micrometastases by transfer of tumour-immune T cells from major-histocompatibility-complex congenic mice. *Cancer Immunol. Immunother.* **32**, 373–381.

21. Müerköster, S., Wachowsky, O., Zerban, H., Schirrmacher, V., Umansky, V., and Rocha, M. (1998) Graft versus leukemia (GvL) reactivity requires cluster formation between superantigen-reactive donor T cells and host macrophages. *Clin. Cancer Res.* **4**, 3095–3106.

25

Green Fluorescent Protein for Metastasis Research

Robert M. Hoffman

1. Introduction

Our understanding of the cancer metastatic process has advanced considerably in recent years. However, the early stages of tumor progression and micrometastasis formation have been difficult to analyze. These studies are hampered by the inability to identify small numbers of tumor cells against a background of many host cells. The visualization of tumor cell emboli, and micrometastases and their progression over real time during the course of the disease has been difficult to study in current models of metastasis. Previous studies used transfection of tumor cells with the *Escherichia coli* β-galactosidase *(lacZ)* gene to detect micrometastases *(1,2,33)*. However, detection of *lacZ* requires extensive histological preparation, and therefore it is impossible to detect and visualize tumor cells in viable fresh tissue or the live animal at the microscopic level. The visualization of tumor invasion and micrometastasis formation in viable fresh tissue or the live animal is necessary for a critical understanding of tumor progression and its control.

To enhance the resolution of the visualization of micrometastases in fresh tissue, we have utilized the green fluorescent protein (GFP) gene, cloned from the bioluminescent jellyfish *Aequorea victoria (3)*. GFP has demonstrated its potential for use as a marker for gene expression in a variety of cell types *(4,5)*. The GFP cDNA encodes a 283 amino acid polypeptide with molecular mass of 27 kDa *(6,7)*. The monomeric GFP requires no other *Aequorea* proteins, substrates, or cofactors to fluoresce *(8)*. Recently, GFP gene gain-of-function mutants have been generated by various techniques *(9–12)*. For example, in the GFP-S65T clone the serine-65 codon is substituted with a threonine codon which results in a single excitation peak at 490 nm *(9)*. Moreover, to develop

From: *Methods in Molecular Medicine, vol. 58:*
Metastasis Research Protocols, Vol. 2: Cell Behavior In Vitro and In Vivo
Edited by: S. A. Brooks and U. Schumacher © Humana Press Inc., Totowa, NJ

higher expression in human and other mammalian cells, a humanized hGFP-S65T clone was isolated *(13)*. The much brighter fluorescence in the mutant clones allows for easy detection of GFP expression in transfected cells *(31)*. We have isolated numerous GFP transfectants of human and animal cancer cells that are stable in vitro and in vivo (**Table 1**) *(17–20,41,42)*. The transfectants are highly fluorescent in vivo in tumors formed from the cells. Using these fluorescent transfectants, orthotopic-transplant animal models *(14–16,41,42)* were utilized for visualizing the metastatic processes in fresh tissue down to the single cell level that heretofore was not possible.

1.1. Isolation of Stable High-Level Expression GFP Transfectants of CHO-K1 and ANIP Human Lung Cancer Cells

The dicistronic DHFR-GFP expression-vector transfected CHO-K1 and ANIP cells were able to grow in levels of methotrexate (MTX) up to 1.5 μM and 50 nM, respectively. The selected MTX-resistant CHO and ANIP cells had a striking increase in GFP fluorescence compared to the transiently transfected cells. A subclone was isolated CHO-K1 GFP 38 (Clone-38), which proved to be stable in 1.5 μM MTX, possibly due to stable chromosomal integration of the amplified GFP and DHFR genes *(17)*. There was no difference in the cell proliferation rates of parental cells and selected transfectants determined by comparing their doubling times. A subclone of ANIP that expressed the strongest GFP was isolated and termed ANIP 973-GFP-Clone-26 (Clone 26) *(17,18)*.

1.2. Stable High-Level Expression of GFP in Tumors in Nude Mice

Three weeks after subcutaneous injection of CHO Clone-38 cells, the mice were killed. All mice had a subcutaneous tumor which ranged in diameter from 13.0 mm to 18.5 mm (mean 15.2 mm ± 2.9). The tumor tissue was strongly fluorescent, thereby demonstrating stable high-level GFP expression in vivo during tumor growth. Extraction experiments showed that GFP expression of the transfectants did not decrease in vivo even in the absence of MTX, as determined by fluorescence spectrometry *(17)*. A >1 cm tumor was formed 5 wk after inoculation of 1×10^7 ANIP Clone-26 cells on the flank of a nude mouse. This tumor fluoresced very brightly in vivo *(17,18)*.

1.3. GFP-Expressing Macro- and Micrometastases in Nude Mice

Six nude mice were implanted with 1-mm^3 cubes of CHO-K1 Clone-38 tumor into the ovary by surgical orthotopic implantation (SOI) *(32)* and were killed at 4 wk *(17)*. All mice had tumors in the ovaries. The tumor had also seeded throughout the peritoneal cavity, including the colon, cecum, small intestine, spleen, and peritoneal wall. The primary tumor and peritoneal metastases were strongly fluorescent. Numerous micrometastases were

Table 1
GFP Transformed Cell Lines Stable In Vitro and In Vivo

Tumor type	Cell lines	Tumor type	Cell lines
Prostate	PC-3	Renal, human	SN-12
	DU-145		A-498
	LNCaP		
		Brain	324
Melanoma, mouse	B16F10		U-251
	B10FO		U-87
Melanoma, human	LOXMIVI	Ovarian, human	CHO-K1
	SK-MEL-5		OVCAR-8
	UACC257		OVCAR-3
			OVCAR-5
Lung cancer, human	H460		RGMI no. 186
	HOP62		
	EKVX	Larynx	HEP2 (CCL23)
	A549/ATCC		
	ANIP973	CNS	SNB-19
	Lewis Lung		SNB-75
Colon cancer, human	HCT116	Tongue	SCC-25
	COLO205		
	SW620	Pancreas	BX PC-3
	LS180		MIA-PACA 2
	HCT15		PACA-1
	KM12		
	HT29	Bladder	HTB-9
	WIDR		RT-4
Breast cancer, human	MDA-MB-435	Fibrosarcoma	HT Z1080
	MDA-MB-231		
	MDA-MB-468	Stomach	NUGC-4
	MCF-7		

detected by fluorescence on the lungs of all mice. Multiple micrometastasis were also detected by fluorescence on the liver, kidney, contralateral ovary, adrenal gland, para-aortic lymph node, and pleural membrane at the single-cell level. Single-cell micrometastases could not be detected by standard histological techniques. Even these multiple-cell small colonies were difficult to detect by hematoxylin and eosin staining, but they could be detected and visualized clearly by GFP fluorescence. Some colonies were observed under confocal microscopy. As these colonies developed, the density of tumor cells was markedly decreased in the center of the colonies.

1.4. Patterns of Lung Tumor Metastases after Surgical Orthotopic Implantation (SOI) Visualized by GFP Expression

Primary tumor grew in the operated left lung in all mice after SOI of GFP-transfected ANIP Clone-26. GFP expression allowed visualization of the advancing margin of the tumor spreading in the ipsilateral lung. All animals explored had evidence of chest wall invasion and local and regional spread. Metastatic contralateral tumors involved the mediastinum, contralateral pleural cavity, and the contralateral visceral pleura. While the ipsilateral tumor had a continuous and advancing margin, the contralateral tumor seems to have been formed by multiple seeding events. These observations were made possible by GFP fluorescence of the fresh tumor tissue *(18,19)*. When non-GFP-transfected ANIP was compared with GFP-transformed ANIP for metastatic capability similar results were seen *(18)*. Contralateral hilar lymph nodes were also involved as well as cervical lymph nodes shown by GFP expression. A cervical lymph node metastasis was brightly visualized by GFP in fresh tissue *(18,19)*.

1.5. GFP-Expressing Metastases after Intravenous Injection in Nude Mice

CHO-K1 Clone-38 GFP transfectants injected via the tail vein were detected and visualized in the peritoneal wall vessels to the single-cell level *(17)*. These cells formed emboli in the capillaries of the lung, liver, kidney, spleen, ovary, adrenal gland, thyroid gland, and brain.

A total of 1.0×10^7 ANIP Clone-26 cells were injected in the nude mice in the tail vein. The mice were killed at 4 and 8 wk. In both groups, numerous micrometastatic colonies were detected in the whole lung tissue by GFP expression *(19)*. Even 8 wk after injection, most of the colonies were not obviously further developed compared with mice killed at 4 wk *(19)*. Numerous small colonies that ranged in number down to fewer than 10 cells were detected at the lung surface in both groups. Brain metastases were visualized in both groups *(19)*. After 8 wk, a mouse had systemic metastases in the brain, the submandibular gland, the whole lung, the pancreas, the bilateral adrenal glands, the peritoneum, and the pulmonary hilum lymph nodes *(19)*. All metastases were detected by GFP expression in fresh tissue. We visualized actively colonizing as well as dormant tumor cells in the lung. Many tumor cells in the lung have remained as small, but live, colonies more than 8 wk after intravenous injection *(19)*. Dormant micrometastasis is one of the most important steps to understand in tumor progression *(34)*. In recent studies, the mechanism of this important phenomenon was studied with regard to angiogenesis and other chemical regulators of tumor colonization *(34)*. However, these experimental models did not allow direct observation of the dormant colonies in fresh live tissue as it occurs over time as do the present studies.

1.6. Isolation of Stable High-Level Expression GFP Transductants of H460 Human Lung Cancer Cells

GFP-Neo^r-retroviral-vector transduced cells were able to grow in vitro at levels of G418 up to 800 µg/mL. The selected G418-resistant H460-GFP cells had bright GFP fluorescence. There was no difference in the cell proliferation rates of parental cells and the GFP tranductants as determined by comparing their doubling times in vitro *(41)*.

1.7. Stable High-Level Expression of GFP in H460 Tumors in Nude Mice

Three weeks after subcutaneous injection of H460-GFP cells, the mice were killed. All three mice had a subcutaneous tumor, which ranged in diameter from 1.5 cm to 2.1 cm. The tumor tissue was strongly GFP fluorescent, thereby demonstrating stable high-level GFP expression in vivo during subcutaneous tumor growth. Lung metastases were found, but no metastases were found in systemic organs in the subcutaneous tumor model of H460-GFP *(41)*.

1.8. GFP-Expressing Lung and Bone Metastases of H460–GFP in Nude Mice

Eight nude mice were implanted in the left lung by SOI with 1-mm^3 cubes of H460-GFP tumor tissue derived from the H460-GFP subcutaneous tumor *(41)*. The implanted mice were killed at 3–4 wk at the time of significant decline in performance status. All mice had tumors in the left lung weighing from 0.985 g to 2.105 g (mean = 1.84 ± 0.4). All tumors (8/8) metastasized to the contralateral lung and chest wall. Seven of eight tumors metastasized to the skeletal system . It was determined that the vertebrae were the most involved skeletal site of metastasis, as seven of eight mice had vertebral metastasis. Three of seven mice had skull metastases visualized by GFP. Metastasis could also be visualized in the tibia and femur marrow by GFP fluorescence. The tumor lodged in the bone marrow and seemed to begin to involve the bone as well.

All of the experimental animals were found with contralateral lung metastases *(41)*. Extensive and widespread skeletal metastasis, visualized by GFP expression, were found in approx 90% of the animals explored. Thus, the H460-GFP SOI model revealed the extensive skeletal metastasizing potential of lung cancer. Such a high incidence of skeletal metastasis could not have been previously visualized before the development of the GFP-SOI model described here which provided the necessary tools.

1.9. Isolation of Stable High-Level Expression GFP Transductants of Human Resistance PC-3 Prostate Carcinoma Cells

The GFP- and neomycin-retroviral-vector transduced PC-3 cells were able to grow in levels of G418 up to 1000 µg/mL. The selected G418-resistant cells had a striking bright GFP fluorescence *(42)*. There was no difference in the cell proliferation rates of parental cells and selected transductants determined by comparing their growth rate in monolayer culture.

1.10. Stable High-Level Expression of GFP in PC-3 Tumors Growing Subcutaneously in Nude Mice

Six weeks after subcutaneous injection of PC-3 cells, the mice were killed. The tumor tissue was strongly fluorescent, thereby demonstrating stable high-level GFP expression in vivo during tumor growth *(42)*. Except for the lung and inguinal and iliac lymph nodes, no obvious GFP fluorescent metastases were found in systemic organs in the subcutaneous tumor model.

1.11. Bone and Visceral Metastasis Visualized by GFP after Orthotopic Tumor Progression of PC-3

Five of five mice developed strongly fluorescent orthotopic tumors after SOI in nude mice. Three of five tumors metastasized to the skeletal system. The skeletal metastasis included the skull, rib, pelvis, femur, and tibia. All the tumors metastasized to the lung, pleural membrane, and kidney. Four of five tumors metastasized to liver and two of five tumors metastasized to the adrenal gland. In two mice, individual cancer cells or small colonies could be seen in the brain and in one mouse a few cells could be seen in the spinal cord by GFP fluorescence *(42)*.

1.12. Fluorescence Optical Tumor Imaging (FOTI)

High-level GFP expression has enabled the real-time external noninvasive whole-body fluorescence optical tumor imaging (FOTI) of the primary tumor and regional and distant metastases in their normal target organs such as brain, bone, lymph node, and liver in live animals *(44)*. The primary tumor and metastasis can be followed in real time in the intact animals by FOTI. A Princeton Instrument charge-coupled device (CCD) thermoelectrically cooled camera is used to collect the optical images from a fluorescence Leica dissecting microscope with a mercury lamp. The images are analyzed and processed with Image Pro-Plus software.

1.13. In Vivo Videomicroscopy to Follow Steps of Metastasis

We took advantage of stable GFP-transfected cells for monitoring and quantifying sequential steps in the metastatic process *(43)*. Using CHO-K1 cells that stably express GFP, the visualization of sequential steps in metastasis within mouse liver, from initial arrest of cells in the microvasculature to the growth and angiogenesis of metastases were quantification by intravital videomicroscopy *(35,36)*. Individual, nondividing cells, as well as micro- and macrometastases could clearly be detected and quantified, as could fine cellular details such as pseudopodial projections, even after extended periods of in vivo growth. The GFP-fluorescent tumor cells had preferential growth and survival of micrometastases near the liver surface. Furthermore, we observed a small population of single cells that persisted over the 11-d observation period, which may represent dormant cells with potential for subsequent proliferation. This study demonstrates the advantages of GFP-expressing cells, coupled with real-time high resolution videomicroscopy, for long-term in vivo studies to visualize and quantify sequential steps of the metastatic process.

1.14. Lung Colony Growth by GFP-Transfected Lung Tumor Cells in Histoculture

ANIP Clone-26-seeded mouse lungs were removed from the mice and then histocultured on collagen-sponge-gels *(20–29)*. Tumor colonies grew and spread rapidly in the lung tissue over time in histoculture *(37–39)*. The progressive colonization of normal lung tissue by the lung tumor cells in individual cultures was visualized at multiple time points. After 6 d in histoculture, the tumor colonies were still classifiable as microcolonies. However, by d 14, very extensive growth of the colonies had occurred with three different areas of GFP-labeled malignant cells being visible. By d 24 of histoculture, the tumor colonies had grown significantly, reaching sizes of 750 µm in diameter and involving approximately one-half of the histocultured mouse lung. By 52 d of histoculture, tumor cells had involved the lung even more extensively and appeared to form multiple layers and histologically suggestive structures on the histocultured lung. Also, by d 52, GFP-expressing satellite tumor colonies formed in the sponge-gel distant from the primary colonies in the lung tissue *(20,29)*.

The tumor host-organ chimeric histoculture system we have developed with GFP-fluorescing tumor cells can significantly advance the ability to understand colonization of normal tissue, which may be the governing step of cancer metastasis *(40)*.

2. Methods

2.1. DNA Manipulations and Expression Vector Constructions

The dicistronic expression vector *(pED-mtxr)* was obtained from Genetics Institute (Cambridge, MA) *(14)*. The expression vector containing the codon-optimized *hGFP-S65T* gene was purchased from CLONTECH Laboratories, Inc. (Palo Alto, CA). To construct the *hGFP-S65T* containing expression vector, *phGFP-S65T* is digested with *Hind*III, blunted at the end. The entire hGFP coding region is then excised with *Xba*I. The pED-mtxr vector is digested with *Pst*I, blunted at the end, and further digested with *Xba*I. The *hGFP-S65T* cDNA fragment is then unidirectionally subcloned into *pED-mtxr (17–20)*.

2.2. Cell Culture, Transfection, Selection

CHO-K1 cells are cultured in Dulbecco's modified Eagle medium (DMEM) (GIBCO) containing 10% fetal calf serum (FCS) (Gemini Bio-products, Calabasas, CA), 2 mM L-gulutamine, and 100 μM nonessential amino acids (Irvine Scientific, Santa Ana, CA). ANIP cells are cultured in RPMI 1640 (GIBCO) containing 10% FCS (Gemini Bio-products, Calabasas, CA), 2 mM L-glutamine, and 100 μM non-essential amino acid (Irvine Scientific, Santa Ana, CA) *(17–20)*.

For transfection, near-confluent CHO-K1 or ANIP cells are incubated with a precipitated mixture of LipofectAMINE™ reagent (GIBCO), and saturating amounts of plasmids for 6 h before being replenished with fresh medium *(17–20)*.

CHO-K1 cells and ANIP are harvested by trypsin–EDTA 48 h post-transfection, and subcultured at a ratio of 1:15 into selective medium that contained 1.5 μM MTX. Cells with stably integrated plasmids are selected by growing transiently transfected cells in the MTX-containing medium. Clones are isolated with cloning cylinders (Bel-Art Products, Pequannock, NJ) by trypsin–EDTA. They are amplified and transferred with conventional culture methods. CHO Clone-38 and ANIP Clone-26 were chosen because of their high-intensity GFP fluorescence and stability *(17–20)*.

2.3. Retroviral DNA Expression Vector

The RetroXpress vector pLEIN is purchased from CLONTECH Laboratories, Inc. (Palo Alto, CA). The pLEIN vector expresses enhanced green fluorescent protein *(EGFP)* and the neomycin resistance (neo[r]) genes on the same bicistronic message that contains an IRES site *(41,42)*.

2.4. Cell Culture, Retroviral Production, Transduction, and Subcloning

PT67, an NIH3T3-derived packaging cell line, expressing the 10 A1 viral envelope, is purchased from CLONTECH Laboratories, Inc. PT67 cells are cultured in DME (Irvine Scientific, Santa Anna, CA) supplemented with 10% heat-inactivated FBS (Gemini Bio-products, Calabasas, CA). For vector production, packaging cells (PT67), at 70% confluence, are incubated with a precipitated mixture of DOTAP™ reagent (Boehringer Mannheim), and saturating amounts of pLEIN plasmid for 18 h. Fresh medium is replenished at this time. The cells are examined by fluorescence microscopy after 48 h. For selection of GFP transductants, the cells are cultured in the presence of 500 μg/mL–2000 μg/mL of G418 (Life Technologies, Grand Island, NY) for 7 d *(41,42)*.

2.5. Retroviral Transduction of Tumor Cells

For GFP gene transduction, 20%-confluent cancer cells are incubated with a 1:1 precipitated mixture of retroviral supernatants of PT67 cells and RPMI

1640 (GIBCO) containing 10% FBS (Gemini Bio-products, Calabasas, CA) for 72 h. Fresh medium is replenished at this time. Cells are harvested with trypsin–EDTA 72 h post-infection, and subcultured at a ratio of 1:15 into selective medium that contains 200 μg/mL of G418. The level of G418 is increased to 800–1000 μg/mL gradually. Clones expressing GFP are isolated with cloning cylinders (Bel-Art Products, Pequannock, NJ) with trypsin–EDTA and are amplified and transferred by conventional culture methods *(41,42)*.

2.6. Doubling Time of Stable GFP Clones

Parental cells and GFP transductants are seeded at 2.0×10^5 in 60 mm culture dishes. The cells are harvested and counted every 24 h using a hemocytometer (Reichert Scientific Instruments, Buffalo, NY). The doubling time is calculated from the cell growth curve over 6 d *(17–20,41,42)*.

2.7. Subcutaneous Tumor Growth

Three 6-wk-old BALB/c *nu/nu* female mice are injected subcutaneously with a single dose of 10^6–10^7 GFP transductants. Cells are first harvested by trypsinization and washed 3× with cold serum-containing medium, then kept on ice. Cells are injected in a total volume of 0.4 mL within 40 min of harvesting. The nude mice are sacrificed to harvest the tumor fragments 3 wk after tumor cells injection *(17–20,41,42)*.

2.8. Surgical Orthotopic Implantation (SOI) of CHO-K1 GFP in Nude Mice

Tumor fragments (1 mm^3) derived from the nude mouse subcutaneous CHO-K1 GFP tumor were implanted by SOI on the ovarian serosa in six nude mice *(17,30)*. The mice are anesthetized by isofluran inhalation. An incision is made through the left lower abdominal pararectal line and peritoneum. The left ovary is exposed and part of the serosal membrane is scraped with a forceps. Four 1-mm^3 tumor pieces are fixed on the scraped site of the serosal surface with an 8-0 nylon suture (Look, Norwell, MA). The ovary is then returned into the peritoneal cavity, and the abdominal wall and the skin are closed with 6-0 silk sutures. Four weeks later, the mice are killed and the lungs and the other organs are removed. All procedures of the operation described above are performed with a ×7 magnification microscope (Olympus).

2.9. Surgical Orthotopic Implantation of ANIP-GFP or H460-GFP Human Lung Cancer in Nude Mice

Tumor fragments (1 mm^3) derived from the ANIP-GFP or H460-GFP subcutaneous tumor growing in nude mouse are implanted by SOI on the left lung in eight nude mice *(18,41)*. The mice are anesthetized by isofluran inhalation. The animals are put in a position of right lateral decubitus, with forelimbs restrained. A 0.8-cm transverse incision of skin is made in the left chest wall. Chest muscles are separated by sharp dissection and costal and intercostal muscles are exposed. A 0.4–0.5-cm intercostal incision between the third and fourth rib on the chest wall is made and the chest wall is opened. The left lung is taken up by a forceps and tumor fragments are sewn promptly into the upper lung promptly by one suture. The lung is then returned into the chest cavity. The incision in the chest wall is closed by a 6-0 surgical suture. The closed condition of the chest wall is examined immediately and, if a leak existed, it is closed by additional sutures. After closing the chest wall, an intrathoracic puncture is made by using a 3-mL syringe and 25G $1/2$ needle to withdraw the remaining air in the chest cavity. After the withdrawal of air, a completely inflated lung can be seen through the thin chest wall of the mouse. Then the skin and chest muscle are closed with a 6-0 surgical suture in one layer. All procedures of the operation described are performed with a ×7 magnification microscope (Olympus).

2.10. SOI of PC-3-GFP Cells

Two tumor fragments (1 mm^3) from a high GFP-fluorescent subcutaneous tumor from a single animal are implanted by SOI in the dorsolateral lobe of the prostate in five nude mice (42). After proper exposure of the bladder and prostate following a lower midline abdominal incision, the capsule of the prostate is opened and the two tumor fragments are inserted into the capsule. The capsule is then closed with an 8-0 surgical suture. The incision in the abdominal wall is closed with a 6-0 surgical suture in one layer (42). The animals are kept under isoflurane anesthesia during surgery. All procedures of the operation described above are performed with a ×7 magnification microscope (Olympus).

2.11. Analysis of the Metastases

Mice are killed when their performance status begins to decline and the systemic organs are removed. The orthotopic primary tumor and all major organs as well as the whole skeleton are explored. The fresh samples are sliced at approx 1 mm thickness and observed directly under fluorescence microscopy. The samples are also processed for histological examination for fluorescence in frozen sections. The slides are then rinsed with phosphate-buffered saline (PBS) and then fixed for 10 min at 4°C in 2% formaldehyde plus 0.2% glutaraldehyde in PBS. The slides are washed with PBS and stained with hematoxylin and eosin using standard techniques.

2.12. Stability of GFP Expression

The subcutaneous GFP tumors from the nude mice are minced for in vitro culture. Cells are subcloned in cell culture medium in the absence of selective pressure. A total of 10^7 parental cells are harvested. Cell extracts are prepared by lysis in 0.1% IGEPAL CA-630 (Sigma) with 1 mM EDTA in PBS *(17)*. The cell extracts are diluted 1:10 with PBS. GFP fluorescence is measured with a fluorescence photometer (Hitachi F-2000; excitation 490 nm, emission 515 nm).

2.13. Microscopy

Light and fluorescence microscopy are carried out using a Nikon microscope equipped with a xenon lamp power supply. A Leica stereo fluorescence microscope model LZ12 equipped with a mercury lamp power supply was also used. Both microscopes have a GFP filter set (Chroma Technology, Brattleboro, VT). An MRC-600 confocal imaging system (Bio-Rad) mounted on a Nikon microscope with an argon laser is also used. Photomicrographs are processed for brightness and contrast with Image Pro Plus, Version 3.0, software (Media Cybernetics, Silver Spring, MD).

2.14. Intravenous Injection

Nude mice are injected in the tail vein with a single dose of 1×10^7 GFP cancer cells. Cells are first harvested by trypsinization and washed 3× with cold serum-containing medium, then kept on ice. Cells are injected in a total volume of 0.8 mL of serum free medium within 40 min of harvesting. After various times, the mice are killed and fresh visceral organs are analyzed by fluorescence microscopy.

2.15. Tumor Progression in Histoculture

Whole lung tissues seeded with ANIP-GFP clone 26 cells are aseptically removed from the nude mice. The lung tissues are divided into pieces of approx 2–3 mm in diameter, which are then placed on prehydrated collagen sponge-gels (Upjohn Co., Kalamazoo, MI). The gels are floated in 24-well plates at the air–water interface in RPMI 1640 containing 20% FCS (Gemini Bio-products, Calabasas, CA), 2 mM L-glutamine, and penicillin. The histocultures are incubated at 37°C in a humidified atmosphere containing 95% air and 5% CO_2. The lung tumor colony growth in the histocultured host lung tissue is repeatedly observed in the same cultures with fluorescence photomicroscopy of the GFP expression at d 6, 14, 24, and 52 of histoculture *(20,29)*.

Using the methods developed described in this review, GFP fluorescence will facilitate the understanding of tumor growth and progression including seeding and target organ colonization that should provide new insights into metastatic mechanisms and treatment of metastatic disease. These developments with tumor cells that stably express GFP in vivo and in vitro provide invaluable new tools for understanding the most important steps in tumor host–organ interaction, tumor progression, and metastasis.

References

1. Lin, W. C., Pretlow, T. P., Pretlow, T. G. 2nd, and Culp, L. A. (1990) Bacterial *lacZ* gene as a highly sensitive marker to detect micrometastasis formation during tumor progression. *Cancer Res.* **50,** 2808–2817.
2. Lin, W. C. and Culp, L. A. (1992) Altered establishment/clearance mechanisms during experimental micrometastasis with live and/or disabled bacterial *lacZ*-tagged tumor cells. *Invasion Metastasis* **12,** 197–209.
3. Morin, J. and Hastings, J. (1971) Energy transfer in a bioluminescent system. *J. Cell Physiol.* **77,** 313–318.
4. Chalfie, M., Tu, Y., Euskirchen, G., Ward, W.W., and Prasher, D. C. (1994) Green fluorescent protein as a marker for gene expression. *Science* **263,** 802–805.
5. Cheng, L., Fu, J., Tsukamoto, A., and Hawley, R. G. (1996) Use of green fluorescent protein variants to monitor gene transfer and expression in mammalian cells. *Nat. Biotechnol.* **14,** 606–609.
6. Prasher, D. C., Eckenrode, V. K., Ward, W. W., Prendergast, F. G., and Cormier, M. J. (1992) Primary structure of the *Aequorea victoria* green-fluorescent protein. *Gene* **111,** 229–233.
7. Yang, F., Moss, L. G., and Phillips, G. N., Jr. (1996) The molecular structure of green fluorescent protein. *Nat. Biotechnol.* **14,** 1246–1251.
8. Cody, C. W., Prasher, D. C., Westler, W. M., Prendergast, F. G., and Ward, W. W. (1993) Chemical structure of the hexapeptide chromophore of the *Aequorea* green fluorescent protein. *Biochemistry* **32,** 1212–1218.
9. Heim, R., Cubitt, A. B., and Tsien, R. Y. (1995) Improved green fluorescence. *Nature* **373,** 663–664.
10. Delagrave, S., Hawtin, R. E., Silva, C. M., Yang, M. M., and Youvan, D. C. (1995) Red-shifted excitation mutants of the green fluorescent protein. *BioTechnology* **13,** 151–154.
11. Cormack, B., Valdivia, R., and Falkow, S. (1996) FACS-optimized mutants of the green fluorescent proten (GFP). *Gene* **173,** 33–38.
12. Crameri, A., Whitehorn, E. A., Tate, E., and Stemmer, W. P. C. (1996) Improved green fluorescent protein by molecular evolution using DNA shuffling. *Nat. Biotechnol.* **14,** 315–319.
13. Zolotukhin, S., Potter, M., Hauswirth, W. W., Guy, J., and Muzycka, N. (1996) 'Humanized' green fluorescent protein cDNA adapted for high-level expression in mammalian cells. *J. Virol.* **70,** 4646–4654.
14. Kaufman, R. J., Davies, M. V., Wasley, L. C., and Michnick, D. (1991) Improved vectors for stable expression of foreign genes in mammalian cells by use of the untranslated leader sequence from EMC virus. *Nucl. Acids Res.* **19,** 4485–4490.
15. Astoul, P., Colt, H. G., Wang, X., and Hoffman, R. M. (1994) A "patient-like" nude mouse model of parietal pleural human lung adenocarcinoma. *Anticancer Res.* **14,** 85–91.
16. Wang, X., Fu, X., and Hoffman, R. M. (1992) A new patient-like metastatic model of human lung cancer constructed orthotopically with intact tissue via thoracotomy in immunodeficient mice. *Int. J. Cancer* **51,** 992–995.

17. Chishima, T., Miyagi, Y., Wang, X., Yamaoka, H., Shimada, H., Moossa, A. R., and Hoffman, R. M. (1997) Cancer invasion and micrometastasis visualized in live tissue by green fluorescent protein expression. Cancer Res. **57**, 2042–2047.

18. Chishima, T., Miyagi, Y., Wang, X., Baranov, E., Tan, Y., Shimada, H., et al. (1997) Metastatic patterns of lung cancer visualized live and in process by green fluorescent protein expression. *Clin. Exp. Metast.* **15**, 547–552.

19. Chishima, T., Miyagi, Y., Wang, X., Tan, Y., Shimada, H., Moossa, A. R., and Hoffman, R. M. (1997) Visualization of the metastatic process by green fluorescent protein expression. *Anticancer Res.* **17**, 2377–2384.

20. Chishima, T., Miyagi, Y., Li, L., Tan, Y., Baranov, E., Yang, M., et al. (1997) The use of histoculture and green fluorescent protein to visualize tumor cell host interaction. *In Vitro Cell. Dev. Biol.* **33**, 745–747.

21. Freeman, A. and Hoffman, R. M. (1986) *In vivo*-like growth of human tumors *in vitro*. *Proc. Natl. Acad. Sci. USA* **83**, 2694–2698.

22. Vescio, R. A., Redfern, C. H., Nelson, T. J., Ugoretz, S., Stern, P. H., and Hoffman, R. M. (1987) *In vivo*-like drug response of human tumors growing in three-dimensional, gel-supported, primary culture. *Proc. Natl. Acad. Sci. USA* **84**, 5029–5033.

23. Hoffman, R. M., Monosov, A. Z., Connors, K. M., Herrera, H., and Price, J. H. (1989) A general native-state method for determination of proliferation capacity of human normal and tumor tissues *in vitro*. *Proc. Natl. Acad. Sci. USA* **86**, 2013–2017.

24. Hoffman, R. M. (1993) To do tissue culture in two or three dimensions? That is the question. *Stem Cells* **11**, 105–111.

25. Hoffman, R. M. (1993) *In vitro* assays for chemotherapy sensitivity. *Crit. Rev. Oncol. Hematol.* **15**, 99–111.

26. Furukawa, T., Kubota, T., Hoffman, R. M. (1995) Clinical applications of the histoculture drug response assay. *Clin. Cancer Res.* **1**, 305–311.

27. Kubota, T., Sasano, N., Abe, O., Nakao, I., Kawamura, E., Saito, T., et al. (1995) Potential of the histoculture drug response assay to contribute to cancer patient survival. *Clin. Cancer Res.* **1**, 1537–1543.

28. Geller, J., Partido, C., Sionit, L., Youngkin, T., Espanol, M., Tan, Y., and Hoffman, R. M. (1997) Comparison of androgen-independent growth and androgen-dependent growth in BPH and cancer tissue from the same radical prostatectomies in sponge-gel matrix histoculture. *The Prostate* **31**, 250–254.

29. Chishima, T., Yang, M., Miyagi, Y., Li, L., Tan, Y., Baranov, E., et al. (1997) Governing step of metastasis visualized in vitro. *Proc. Natl. Acad. Sci. USA* **94**, 11573–11576.

30. Fu, X. and Hoffman, R. M. (1993) Human ovarian carcinoma metastatic models constructed in nude mice by orthotopic transplantation of histologically-intact patient specimens. *Anticancer Res.* **13**, 283–286.

31. Levy, J. P., Muldoon, R. R., Zolotukhin, S., and Link, C. J., Jr. (1996) Retroviral transfer and expression of a humanized, red-shifted green fluorescent protein gene into human tumor cells. *Nat. Biotechnol.* **14**, 610–614.

32. Hoffman, R. M. (1994) Orthotopic is orthodox: Why are orthotopic transplant metastatic models different from all other models? *J. Cell. Biochem.* **56**, 1–3.

33. Lojda, Z. (1970) Indigogenic methods for glycosidases. I. An improved method for β-galactosidase and its application to localization studies of the enzymes of the intestine in other tissues. *Histochemie* **23**, 289–294.

34. Holmgren, L., O'Reilly, M. S., Folkman, J. (1995) Dormancy of micrometastases: balanced proliferation and apoptosis in the presence of angiogenesis suppression. *Nat. Med.* **1**, 149–153.

35. Chambers, A. F., MacDonald, I. C., Schmidt, E. E., Koop, S., Morris, V. L., Khokha, R., and Groom, A. C. (1995) Steps in tumor metastasis: new concepts from intravital videomicroscopy. *Cancer Metastasis Rev.* **14**, 279–301.

36. Koop, S., MacDonald, I. C., Luzzi, K., Schmidt, E. E., Morris, V. L., Grattan, M., et al. (1995) Fate of melanoma cells entering the microcirculation: over 80% survive and extravasate. *Cancer Res.* **55**, 2520–2523.

37. Margolis, L. B., Glushakova, S. E., Baibakov, B. A., Collin, C., and Zimmerberg, J. (1995) Confocal microscopy of cells implanted into tissue blocks: cell migration in long-term histocultures. *In Vitro Cell. Dev. Biol.* **31**, 221–226.

38. Leighton, J. (1957) Contributions of tissue culture studies to an understanding of the biology of cancer: a review. *Cancer Res.* **17**, 929–941.

39. Hoffman, R.M. (1991) Three-dimensional histoculture: origins and applications in cancer research. *Cancer Cells* **3**, 86–92.

40. Kuo, T., Kubota, T., Watanabe, M., Furukawa, T., Teramoto, T., Ishibiki, K., et al. (1995) Liver colonization competence governs colon cancer metastasis. *Proc. Natl. Acad. Sci. USA* **92**, 12085–12089.

41. Yang, M., Hasegawa, S., Jiang, P., Wang, X., Tan, Y., Chishima, T., et al. (1998) Widespread skeletal metastatic potential of human lung cancer revealed by green fluorescent protein expression. *Cancer Res.* **58**, 4217–4221.

42. Yang, M., Jiang, P., Sun, F. X., Hasegawa, S., Baranov, E., Chishima, T., et al. (1999) A fluorescent orthotopic bone metastasis model of human prostate cancer. *Cancer Res.* **59**, 781–786.

43. Naumov, G. N., Wilson, S. M., MacDonald, I. C., Schmidt, E. E., Morris, V. L., Groom, A. C., et al. (1999) Cellular expression of green fluorescent protein, coupled with high-resolution in vivo videomicroscopy, to monitor steps in tumor metastasis. *J. Cell Sci.* **112**, 1835–1842.

44. Yang, M., Baranov, E., Jiang, P., Sun, F.-X., Li, X.-M., Li, L., et al. (2000) Whole-body optical imaging of green fluorescent protein-expressing tumors and metastasis. *Proc. Natl. Acad. Sci. USA* **97**, 1206–1211.

Index